Modernity and Malevolence in the Psychiatric Clinic

Modernity and Malevolence in the Psychiatric Clinic

Anxious Selves in Urban and Rural South India

Andrew C. Willford

HAWAI'I

University of Hawai'i Press
Honolulu

Printed in the United States of America
First printed, 2025

Library of Congress Cataloging-in-Publication Data

Names: Willford, Andrew C. (Andrew Clinton) author
Title: Modernity and malevolence in the psychiatric clinic : anxious selves in urban and rural south India / Andrew C. Willford.
Other titles: Anxious selves in urban and rural south India
Description: Honolulu : University of Hawaiʻi Press, 2025. | Includes bibliographical references and index.
Identifiers: LCCN 2025010864 (print) | LCCN 2025010865 (ebook) | ISBN 9798880701377 hardback | ISBN 9798880701407 epub | ISBN 9798880701414 kindle edition | ISBN 9798880701391 pdf
Subjects: LCSH: NIMHANS (Institute)—Case studies | Mental health—Social aspects—India—Case studies | Psychiatric clinics—India—Case studies | Mental health services—India—Case studies
Classification: LCC RA790.7.I5 W57 2025 (print) | LCC RA790.7.I5 (ebook) | DDC 362.2/20954—dc23/eng/20250721
LC record available at https://lccn.loc.gov/2025010864
LC ebook record available at https://lccn.loc.gov/2025010865

Front cover and spine: A corridor in the NIMHANS Psychiatry Department. Back cover: The Department of Psychiatry building seen from inside the NIMHANS campus. Both photographs by Andrew C. Willford.

Cover design by Melissa Olaivar Wong

University of Hawaiʻi Press books are printed on acid-free paper and meet the guidelines for permanence and durability of the Council on Library Resources.

Modernity and Malevolence in the Psychiatric Clinic

Anxious Selves in Urban and Rural South India

Andrew C. Willford

University of Hawai‘i Press
Honolulu

Printed in the United States of America
First printed, 2025

Library of Congress Cataloging-in-Publication Data

Names: Willford, Andrew C. (Andrew Clinton) author
Title: Modernity and malevolence in the psychiatric clinic : anxious selves in urban and rural south India / Andrew C. Willford.
Other titles: Anxious selves in urban and rural south India
Description: Honolulu : University of Hawaiʻi Press, 2025. | Includes bibliographical references and index.
Identifiers: LCCN 2025010864 (print) | LCCN 2025010865 (ebook) | ISBN 9798880701377 hardback | ISBN 9798880701407 epub | ISBN 9798880701414 kindle edition | ISBN 9798880701391 pdf
Subjects: LCSH: NIMHANS (Institute)—Case studies | Mental health—Social aspects—India—Case studies | Psychiatric clinics—India—Case studies | Mental health services—India—Case studies
Classification: LCC RA790.7.I5 W57 2025 (print) | LCC RA790.7.I5 (ebook) | DDC 362.2/20954—dc23/eng/20250721
LC record available at https://lccn.loc.gov/2025010864
LC ebook record available at https://lccn.loc.gov/2025010865

Front cover and spine: A corridor in the NIMHANS Psychiatry Department. Back cover: The Department of Psychiatry building seen from inside the NIMHANS campus. Both photographs by Andrew C. Willford.

Cover design by Melissa Olaivar Wong

University of Hawaiʻi Press books are printed on acid-free paper and meet the guidelines for permanence and durability of the Council on Library Resources.

For Vasantha

Contents

Acknowledgments

My JOURNEY INTO THE WORLD of Indian psychiatry and neurology would not have been possible without those who encouraged me in this direction and opened doorways that would have otherwise remained closed to me. First, I thank A. R. Vasavi for her encouragement, sharp intellect, and necessary introduction to a colleague at NIMHANS. Tanya Luhrmann offered encouragement in the very early stages when this was just a vague idea for a project, as well as introducing me to young scholars working in this field. In upstate New York, David Halpert and Mike Berg provided an important window into the world of clinical neurology. Friends and colleagues in Bangalore provided both intellectual and social nourishment over the years. I thank Gayatri Menon, Linda Carlos, S. Carlos, and Cohan Sujan Carlos for their kindness, generosity, and stimulating company over the years. My colleagues at Cornell, particularly Lucinda Ramberg, Stacey Langwick, and Rachel Prentice, were sympathetic and insightful ears and eyes when I shared early thoughts on this work. Lucinda overlapped with me in Bangalore, comparing research experiences with me from time to time.

I benefitted greatly from the intellectual comradery of Sarah Pinto, Aidan Seale-Feldman, Jocelyn Marrow, Saiba Varma, and Sharika Thiranagama. Our conversations regarding a rethinking of "hysteria" in South Asia influenced me greatly, and always for the better, opening my eyes to new frontiers in psychological and medical anthropology. Lawrence Cohen's enthusiasm about, and commentary upon, the aforementioned dialogue was characteristically brilliant and helpful. Jim Siegel was his usual sharp interlocutor self, and was a particularly sympathetic friend as I fumbled around with some early ideas about this project. His subtle encouragement and provocations were always greatly appreciated.

Sanjeev Jain profoundly influenced my understanding of psychiatry in India, along with its broader social, cultural, and historical context. I am forever grateful for his assistance and friendship. I must also thank Mathew Varghese for intellectual stimulation, friendship, and logistical assistance.

Others in India who were instrumental in making this project possible include: Pratima Murthy, Srikala Bharath, Sydney Moirangthem, Vandana Gopikumar, Sanjib Sinha, and Mrinalini Ravi, among many others.

I am eternally grateful to all the doctors, patients, residents, fellows, students, clinical psychologists, nurses, counselors, and staff at NIMHANS for making this study possible. Without their generous support, patience, and unique access to all parts of NIMHANS clinical life, this project would never have reached fruition.

My research was supported by a Fulbright-Nehru Senior Research Fellowship, as well as an American Institute of Indian Studies Senior Research Fellowship. Additional support was provided by Cornell University's College of Arts and Sciences, the Department of Anthropology, and the South Asia Program.

I must thank Masako Ikeda, my editor at the University of Hawai'i Press, for her savvy and deft editorial guidance, as well as for her support for this project. She also had the good sense of breaking this study into two parts, the first of which is offered here. I am grateful to Jehanne Moharram for her eagle-eyed and skillful copyediting. I also benefitted greatly from the two anonymous readers, and am grateful to them for their detailed, serious, and thoughtful suggestions. I absolve them, however, of any shortcomings in the present work.

Finally, to my children, Anisha and Rabindra, who kept me grounded in reality, a huge debt is owed. Anisha inspired this research in ways she will never understand, but was, nevertheless, a guiding light. Rabin became an anthropologist himself between the time this project commenced and its completion. We often overlapped in India in recent years, which always brought me happiness. Lastly, I must offer my most heartfelt and loving thanks to my wife and partner, Vasantha, who has made enormous sacrifices to make this work possible. Without her love and support, I could not have carried on with this work. To her goes all the credit.

Introduction

Two Deaths

I awoke on a Sunday in August 2015 to see in the local news that a patient at NIMHANS (National Institute for Mental Health and Neurosciences) had been shot to death after he "posed a danger" to other patients and staff. It was reported that he was armed and threatening to harm others. This was the first serious violent episode I had heard about, let alone witnessed, in my year-long residency at this esteemed hospital and research institution in Bangalore. While shocked to hear the news and wondering to myself if I had seen this particular patient before, the media portrayal of the killing was salutary, indicating that the police had acted bravely to protect the safety of others in subduing a violently unstable individual. The dead man, it was said, was a prisoner who was being treated at NIMHANS, not a long-term patient living within one of its wards.

I came to the office the next day after this incident. At the end of the corridor where my office was located, a blood stain was visible on the side-walk, evidently left after the prisoner was removed from the building where he was killed. The prisoner had stolen a gun from a guard and had begun shooting into the ceiling and walls of a room he had holed himself into. The room was also a small gunnery the police used at NIMHANS. Therefore, the police were concerned about the danger this posed to the public and staff. The prisoner reportedly refused to surrender and was approached by a special operations unit, akin to a SWAT team. The team, a doctor at NIMHANS told me, shot him in the head and chest upon entering the room, though the victim "had not actually threatened any-one." The doctor felt the violent death was senseless as this was "not a hardened criminal," just a confused, and perhaps panicked, individual. He suggested that the police were poorly trained and unmotivated to resolve the situation peacefully.

The broader question that lingered among the doctors I spoke with that day was whether this was yet another instance of "criminalizing the mentally ill," albeit in starker, more visible terms than the usual, more subtle, means through which the mentally ill in India were mistreated, sometimes chained to their beds and abandoned in traditional healing centers. A media frenzy surrounding the "crisis" of mental health in India was sensationalized in stories like this one, coupled with alarming suicide rates, addiction, and other social vices that accompanied depression and anomie within the country. To the psychiatrists I had spent the previous year observing at NIMHANS, there was urgency in adding nuance to the emergent public narrative about the so-called crisis, on the one hand, and a desperate need to address the structural violence that precipitated it on the other.

In February 2018, in the Nilgiris town of Attapadi, in Kerala, Madhu, a Kurumba Adivasi (tribal) man, twenty-seven years old, was beaten to death by group of men who took "selfies" of themselves in the act. Madhu, who was believed to suffer mental illness, was said to be living alone in a cave within the forest. He was accused of stealing rice from a local shop, which prompted the mob to drag him from his cave, bind, strip, and beat him. In his possession was a packet of chili powder, a bit of coriander powder, and a small amount of rice. In the photos and videos that surfaced of this heinous act, Madhu appeared confused and terrified, not understanding why he was being beaten. By the time police arrived and he was transported to a local hospital, he succumbed to internal injuries and died. The shocking brutality of this event appeared in all the major newspapers in the country. It was particularly jarring giving the laughter and smiles of the perpetrators as they filmed the murder. Outrage was swift, as sixteen men were soon charged for murder, though the case had yet to, as of 2022, come to trial.[1]

Both of these tragic cases point to figures of malevolence, be they that of the tribal person, the mob, or the criminal; or more pointedly, for our purposes, the mentally ill. While deadly violence will not be the focus of this study, these two dramatic examples notwithstanding, the treatment of the mentally ill, and the purported sense of crisis around mental health in India, is my concern. Beyond containment of the "ill" from the wider society through stigma, or normalizing the patient through pharmaceutical fixes or demonological exorcism, it is critical to address the wider social and cultural canvas in the nation, which requires different vantages on the purported crisis surrounding mental health. These can take the form of public health studies addressing access to care, epidemiology, patient rights, psychiatry, education, etc. In my two-part work, I offer two separate vantages, both of them ethnographic: one from a rural and Adivasi area within the Nilgiris Biosphere

Reserve; and the other, the present study, within a major research hospital, NIMHANS, that treats hundreds of patients from all over the country every day in Bangalore. The comparison, I argue, illuminates a larger canvas of malevolence shaped by politics and modernity, though important distinctions between the two sites also reveal local and regional variation and, with this, a need to oscillate between macro- and micro-perspectives in addressing a purported mental health crisis at the national level. The present book concerns the latter site, the urban hospital setting. A separate book on the Nilgiris indigenous context is forthcoming.

Providing symptomatic relief to acute sufferers was an overwhelming and all-consuming challenge at NIMHANS. At the same time, the psychiatrists I worked with, taken as a whole, were themselves acutely sensitive to the risks of medicalization and diagnostic certainty, coupled with pharmaceuticalization as a "quick fix" or "Band-Aid" upon deeper social wounds. The enduring stigma attached to mental health, the paucity of quality providers—particularly therapists who might offer more than a medication—and financial considerations, as drug treatment was less costly for poor patients than long-term psychotherapy, brought two temporalities into play within the clinic. Quick relief for patients was essential, on both humane and social grounds. In the longer term, slowing down diagnostic certainty and opening up questions of structural violence, precarity, and stigma were central to combatting society's ills as manifested in mental health problems. Beyond questions of economic precarity and its relationship with mental illness, particularly depression, as in the well-publicized cases of "farmer suicides" (Vasavi 2012), the psychiatrists I observed at NIMHANS were concerned about an increasing literalism and intolerance of ambiguity around social identities in the country. As social and cultural analysts, they found that the increasing political divisions around religious and ethnic identities were becoming impactful at the level of individual psychopathology, leading those already vulnerable to become increasingly judgmental towards themselves and others, where displaced fears, aggressions, and intolerable others were perceived as a malevolent presence. In short, paranoia was not just a clinical feature, but a political one, with the two being somehow related. The term "hysteria" was, in turn, often deployed informally in the clinic when talking about the intractable feelings of malevolence and othering, coupled with somatic and occasional paralyzing symptoms.

To briefly foreshadow the second book, in the context of the Nilgiris, and within Kurumba and Irula indigenous communities, affects of malevolence came from many sides. On the one hand, racialized stigmas, owing to complex historical forces, led to tragedies of neglect, abuse, and precarity, most dramatically illustrated in the killing of Madhu, mentioned above. On the other hand, within the communities I worked with, there was a growing feeling of unease, an "ill wind," that seemed to sweep through the Nilgiri hills, haunting individuals and their communities. Malevolence in both cases had a social provenance, and spoke to forms of structural violence that exacerbated psychological distress. Looking at these social forces, or what we might call the "violence of the social," following Siegel (2006), from the top down, within a psychiatric hospital and research center, and from the bottom up, from a rural and tribal area underserved by biomedical specialization, provides a unique optic upon mental wellbeing within a larger social, indeed, national framework.

Malevolence

The term "malevolence," as used in this study, points to four dimensions of experience, with some overlap between them. The term as commonly defined speaks to doing harm, ill intent, or a sense or perception of harm being done to individuals and groups. In the first instance, many of the cases within the ethnography that follows speak to spirits and supernatural entities that are causing harm and/or haunting afflicted individuals through sorcery, possession, and other spiritual maladies. This relates to the second usage (or invocation), which indexes structural violence and social violence, not to mention symbolic violence, within India around caste, poverty, and patriarchal forms of gendered hierarchy. These two categories of malevolence are etiologically related, as the second often produces hauntings of the first.

Thirdly, and pointing to projects of modernity, statecraft, and identity politics, I describe how social othering, themes of betrayal, judgmental attitudes, and totalizing and excessive fantasies of the other are taking hold of fragile subjects in clinical cases, exacerbating pre-existing insecurities and social traumas, now figured as caused by the inscrutable and malevolent traits of cultural others, oftentimes figured in religious terms. This disentangling of more protean and fluid cultural words within political imaginaries makes impossible demands upon subjects already experiencing precarity and vulnerability, be it from the social violence (my second usage above), or by organic biological factors, or in combination. That is, being forced into modern identity categories around language, ethnicity, and religion, the stuff of nationalism, causes feelings of inward betrayal manifesting in othering and hauntings as a form of displacement. This, in turn, relates to the first usage, described above. For instance, I describe individuals who, in the name of reformed religion, or conversion to a more "orthodox" path influenced by modernist projects, have renounced part of their culture and self-identity, which, in turn, produces haunting displacements and/or excessive othering. In one chapter, I also describe the singularities and monotony demanded within the IT workplace sector, another kind of singular identity that exacts a psychic and physical toll on individuals, though not necessarily productive of spiritual hauntings of social othering.

And fourth, I illustrate the ambivalence and perceived malevolence of biomedicine as perceived by psychiatrists, who understand the double binds caused by social pressures for the "normalization" of patients, as fueled by stigma, as well as social and cultural attitudes (i.e., the second factor discussed above, around socially prescribed and proscribed roles). This is the proverbial "Band-Aid," as doctors described it at NIMHANS, provided by pharmaceuticals and the bureaucratization of biomedical psychiatry, over and against "gaping social wounds," as one interlocutor described it to me. The physicians I describe are grappling with two types of potential malevolence, in that sense: the social violence that leads patients to their clinic, on the one hand, and the demands for quick fixes from patients on the other. This is fueled by the pharmaceutical industry coupled with limited resources, producing a lament, or at a minimum, an inextricable ambivalence enveloping clinical care as a type of malevolence, located within particular ecologies of biomedicine, culture, bodies, and materiality (Lang 2018; Cohen 2012).

In sum, malevolence, in this study, assumes a floating quality, as it appears in multiple registers and is felt but inscrutable at times (Massumi 2002). But I argue that these four factors (and probably more than just four, but these are the main categories) are closely intertwined and co-productive of haunting affect and the violence embedded within the social.

The "Crisis"

A purported and brewing mental health crisis in India has been driven by journalists and physicians, and has called attention to alarming rates of suicide, depression, alienation, addiction, and burnout. These disturbing trends generally point to urbanization and anomie, a lack of infrastructure, stigma and the need for education, and the dangers of social change. But the underlying animus of this discourse is the potential for social upheaval, conflict, and slowed economic growth that a crisis might precipitate. A detailed analysis of this discourse is warranted but not possible here, though numerous magazines and newspapers, too ubiquitous to cite, have discussed the "crisis" as worsening (Lang 2018).[2]

On the one hand, discussions of cultural dislocation, anomie, and social vices are deployed, sometimes romantically, to imagine a less pathological past when religion, traditional values, and sociocentric collectivities were uncontaminated by Western materialism and individualism (Lang 2018; Addlakha 2008). This is a long and complicated discourse within twentieth-century Indian and Hindu nationalisms (Langford 2002). But more pointed, in terms of health care, the allocation of 20 percent of the national health budget for AYUSH revitalization, treatment, and research,[3] which is now instituted in most major hospitals, including NIMHANS, reflects notions of context specificity and cultural uniqueness (Sujatha and Abraham 2012).

On the other hand, a glaring gap in care has opened, with the perceived need for more specialists far outpacing patient demand, hospital beds, and institutions of care. After a tragic fire took twenty-six lives in Erwadi, Tamil Nadu, in 2003, as "mad" people within a *dargah* (saint's tomb) were chained to their beds and died as a result, the public and government have demanded reform and increased spending on mental health (Sebastia 2009a). One consequence, however, of legal reform for the mentally ill has been the disqualification of many traditional forms of faith-based care, such as leaving the mentally ill within *dargahs*, temples, and other places of worship. Legislating that medical licensing was required to house and treat the mentally ill was meant to protect patients from abuse, abandonment, and neglect, but it also exacerbated the shortage of care by closing traditional care centers whilst not offering sufficient biomedical care. Therefore, homelessness among the mentally ill increased (Nagaraja and Murthy 2008; Sebastia 2009a).

The Mental Health Care Bill was passed by the Rajya Sabha in 2013, and promised to address the rights of patients to quality mental health care within accredited mental health facilities. Still, a glaring lack of psychiatrists and budgetary constraints exists, making the bill aspirational in name, but not in reality. A mere 1 percent of the health budget, which comprised a mere 4 percent of the total national budget, was used for mental health. In the year 2000 there were only 2,000 psychiatrists in India (Goel, Agarwal, Ichhpujani, and Shrivastava 2004), though by a decade later, there were 3,000 with an uptick in graduates. Many districts, despite a District Mental Health Programme stipulating that there should be at least one psychiatrist per district, have no specialists in neurologic and psychiatric care, an issue I will examine in the second volume on the Nilgiris. In the rural context, psychiatrists are often put in the role of treating epilepsy, for instance, because there are even fewer clinical neurologists than there are psychiatrists.

Patients are forced to travel long distances to major tertiary centers such as NIMHANS, or AIIMS (All India Institute of Medical Science) in Delhi.

Suicide has increased by 22.7 percent in the last decade, according to official statistics (NIMHANS 2009). While statistics, especially suicide rates, are not necessarily reliable "social facts" given the many controversies of reporting, still the general trend has been alarming. India has the 11th highest rate of suicide globally, at 22/100K (NIMHANS 2009; Iype 2004; Datta 2015). Suicides among farmers are blamed on spiraling debt and are thus explicable, though disturbing. Urban suicides, though they are not divorced from economic hardships, seem to suggest other forces at play. Specifically, cultural and social dislocations associated with a kind of anomie that rapid change is believed to produce suggest that addictions and depression caused by job burnout and stress are the culprits. These, in turn, are blamed often on a loss of values, the breakdown of the joint extended family, and Western cultural influences (Lang 2018; Cohen 1998).

One focus in the aforementioned Mental Health Care Bill has been on "advance directives." This concerns the patients right to determine the form of treatment that they will receive. The notion behind this part of the legislation is that social abandonment is one of the primary causes and concerns within the institutionalized context (Pinto 2014).

Decriminalizing suicide is also part of the bill, which means treatment would replace prosecution after a failed suicide attempt. Penal and institutionalized abandonment, more generally speaking, is to be phased out, replaced by a more efficacious and less stigmatizing community-based model of care, utilizing lay caregivers. Dealing with stigma, superstitions (e.g., demonic possession, exorcism), and prevention/postvention care are the new watchwords in building community awareness and support. And while these moves are not without obvious merit, the emergent discourse surrounding mental health in India pathologizes a percentage of the population, which, in turn, is a public target for rescue, reform, and "healing."

As Foucault observed in his *History of Madness* (2006), the homeless wandering madman, tolerated for centuries in the classical age, became an intolerable presence within a reasoned post-Enlightenment Europe, and is similarly tolerated less in modern India. This is not to suggest that the crisis is not real; indeed, the reality measured in terms of human suffering is palpable to anyone visiting NIMHANS. This point notwithstanding, the conditions that make this discourse possible deserve greater scrutiny. This is particularly so given that the risks within the "crisis" so clearly identify symptomatic behavior associated with volitional and moral fault lines (even criminal) such as addiction, suicide, and depression.

These illnesses bring to the fore the social at a moment when biomedical diagnoses weigh less on psychosocial causation, despite the latter's critical importance. Moral defects are refigured as chemical imbalances and neurological misfirings. These, in turn, can be magically remedied with "tablets" (pills), and not, in most cases, with psychotherapy. Moreover, the historical silences and amnesia of past traumas, particularly the Partition of the subcontinent, have been insufficiently studied; and, as two leading psychiatrists in India, Alok Sarin and Sanjeev Jain, argue (2018), the social provenance of much psychological suffering in India in the twentieth century has drawn scant attention within the field of psychiatry itself, despite it being the arena of care and symptomatic treatment:[4] "We realised, as clinical psychiatrists, that the issue was almost absent from our textbooks and clinical work. By contrast, in the wider context of literary theory, gender studies, and political analysis, however, there was a constant reiteration of the negative consequences, emotional and cognitive, on both individuals and communities. . . . Do political trauma and social distancing, whether by fascism in Germany or by colonialism and racism or other forms of social oppression, contribute to psychological symptoms?" (Sarin and Jain 2018, 10–11). Echoing the concerns of Fanon, the great anti-colonial psychoanalyst, they go on to ask the question that biomedical psychiatry all too rarely asks: "The seeming retreat of universal humanism and the resurgence of identity politics, as well as the perpetual creation of a 'demonic other,' is perhaps a sign of psychological malfunction" (Sarin and Jain 2018, 11).

By extension, we might then ask whether madness is located with the individual or within the realm of the social itself, with its sometimes arbitrary and cruel demands. In Saadat Hasan Manto's famous short story "Toba Tek Singh," the impossibility of finding the exact location and identity of an apparent mad person's place of origin after Partition, as patients in a mental health institution located on the border are being transferred to either India or Pakistan, illustrates the impossibility of identity subsisting within the randomness of political demarcations. The protagonist of the story ends up lying face down between the barbed wires separating the two young nations, unable to find "home" and an identity in either. His refusal indexes not his personal madness, but that of drawing arbitrary borders in the sands of time, disentangling memory and affect from politics. A psychiatry to come, its radical promise, seems to urgently cry out in the clinical and intellectual work being done at NIMHANS, precisely as the dangers of medicalization and partitioning the insane or "mad" from the rest of society is felt by those on its front lines. While a crisis of mental health may, indeed, exist, it is a far more nuanced and complicated problem than is capable of being resolved through biomedical treatment alone. As another important psychiatrist based at NIMHANS, Pratima Murthy, writes, "The practice of psychiatry in India, in its fervour to emerge as a scientific, empirical, and universal science, has, in the process, become sterile and devoid of the richness of human experience. Human experience is both universal and, at the same time, highly personalized. The importance of understanding individuals in their personal, social, and larger-world contexts in this helping profession has given way to looking for sterile biological explanations for underlying conditions, and an enthusiasm to fix the human condition with a 'pill for every ill.' This, in some ways, is the sequestration or partitioning of professional minds" (Murthy 2018, 233).

While drawing direct insights from psychiatrists, such as the ones quoted above, as well as others I observed in India with similar insights and concerns, I also draw significantly upon the anthropological work on mental health and wellbeing in India, particularly work that looks at the nexus of socioeconomic precarity, familial constraints and demands in a changing economy, and the spiritual hauntings and idioms of distress through which these tensions are expressed (e.g., Nichter 1982; Obeyesekere 1981; Kakar 1982; Ecks 2013; Halliburton 2009; Sebastia 2009a; 2009b; Fabrega 2009; Corin 2007; Corin, Thara, and Padmavati 2004), particularly in the pathbreaking work by Sarah Pinto (2014; 2020a), Claudia Lang (2018), Lawrence Cohen (1998), Saiba Varma (2020), Renu Addlakha (2008), Jocelyn Chua (2014), Luhrmann and Marrow (2016), Marrow (2022), and Veena Das (2006), all of whom look to the fractures, wounds, and everyday violence that mark the lives of those deemed mentally ill in oftentimes brilliant and provocative analyses grounded in local culture and context, but theoretically broad enough to connect their work to other parts of the world.

Troubled Identities

I had the opportunity to spend hundreds of hours at NIMHANS during twelve months of fieldwork in 2014–2015. Most of my time was spent discussing mental health concerns in today's India with psychiatrists, as well as spending much time in the outpatient and inpatient clinics at NIMHANS, observing patients interacting with physicians. I highlight here a few patterns that I observed that helped to frame the key questions of the book.

First, it should be noted that there is still a significant stigma attached to biomedical mental health treatment in India, though this has been slowly changing within the urban context due to outreach and education. NIMHANS has played a pivotal role in disseminating information about mental health, as well as dispelling popularly held beliefs about mental health that oftentimes involve demonologies that can harm the afflicted (Chandrasekhar 2008; Ram 2013). In the rural context, belief in supernatural causation is still quite strong, whereas in the urban, and particularly middle-class, sectors, these beliefs are slowly changing towards the biomedical and/or Ayurvedic or AYUSH explanatory models.[5] One consequence of the stigma (Koschorke, Padmavati, Kumar, et al. 2014) still attached to mental health care has been a patient desire for quick pharmaceutical fixes rather than sustained forms of therapy, such as in undergoing psychotherapy (Ecks 2013). Physicians oftentimes lament the structural position they find themselves in, having to send patients home with ameliorative medications but knowing that psychosocial stress owing to various forms of social and cultural precarity has been left unchanged. That is, doctors are often cognizant that a high percentage of a patient's symptom presentation is rooted in structural conditions that cannot be remedied in the fast pace of the clinic, given both the heavy patient loads and the commitments of time by the patients to stay and be admitted into the hospital. Another aspect of stigma that I encountered several times throughout the year concerned the concealing of a mental illness before marriage by one or the other party involved. The consequences of this deception could be felt in the marital complications that inevitably ensued, leading to greater psychosocial stress within the family.

Hundreds of patients come each day to NIMHANS's Outpatient Department (OPD), sometimes having traveled a long distance from other parts of the country. While the majority come from the tri-state areas of Karnataka, Tamil Nadu, and Andhra Pradesh, and the most from Bangalore itself, patients from North India are commonly seen and treated.[6] It is not uncommon for a doctor at NIMHANS to treat twenty-five patients or more in one OPD session that might last six to eight hours.[7] While social workers, residents, and fellows perform fairly detailed intake interviews, the attending psychiatrists must still review and query each case history before making a recommendation for treatment and follow-up visits. Given the combination of this structural reality and constraint upon both patient and doctor time, as well as the stigma attached to mental health, patients and their families are often very eager to receive a (magical) "tablet," as Murthy had suggested above, with the promise of symptom alleviation. Being admitted or recommended for extended care or psychotherapy sessions raises the specter of revealing oneself as "ill" to the extended family and community, with consequences for one's social standing or that of one's family or community. This is a profound problem doctors and patients deal with, and one that constrains treatment options.

The mainstream print media oftentimes highlights the nature of the stigma and necessity of combatting it to meet the demands of mental health care in contemporary India. Another theme that emerges ubiquitously in the

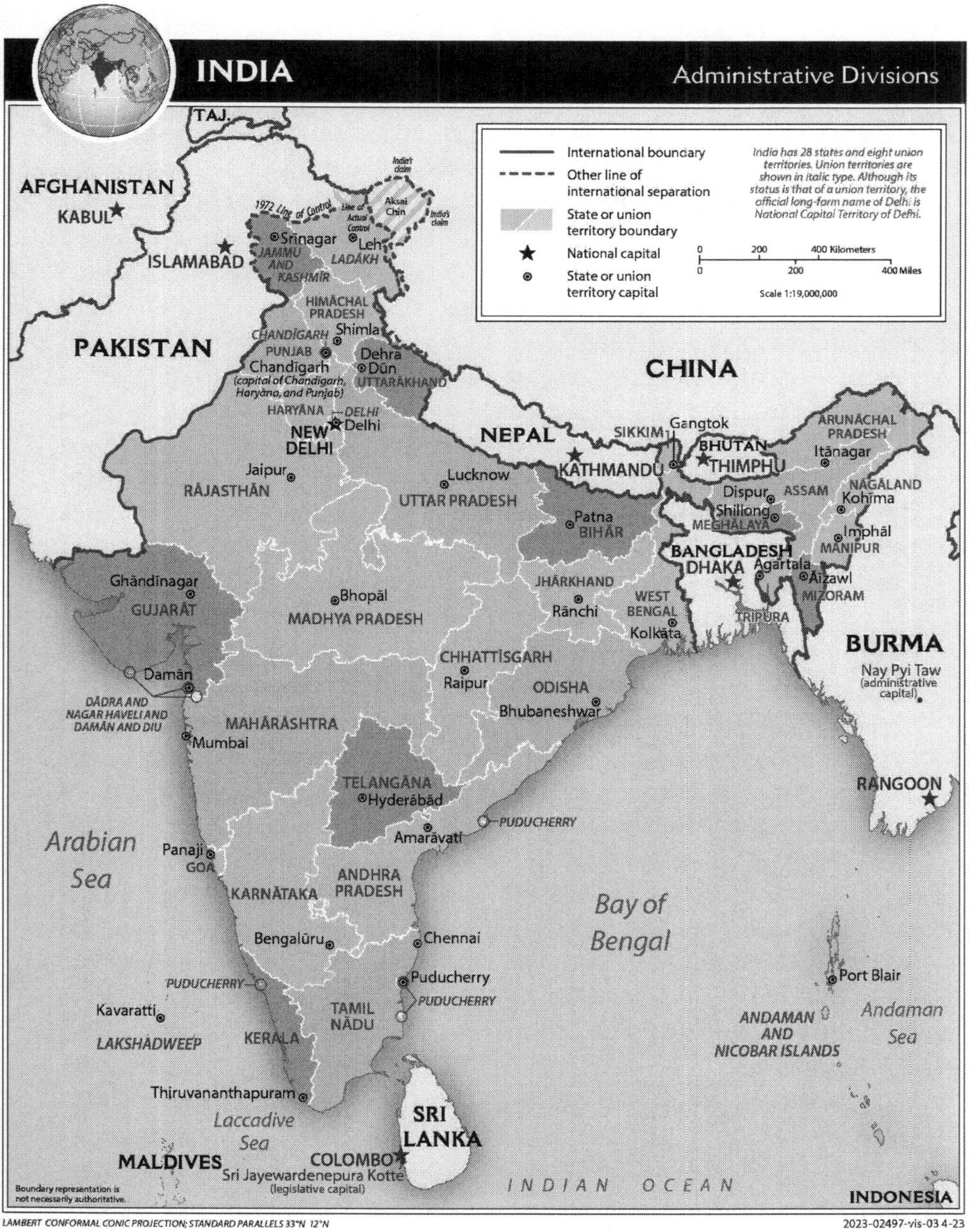

Map of modern India. (Digital Maps, Geography and Map Division, Library of Congress Online Catalog.)

media concerns the "crisis" of depression and burnout that is thought to be enveloping India's most vibrant urban centers. This discussion points to high stress levels within the competitive workplace and the breakdown of social institutions, such as the extended family, to mitigate against this modern-day malaise associated with urban life (Lang 2018; Chua 2014). Bangalore is thought to exemplify this crisis with its very large and itinerant population working in IT, as well as its very large low-skilled call centers and factories run by multinationals (Upadhya and Vasavi 2008; Mankekar and Gupta 2017). At NIMHANS I was oftentimes told that Bangalore's suicide rate is the highest in the country and ran in the tens of thousands annually, an astonishing figure (Nanjappa 2008).[8] I will discuss this burnout and depression phenomenon as one of the main patterns of clinical observation witnessed in the OPD in chapter 5.

There are two other significant patterns relevant to this study of troubled identities as they relate to sociocultural changes and new imaginaries. One concerns the changing relationship between gender roles and modernist and/or reformed versions of Islam, Hinduism, and Christianity. In short, and I will elaborate later, women with aspirations for education and careers have felt their dreams and aspirations clipped by increasingly rigid patriarchal values associated with religious reform and, perhaps ironically, modernity (Addlakha 2008; Pinto 2014). These frustrated aspirations have produced somatizations and/or possessions by forces unseen. We examine the role of gendered suppression and somatization, particularly as colloquially diagnosed within the clinic as "hysteria" in chapters 2 and 3, including cases of male "hysteria" and somatization and possession.

The other clinical pattern, according to the doctors I shadowed, was an increasing inability to think flexibly or contextually about categories of right and wrong, good and bad, and self vs. other, again echoing the points raised by Sarin and Jain regarding the political in relation to madness. Patients often presented with symptoms of feeling betrayed by significant others in their lives, and a very rigid legalistic perspective when it came to judgements. This iron cage of thinking, to paraphrase Weber, was apparently increasing and was fostered by experiences of flux and rapid change (Appadurai 2000). Psychiatrists at NIMHANS suggested, through clinical case studies and their accompanying commentary, a parallel between these patterns and the overzealous attachments to particular religious and/or linguistic and ethnic identities. I suggest that madness in these cases, like in the semi-fictional case of "Toba Tek Singh," is produced by impossible demands for singular identities that suppress more fluid traces of subjectivity and the complex histories that produce them. While this is an argument and observation that weaves throughout the book, this receives more detailed analysis within the clinic in chapters 3 and 4.

On this last point, I have elsewhere (2006; 2014; 2018) argued that the psychology and phenomenology of excessive identity attachments can be understood in the particular demand that modern statecraft and nationalism makes of its citizenry (Hansen 2001; Siegel 2006; Menon 2022). And here, Anderson's less heralded contribution to the study of modern identity is relevant. Anderson (1998) identifies two modes of serial identification that develop within the politics of imagining community. "Unbound" serialism allows for a more expansive and inclusive form of community imagining. Though boundaries exist within the nation's idealized image, it is not exclusively defined by a linguistic region or cultic practice. On the other hand, "bound" serialism is framed around the bureaucratic measurement of types, facilitated by the census. Bound serial types are sustained, in turn, through a disentangling of identities that might be otherwise more complex, bearing traces of otherness, fluid and permeable. But as I have argued (2014; 2018), these "types" or bound identities are, in turn, troubled by the displacements and disavowals that sustain them, as a form of "archive fever" (Derrida 1995) or fetishism (Morris 2017; Willford 2006). This is not to imply that bound identities are a pure fiction or invention. Rather, it is to suggest that modern forms of state politics can engender a fetishizing of such types, precisely in an attempt to cover their contingent origins through law and statecraft (Comaroff and Comaroff 2006; 2009). The demands of nationhood, ethnicity, or a particular singularized identity and/or modality within the workforce can produce the Kafkaesque effect in which the circular madness of referencing a principled truth only occurs through its supplement (Zizek 1993; Aretxaga 2008). Under these conditions, life-negating principles or Freud's *thanatos* (1961) meets its sociocentric counter, as either the latter is symptomatic of the former or the latter requires the supplement of the former, ironically, to sustain itself. This is not a study of politics, revivalism, or nationalism, however. For an analysis of these singularizing nationalistic or religious forces, we can turn to other works that inform and provide a political context for the present study of the psychiatric clinic (e.g., Hansen 1999; 2001; Menon 2010; 2022; Jaffrelot 2021; Willford 2018).[9] That is, in this political and social context, a discourse around modernity and a loss of social values around family and faith act as symptomatic supplements, displacing other causal factors (Lang 2018). In either case, an intimacy inheres in the madness and its treatment in modern psychiatry, particularly when labeled as "hysteria," the history of psychiatric biomedical orientation in India notwithstanding.

Burnout and depression were evidently increasing at an alarming rate, according to clinicians that I knew, as well as media discussions that I observed (see Upadhya and Vasavi 2008; Mukherjee 2008; D'Mello and Sahay 2008; Datta 2015; Sen 2015). The high stress placed on employees of IT companies in order to remain competitive included working long hours that exceeded the normal workday, as well as dealing with firm deadlines and job insecurities. Some of the patients who came to NIMHANS would complain of feeling numb, depressed, or inadequate at their jobs and in their home lives. Many, particularly younger employees far from their hometown, felt isolated, suffering a lack of meaningful social connections. Others felt culturally estranged, working alongside individuals from all over the country, if not the world, with different languages, culture, and food habits. Though all major IT centers and tech parks had food courts offering a range of food choices, the absence of home-cooked food was an issue for some. But it was, in many instances, a combination of the quotidian day-to-day life, requiring repetition and routine, coupled with the expectation of producing a certain product under the duress of time that led to a kind of burnout and enervation, if not exasperation and depression. Moreover, familial expectations could also prove stress-inducing, with hopes pinned on a recent college graduate's potential but oftentimes unrealized earning power. While many were drawn into the IT-related fields with hopes for upward mobility and the promise of novelty and creativity, those that experienced burnout and depression found that they were simply going through the motions of a set routine, becoming, in a word, automatons. Such alienation would not surprise most readers, but the specific cultural shape with which it presented in Bangalore is interesting to note, particularly as the search for meaning in this context might take the form of a heightened sense of religiosity and, akin to the singular demands of religion and ethnicity, an impossible and social demand. In this case, specialized yet highly stressful labor conditions seemed to call forth symptomatic refusals and excesses of identification, or in some cases, a withdrawal from social life altogether.

Paralysis or affective disorders were also common responses to the stresses of this new economy, even resulting in conversion disorders that mimicked epilepsy, the so-called "pseudo seizure" phenomenon. Here the lines between neurology and psychiatry at NIMHANS were sometimes blurred, as indeterminant symptoms of seizure-like activity might lead to a neurological workup, complete with EEG (electroencephalogram) and video monitoring of seizures. This blurred line is examined in chapter 6, through the vantage of the neurology OPD and observing patients with sometimes clear neurological symptoms, whereas in other cases the blurred line with psychiatry suggested an ambiguity that lies at the heart of both clinical traditions.

Arrival at NIMHANS

Upon a pilot visit to NIMHANS in early 2014, prior to my fieldwork proper, I was able to spend a few days observing life on its campus, witnessing outpatient clinical care, and speaking to clinicians. One doctor was particularly interested in my presence and questions, himself drawn to social and cultural aspects of mental health, symptom presentation, and specifically to two kinds of "hysteric" presentations that were common in India, spirit possession and somatization. To this physician, the consequences of power, inequality, and dispossession among the poor were central to these symptoms. Though biomedical treatments were palliative, they did not address these underlying structural conditions, genetic vulnerabilities notwithstanding. When I mentioned the enduring stigma around mental illness in North America, and in describing some of my own research on psychogenic seizures in New York state, during which I had learned that roughly 25–30 percent of intractable seizure disorders at epileptology centers of care in the US were, in fact, nonepileptic conversion disorders, according to the American doctors I had interviewed, my NIMHANS colleague said that this was "remarkable, as 'hysteria' was thought to have disappeared in the early twentieth century in Europe and America. You have rediscovered hysteria!"

I had not thought much about the term "hysteria" when learning about conversion disorders, paralysis, and psychogenic seizures, though when rereading the older literature on hysteria, there was an uncanny resemblance of symptoms described under the broad rubric of hysteria (hemiparalysis, catatonia, seizures, etc.). Moreover, while hysteria was a gendered term, fraught with images of patriarchal normalcy and the suppression of the iniquities and familial violence in the European and North American contexts in which it became clinically salient, its usage in this context at NIMHANS seemed to open, rather than foreclose, an analysis of structural violence. And in the year that followed, while this term was not exclusively hegemonic, given that new diagnostic frames had complicated the gloss of this now unofficial clinical term, I was to see just how much of an opening into the psychosocial and cultural this term would afford, as well as what it may have foreclosed as it bore older traces and meanings, some undoubtedly lost in translation (Pinto 2022).

NIMHANS is a very large government institution near the sprawling neighborhood of Jayanagar, right in the heart of Bangalore, now officially named Bengaluru,[10] one of India's great megacities. Its sprawling campus is said to serve a population within a 300 km radius extending into the states of Karnataka (where it is located), Andhra Pradesh, Kerala, and Tamil Nadu. As specialized psychiatric and neurological care is relatively scarce in India, referrals are quite far and wide, extending to the entire nation, though the majority of patients come from within this radial catchment zone.

The doctors at NIMHANS are, generally speaking, highly articulate professionals who often comment in the national and local media. Yet they work in a government hospital, where most patients are working-class and poor, on the front lines of mental health care, whereas in the private medical sector they might earn more. NIMHANS is highly regarded as a national center for research and care, and, along with AIIMS in New Delhi (Ruddock 2021), has a reputation that allows the physicians, both psychiatrists and neurologists, along with the many counselors, therapists, psychologists, and technicians who work there, to enjoy a certain prestige that they would not hold within a private hospital or practice. As an academic center for research and a medical school for residents and fellows, its doctors are also engaged with research and publishing on a regular basis. Salaries are, as such, substantially higher than would be the case for general practitioners at other government hospitals.

The aforementioned doctor, who would become a close colleague and mentor in the subsequent year, and in continuing with the topic of conversion disorders or hysteria, said that he saw many patients who suffered from "fits" (seizures) that were nonepileptic. "Teeth-clenching" and "thrashing about" were the typical symptoms, he said.[11] To my surprise, he mentioned that while a vast majority do in fact enact symptoms of possession, following cultural models, there are a number who do mimic epilepsy, and believe they have the disease. In a word, these are "pseudo seizures" or psychogenic events, a type of conversion disorder in contemporary psychiatric language, which has formally abandoned the term "hysteria."

I was startled to learn that only fifty psychotherapists were trained in a year at the major medical schools in India, as the doctor informed me. The doctors at NIMHANS would explain, somewhat ruefully, that as in much of the developing world (Reyes-Foster 2019; Kilroy-Marac 2019), a pharmacological approach to psychiatry had supplanted psychotherapy. The new generation of psychiatrists, I was told, were being trained in neuroscience and pharmacology, but were not taking the "holistic approach to the person," a refrain I often heard, regardless of the age and gender of the psychiatrist. Consideration of the person's experience of everyday violence (Das 2006; Pinto 2014), their class oppression and position in society—that is, the structural and psychosocial determinants of mental health—was not given sufficient weight in India, according to my NIMHANS interlocutors. This persistent theme, as amplified at NIMHANS by physicians and by some psychiatrists I met at other institutions, surprised me to the extent that I assumed this was a critical anthropological position (e.g., Young 1995; Kirmayer, Lemelson, and Cummings 2015; Kleinman 1988; 2009; Rose 2018; Biehl and Thomas 2009; Good, Subandi, and Good 2007), and not necessarily the view of biomedical psychiatry at the most esteemed biomedical psychiatric and neurological hospital in South India. And while there might be a bias in my methodology and sample, given that the circle of psychiatrists and social workers I met, both within and outside of NIMHANS, came through recommendations I received from my faculty mentors who were sympathetic to anthropology and the holistic perspective, the ethos of and clinical care in the institution seemed to call out its own limits on a daily, and sometimes despairing, basis. This indictment of biomedical psychiatry from within its deepest navel caught my attention, though of course, my surprise was unwarranted, given that only those deeply embedded within the complexity and temporality of clinical care would have the most salient insights as to its fissures and failures. Moreover, only the brightest physicians would be offered a position at this prestigious institution, with a tremendous degree of competition for top postings. NIMHANS was the center of psychiatry and neurology in the nation, attracting those with the academic pedigree and training to see beyond narrow specialization. Moreover, it was a progressive institution in its founding principles, against the asylum model of care, a history I will return to shortly.[12]

The aforementioned doctor estimated that 30–40 percent of patients who suffered from seizures or possession went to "native healers" of one sort or another, in addition to psychiatric care. That statistic did not include alternative medical systems like Ayurveda or yoga. Rather, these were the *dargahs* (Sufi saint shrines), temples, and within them various traditional healers and mediums. He went on to speak about R. L. Kapur, a pioneering psychiatrist in India who advocated training native healers in basic psychotherapy, given the problems of health care delivery in India, with its limited specialist resources. A partnership system between psychiatry, neurology, and traditional healers was more appropriate, according to Kapur, given the demonstrable efficacy in traditional medicine (which he was also researching), as well as the paucity of clinicians and their limited knowledge of the local cultural psychology within local communities (Fabrega 2009; Murthy and Jain 2009; Kapur 2004; 2012; Kapur and Carstairs 1976).[13] This medical care delivery model, however, was rejected, the doctor said, by the government in favor of an "antidepressant" model, which was seen as more scientific. The problem now, he maintained, was that antidepressants were overused and, as a result, there was little understanding of the structural causes of depression and suicide (Kleinman and Patel 2003).

A history of the lunatic and criminal asylum in colonial India is beyond the scope of this study (see Murthy and Jain 2009; Sarin and Jain 2018; Murthy and Jain 2015; Pinto 2020a). But the emergence of a new kind of mental hospital in the late nineteenth century mirrored events that had occurred in Europe as described in Foucault's *History of Madness* (2006). Mysore, an independent princely state in South India, was the epicenter of change. Mysore's Dewan and the policy of the enlightened kingdom was to emulate Europe's model. Dr. Francis Noronha, a doctor in the Mysore Medical Services, was trained in England. He sought to build a state-of-the-art facility in Bangalore. In 1932 the new buildings—a series of pavilions and enclosed gardens—were constructed (Murthy and Jain 2009). This style of architecture and gardens were believed by reformers to be conducive to recovery.

Later, Dr. M. V. Govindaswamy collaborated with Dr. Willi Mayer-Gross from the famous Heidelberg school of psychiatry. Despite the presence of one of Freud's early students, Girindrasekhar Bose, starting a psychoanalytic school in India influenced by Indian philosophy and ontology—themes that would later be developed by clinicians and scholars such as Sudhir Kakar, Horatio Fabrega, and Alan Roland, among others—the development of modern biomedical psychiatry at the All India Institute for Mental Health, later named National Institute of Mental Health and Neurosciences, followed the Emil Kraepelin school of thought that Mayer-Gross had brought from Heidelberg. That is, mental illness was viewed as an organic and neuropsychiatric problem. Govindaswamy himself felt that psychoanalysis was a "strain on one's credibility" (quoted in Murthy and Jain 2009, 226). Indeed, Dr. Edwin Mapother, a British psychiatrist advising Govindaswamy and others, argued that Bose's psychoanalysis "represented the greatest danger to the development of psychiatry in India" (Murthy and Jain 2009, 226–227).

This dim view of psychoanalysis persisted through the history of NIMHANS; and unlike in the US, the emphasis of neuropsychiatry and psychopharmacological therapeutics did not represent a more recent shift. As one psychiatrist trained and practicing at NIMHANS told me, "We were not allowed to read Freud." And as Murthy and Jain put it, "All attempts to describe fundamental etiologies of psychiatry disorders in purely mentalist terms were thus viewed with suspicion and phenomenological approaches were given more prominence" (Murthy and Jain 2009, 213).

Interestingly, Govindaswamy was a Sanskrit scholar and believed Indian philosophy should be studied—a point to bear in mind. NIMHANS developed along Kraepelinian lines of psychiatry, but simultaneously encouraged research in Ayurveda, yoga, and other "traditional" systems of medicine. For the most part these remained separate streams from biomedicine. They were, however, viewed as complementary, owing to the sociocultural context of patient beliefs. Indeed, while psychoanalysis was derided, community-based health care was encouraged, owing to a tolerance of, and complementarity between, traditional medicine and psychiatry (Corin and Bibeau 2009; Kapur 2004) as accepted by Indian psychiatry, as well as the fact that the majority of Indians sought traditional and faith-based therapies and counsel (Kapur 2004; Kakar 1982; Fabrega 2009).

One result of this trajectory at NIMHANS was a very undeveloped psychotherapeutic tradition (Murthy and Jain 2009). "Pastoral" care for the Self, in Foucault's (2003) terms, remained the traditional healer's domain. The social, as the scene of psychic troubling and healing, was mediated by the gods, by the traditional healers, and, through the back door, as we will see, by psychiatrists, though not without their own resistance to normalizing strategies of care.

Sociocentric Selfhood

While "charlatans" were often decried, the normalizing of the patient within the sociocentric order was a frequent occurrence, yet troubled the psychiatrists I observed. Though this should be developed more fully and critically in a longer review, let us describe, for parsimony's sake, what is meant, broadly speaking, by the sociocentric self. Utilizing Edward Sapir's (2010) terms we could describe this as an idealized "as if" psychology—a collective self-image of a culture acting as a kind of Freudian ego-ideal, and, of course, interpolated by individuals within that society. In this instance, it is a self with permeable and porous boundaries that exists only through and in its relations to others. This notion of ideological holism, associated most famously with Dumont's (1970) analysis of caste and hierarchy in India, argued that individuals do not exist as automatous beings, but rather, in their being-for-another, hierarchically organized and "organically" or structurally constituted. The ordering principle of this "dividual" being (Marriott 1976), or the collective to which he or she belonged, was the relationship between the pure and the impure. Not only regulating sociality through caste, but also cosmologically, the principle ordered through isomorphisms or mimesis between macrocosm and microcosm, or between the self and the environment (Halliburton 2009; Lang 2018; Zimmermann 1987; Daniel 1984).

Ironically, contra to the "dividual" argument, to some extent, was the isomorphism of hierarchy within each person. Hence mental discipline and yoga were developed to "balance" the proper hierarchy within, whilst also simultaneously destroying the sociocentric hierarchy—an archivic and anarchivic principle coexisting in perpetual tension (Derrida 1995), grounded, in this case, in speculative philosophy (e.g., Buddhism, Vedanta, etc.). This principle deconstructs notions of individual self-existence, and that allows us to see, arguably, a back door to psychodynamic approaches and etiology, despite the biomedical orientation of Govindaswamy (Corin, Thara, and Padmavati 2004). We might recall, too, that Lacan (1977) often cited Buddhist and Vedantic verses to illustrate the illusory nature of the "imaginary" self or ego.

Returning to the question of suicide and depression, the doctor spoke of the skyrocketing rates, and related this to neoliberal transformations in the agricultural sector (Vasavi 2012). There were, he claimed, 14,000 suicides in Bangalore alone in one year. Countrywide, the rates ran in the hundreds of thousands, and most went unreported, he claimed. The primary issue concerned investments and price fluctuations in a volatile commodity market that had been deregulated. With unexpected losses and staggering debts, farmers saw no other options than suicide. In urban contexts, stress and loneliness were key factors, as was burnout within certain sectors of the workforce, particularly within the IT fields that were dominant in Bangalore, India's "Silicon City" (Upadhya and Vasavi 2008). Therefore, whether it be in rural or urban settings, "class is at the heart of psychiatry" with the "petty cruelties" that people endure in their daily lives, according to this doctor.

Aside from suicide and depression, coupled with increasing rates of addiction, "hysteria" came in the form of possession, dissociation, and somatic symptoms like paralysis and "fits" (seizures). Possession was more common among women, and often appeared collectively through ritual means. The Goddess, for instance, allows for the unspoken and unsaid to be expressed in Hinduism (Obeyeskere 1981; Kakar 1982; Nabokov 2000; Addlakha 2008; Ram 2014; Ramberg 2014). But there were also malevolent *jinn*, *bhut*, *pey*, and other spirits that speak through symptoms such as hearing voices, paralysis, and "fits" (seizures). Among adolescents, conversion disorders can provide symptoms of a more individuated sign of distress. Possession, on the other hand, can be more collective and speak to shared idioms (e.g., the role and status of a newly married woman in the joint patriarchal family).

The doctor suggested that the "modernist mindset" never took root in India completely. The separation of religion and science was not absolute in India. Scientists happily practiced their yoga and prayed in the temples while doing material science following a "rational method." "There is no conflict between the two, as has developed in the West," he claimed. The possibility of a layered self existed, as indicated by Kapur's fascination with traditional forms of healing (2004; 2012) coupled with Indian speculative philosophy. On the other hand, people, he maintained, especially patients with mental health issues, had a hard time imagining themselves as more than the position or status into which they had been born. Their very sense of being was defined in multiple ways by the interlocking ways the land, kin, and caste status were imprinted onto a person's very being. Social placement and rootedness gave people an identity and a sense of social support; but this also limited the possibility of Indians imagining themselves as otherwise when things turned bad. Hierarchy and space seemed immutable. The autonomy and horizon of mobility for the person was quite different than it was in the West, he maintained. In saying this about spirituality and identity, he reiterated notions of the sociocentric and hierarchic self that marked the anthropological literature on Indian and South Asian selfhood and personhood. But what was pivotal here, and as will be unfolded in the varied cases that will pass through the clinic in the following pages, was the disjuncture between the cultural ideals and the conflicting, and at times impossible, demands they made upon people. It was this tension between what Edward Sapir famously called the "as if" psychology of a culture, and the individual psychology of persons who were interpolated into that cultural ideal or personhood, which, in turn, may clash with their internal selfhood (Corin, Thara, and Padmavati 2004). An emphasis, in short, on filial and community harmony acted as a source of both support and stress (Kleinman 1988) within the selves of individuals. This essential, and arguably Freudian, insight that normative ideals ("ego ideal") do not constitute the self without resistance and fracture was to manifest itself repeatedly during the clinical case observations and discussions I participated in during the year that followed. While the sociocentric ideology exerted normative pressures within a behavioral environment, a fissure or resistance marked individuals in different ways, depending upon their social predicament (Pinto 2014). The classic psychoanalytical notion of the "split subject" carried currency, despite the anti-Freudian legacy within Indian psychiatry.

The OPD

My first experiences within the Outpatient Department (OPD) at NIMHANS were overwhelming to my senses. There were over one hundred individuals in the waiting room at any given time. Less than ten offices occupied by different psychiatrists attempted to serve this large crowd. The aforementioned doctor mentioned that he had read about Western doctors complaining about their working conditions and case load. He said they "couldn't imagine India's conditions for doctors." I agreed that this intensity and volume would be unimaginable in psychiatric clinical care in the United States. The psychiatrists at NIMHANS would only take very short breaks for tea/coffee, mid-morning and afternoon, as well as a lunch break, during what could easily be an eight-hour shift, potentially seeing more than twenty-five patients each day.

In addition to the heavy volume of patients, I was mildly surprised to see a near total absence of patient confidentiality. Not only did most patients come accompanied by family, most of whom were brought into the conversation and queried about their relatives, but treatment rooms always had their doors open, allowing people to stroll in and out when patients were being seen. The doctors sat behind desks and performed little if any physical examination, though they did note physical features that were visible on the patient. Questions by the doctors and comments by the patients were evaluated for their emotive and cognitive response. The clinical visit was mainly an interview wherein the doctor viewed the chart of the patient very rapidly, asked questions of the patient and their accompanying family members, and then prescribed medications along with offering some brief practical advice, whilst also recording notes in the patient's chart. In many cases, the doctor had to ascertain whether the names in the chart matched with a medical identification card. Naturally, new patients received more time with the doctors than did follow-up patients. While most visits were in the ten-minute range, some new patients might receive thirty minutes of care from the doctor.

A hospital bed was placed in each OPD examination room, though I rarely saw patients make use of it. In one instance, a patient took a nap while the doctor continued to see other patients. Sometimes patients would stand and wait behind another patient unconcerned about whether the patient might want privacy or not. Clearly there was no expectation of privacy, whatever the patient may have preferred.

After my first day in the OPD it was already clear that poverty and family strife were ubiquitous problems that contributed to the worsening symptoms faced by patients and their families. Indeed, many of the family problems related directly to poverty and precarity, and the stress it caused. At the end of the shift, and after my first day witnessing the OPD, the doctor I had interviewed said, in a matter-of-fact tone, that what I saw was quite typical, and that he had seen over one thousand patients in the last three months! Of these, one hundred and fifty patients had been ongoing patients for past twenty-five to forty years.

It is these everyday forms of violence and precarity, and the rhythms and flows of the OPD's unique phenomenology and velocity of care, that this book attempts to capture, rather than the deep case histories of patients, which were largely inaccessible to me. In the velocity of care, the modalities of clinical life and the interpretative frames and interruptions to those same frames are discussed and highlighted, though patient case studies are not the extended biographies of the patient one might find in deeper case-oriented institutional studies (e.g., Pinto 2014; Biehl 2005; Addlakha 2008).

This study is bracketed by the institutional flows and restrictions imposed upon the fieldwork method. I would use shorthand notes during the day to capture case details and commentary by physicians, followed by write-up in the evenings. Analysis was done later through thematic and terminological content indexing, with those most frequent and prominent themes then organized into chapter headings. To maintain confidentiality, no identifiers were collected. Moreover, and perhaps against the grain of conventional ethnographic accounts of professionals, I chose to not personify the doctors I interacted with in an effort to also preserve their anonymity. Therefore, they do not come across as distinct and complex characters, except in their clinical interventions and commentary. Pseudonyms are used only for patients, whereas doctors are simply quoted, but not given personality profiles or names. This may seem paradoxical in that this is an ethnography of the modalities of care I observed. But I felt this was necessary to protect the doctors who were often outspoken and sometimes critical in matters of politics and policy.

While the pragmatic temporalities, constraints, and limits of care are described in the chapters that follow in the NIMHANS context, inevitably, questions of theory emerged when trying to make sense of the malevolence that seemed to be figured excessively. In what follows, as I became enmeshed in this research, I turned to psychoanalytic and deconstructive tools that emerged as relevant, and away from the more urgent pragmatic concerns. This was in the hope that ethnography can speak to theory, and reopen some of the perennial questions concerning mental health and subjectivity, and, indeed, the human condition, that seemingly cry out for renewed discussion in the age of neuropsychiatric determinism (Rose 2018; Luhrmann and Marrow 2016; Patel and Kleinman 2003; Kleinman 2009), empirical historicism, and much concern over ontological pluralism. While the latter objects of inquiry are undoubtedly important, the former, that is, theories of selfhood more broadly, have come out of focus in recent times.

The Violence of the Social and "Hysteria"

The sense of crisis surrounding the question of mental health care in India has focused upon expanding coverage and educating the public about the potentials for increased risks of illness in times of increasing stress, as well as the need to combat the stigma associated with mental illness (Datta 2015). The key debates in the media and academy, as mentioned above, have taken as given the preponderance of mental illness as statistically underreported and the need for the expanded reach of biomedical psychiatric care, given the paucity of psychiatrists relative to the population size. But the question of just how stigma produces its pathological object, the mentally ill patient, requires an opening up of the cultural and social forces that, in the name of normalizing and harmonizing relationships, enact regimes of power, oftentimes gendered, and quell creative and rebellious resistances to these hierarchy-enacting forces. How modern psychiatric clinical practice fits into, or resists, the violence of the social in producing the "normal" moral subject is the question I address.

Much has been written about the "sociocentric" self in India and other parts of Asia, in which, as many analysts have suggested (Kakar 1982; Obeyesekere 1981; Nichter 1982; Roland 1988; Fabrega 2009, etc.), the individual is healthy insofar as they are in harmony with the collective, simply speaking. To "know thyself," as Kakar (1982) has argued, is to shift one's internal states to harmonize with the social and, by extension, the universal, and to dissolve the individual ego, in normative Hindu terms. Whereas, stereotypically, in the West, to "know thyself" is to surmount external constraints and to maintain a constant sense of identity as unique and bounded. Taking a constructivist position, the experience of selfhood and normalcy is culturally defined, making universal claims about disease and illness impossible. Foucault (2006) takes this argument in one direction, claiming that madness is the thinking of power and the defining of normalcy based upon its workings through cultural discourse and social practice (Rose 2018). Within anthropology, cultural determinists, on the other hand, committed to the idea of greater plasticity as an adaptive capacity, claim the mantle of relativism in shaping the human experience (e.g., Geertz 1973; Rosaldo 1984; Benedict 1934; Shweder 1984), denying that a common transhuman species-being can be operationalized in a singular and universal psychiatric paradigm. On the other end of the spectrum, a universalized biomedical diagnostic psychiatry would argue that while symptom expression may vary according to cultural content, the underlying brain pathology behind, for instance, schizophrenia, is more or less the same, despite its varied expression. In early psychoanalytic anthropology, similarly, the cultural content is merely a secondary institution or elaboration of defenses arising out of particular socialization practices (Spiro 1984; Devereux 1980; Kardiner 1939).

An indeterminate middle ground is important, if we are to avoid the romanticism of extreme constructivism on the one hand, and the reductionism of biomedical etiology on the other, which ignores the social and cultural forces that impact upon wellbeing and give conscious meaning to life (Kakar 1981; Obeyesekere 1981; 1985; Kleinman 1988; 2009; Good, Subandi, and Good 2007). Moreover, despite the apparent hegemony of Kraepelinian biomedical psychiatry in India (Murthy and Jain 2009), the doctors, I found, are much more biocultural in their thinking and approach to caring for their patients than one might expect, particularly in the age of genomics and psychopharmaceutical dominance. Indeed, my observations, of which I will share a few examples in broad representative strokes, suggest patterns of presentation and care that were deeply shaped by cultural and social forces.

The ranges of stigma, rebellion, and pathology versus normalcy within the NIMHANS clinical context are vast and varied, given its status as a major tertiary center. While dozens of patients pass through the OPD each day with a myriad of illness presentations, these patterns are both a function of the cultural and social shaping of illness within families and communities, as well as clinical modalities shaped by the physicians at NIMHANS. These doctors struggle, oftentimes valiantly, against the pressures of high patient loads, coupled with a need to mitigate symptoms, indeed, to normalize and harmonize patients within their families and communities.

Though the case particularities suggest patterns and social causation, to some extent, underlying biological vulnerabilities certainly vary substantially from case to case. My aim is not to add another layer of diagnostic interpretation to the patients' diagnosed psychopathology, based upon an oblique metacommentary of both patient distress and medical diagnosis. Rather, my intervention is to observe how the violence of and within the social is manifested in particularly patterned psychosocial symptoms, rather than to determine individual etiologies which are, of course, quite complex, and would require a manner of depth interviewing I was not able to undertake. With breadth, I could thematize prevalent patterns of distress, as well as modalities of diagnostic and pragmatic aspects of clinical care.[14] This patterning, paradoxically, and arguably forensically, can only be made visible through individual case histories, albeit truncated, involving a kind of double hermeneutic: that of the patient's individual narrative, an artefact of the OPD encounter, as well as the larger social field of discourse in which it was embedded.

In most cases, the acute nature of the illness and the social violence that might have been its primary symptom, and perhaps, in some cases, its traumatic cause, the ideal of patient insight, was sometimes buried under the weight of urgency and the need to offer only a salve to deeper structural problems. Symptoms that led to abuse perpetrated by the patient, or its reverse, as caused by the social context in which the patient was traumatized, were subject to biomedical interventions. This, moreover, demonstrated to me that the romantic constructivist view of mental illness as protest, or simply labeling, that is, the thinking of power, proved inadequate in addressing the acute and very palpable suffering patients and their families endured as a result of their illness.

There would be little analytic substance to the OPD session if not for some psychotherapeutic techniques employed. Usually, however, advice was immediate and geared towards behavioral modifications that were thought to be "healthy" for the patient, given their specific distress. For example, a person who would spend too much time on the computer or TV would be advised to keep themselves occupied with other activities. Or a person prone to depression or schizophrenia might be advised to have a structured daily schedule, leaving less room for rumination, and apparently, delusions, to harden and take hold of the mind. Diaries were not encouraged among those with severe delusions or hallucinations. Family issues might be hinted at, but provocation and probing in great depth were rarely witnessed in the OPD. Sometimes, the doctors, however, would ruminate and speculate further on the psychosocial and cultural dimensions of the patients they were treating once the patients had left the room.

Whatever its biological or neurological underpinnings, the violence of the social was brought into the causative formation of symptoms in most cases. These oftentimes involved gendered norms that coerced a kind of normalization within the familial and social, inducing symptoms of protest or resistance, which, in turn, were then partially normalized within the clinical context through the desired "cure" offered by medications. But the doctors, though varied in style, often resisted patient or familial desires for a kind of normalcy that suppressed symptoms but did not get to their provenance in everyday forms of social violence (Das 2006).

Factors such as the patrilocal joint family, the tensions caused by the increasingly competitive forces of education and labor, and the increasing legalism or literalism that are both symptomatic of a more bureaucratized society, as well as the causal force of today's demands upon identity and self-worth, have, to some extent, exacerbated the shame surrounding mental illness (Martin 2009; Biehl 2005). The venue of the OPD, with its heavy patient loads and limited clinical durations, focused upon symptom alleviation, despite doctors harboring more complicated understandings of case histories and illness presentations than they were able to effectively treat.

Shame and stigma, however, in most cases did not lead families to reject the person possessing the illness. Rather, conflicts that were difficult and strained familial relationships seldom led to the abandonment or institutionalizing of the afflicted. The lives of patients and their families were entangled in complicated ways, both in terms of the etiology of illness (the psychosocial causative factors) and their attempts at resolution (Pinto 2014).

When thinking about psychic resistance, we can recall that to Freud, the symptom always resists against the disclosure of the psychic tension that prompted it. Therefore, there is much resistance the closer one approaches the scene of trauma, division, and anxiety. Repetitive and compulsive behavior can be, even in masochistic displays, a form of resistance against the normative order, as much as it seems to be a "resistance without resistance," or a subjection to this order through its ostensible and relentless punitive face. As Derrida notes in his *Resistances to Psychoanalysis*, "the repetition compulsion, hyperbolic resistance of nonresistance, is in itself analytic . . . in the surest form of its ruse: disguised as non-resistance" (1998, 24). And for Deleuze (1997; 1987), acts of resistance can be a creative disarticulation of the arboreal orderings of things, a defiant and creative impulse. To Derrida, resistance marks the edge of intelligibility and meaning (Corin 2007), which, in turn, also indexes a suffering and division that cannot be aestheticized without violence. But sometimes, rebellion or resistance, as an explanation, was not countered, contradicted, or denied. There were numerous cases of addiction, particularly substance abuse of alcohol and ganja (marijuana) that passed through the halls of NIMHANS. Oftentimes, these were working-class males who used substances to cope with the pressures of making ends meet, working in arduous and physically demanding jobs, or even due to peer pressure. But in other cases, particularly among the young and more affluent, addictive behaviors could mark a rebellion against the normative order, or even mark a boredom and fatigue with the increasingly hectic pace of life in the urban metropolis (Simmel 1971). But resistance took other, more dramatic, refractory, and somatic forms as well. The term "hysteria" would often be used to refer to dissociative possession states, somatizations, and other "conversion disorder" symptoms that were not clearly identifiable as schizophrenia, acute psychosis, or bipolar affective disorders. Hysteria, while not, technically speaking, a clinical diagnosis anymore, retained valence within clinical discussions of social tensions and violence. It marked a political grey zone demanding more explication.

Hysteria's Others

Hysteria connotes a myriad of emotions, symptoms, and resistances. Though an imprecise, shapeshifting, and gendered term (Mitchell 2000) when approached genealogically, in the Freudian, Kleinian, and Lacanian traditions it indexes the "bad object's" overbearing presence (Klein), or the excess of the Other's desire (Lacan, Freud) manifested as an embodied yet non-symbolizable resistance. In short, it concerns a corporeal and immobilizing subjection under the sign of the Other's power to constitute the self. As such, it is a political symptom on both the micro- (e.g., familial, filial) and macro-levels (e.g., ideology, the symbolic, law).

In Deleuze and Guattari (1972; 1987), in contrast, hysteria's morphings represent a "becoming," not a paralyzing regression or repression; but rather, a transformation through a "deterritorialized" selfhood, away from the "molar" structures of patriarchy and capitalism, and into new machinic interconnections or rhizomic intensities. These becomings are open possibilities, so long as they are not re-Oedipalized through psychoanalytic cures (Deleuze and Guattari 1972). While a provocative and destabilizing critique of institutionalized psychoanalysis and normalizing pathologizations within psychiatry, more generally, the politics of hysteria in the psychoanalytic and Derridean understandings of the symptom, I suggest, speaks more to the intimacies, ambivalence, and, most importantly, a sense of betrayal or violence within the social. This, in turn, divides signification, consciousness, and the unconscious process within itself, and against a monadic, vitalist, and transcendent life-force, which risks effacing these fissures and the negations they generate (Morris 2017).

In the Indian psychiatric clinical context, and arguably beyond it, the themes of betrayal are increasingly witnessed in a growing sense of malevolence that is marked by the Other's failure to be as idealized. In this sense, the "good object" of desire is increasingly revealed, through an incapacitating literalism that cannot subsist within ambivalence, to be lacking. The trauma of this failure is, in turn, masked by a "hysteria" of somatic and possessive overcoming, repetitive, inarticulate, and traumatic. Hysteria as a clinical diagnosis marks this stasis and paralysis, though it is sometimes figured, at least partially, by a range of malevolent spirits (*jinn*, *bhut*, *pey*, etc.), as well as by deathlike catatonic fugues and conversion-disorder symptoms. Though often framed in terms of tradition and cults of possession, it is increasingly symptomatic of a modernity that flattens difference in the name of singular identities and modalities of life within capitalist modernity.

The animus of betrayal within these most social of symptoms suggests two forms of what Derrida calls "archive fever" (1995). Archive fever is the invocation of a judgement, buttressed by knowledge claims that exceed containment, revealing fissures within a discourse marked by internal inconsistency and division. The archive is constructed to efface this division and contradiction, and is most feverish when the arbitrariness of the Law, in

Derrida's and/or Lacan's sense, and its literalism are carried to greater ossifying lengths, in a fetish-like fashion, masking a division between wish and perception (Morris 2017).

The homogenizing malevolence of modern, serialized, categorical distinctions, against a more fluid and protean past in India, I suggest, fuels archive fever, which, arguably, is its hysteric symptom, attempting, as Lacan might say, to fill the hole within the Other's whole, or lack (Willford 2018; Hansen 2001; Fink 1996; Zizek 1993; Aretxaga 2008). And while, in the cases discussed in this book, intimacies, care, and betrayals are located within the bonds of kinship and family, these forces of betrayal index wider social totalities and the growing intolerance of literalisms against metaphor and ambiguity. Hysteria, as a resistance against resistance, immobilizes and paralyzes, bringing a victim's discourse into public view as the patient approaches proximity with a death-like existence, mastering a trauma through a horrible psychic cost (and social cost, when ostracized or accused of witchcraft, for instance).

On the other hand, and in following Lacan (1977), the hysteric's or victim's discourse is also generative of the master's discourse, fueling a diagnosis and pathologizing of the hysteric as one of "modernity's figures," as aptly described by Sarah Pinto (2020b). In that sense, archive fever, as the logic of the supplement, catalogues the symptoms of the hysteric in order to normalize, and to respond to the political challenge posed by this proximity with a living death that threatens to reveal the effaced arbitrariness of the Law. The twin discourses can become co-generational, each divided within the presence of the other. The horrors of the unfilial, the "witch," the mentally ill, and the dangerous disable, under conditions of precarity and hierarchy, the radical becomings that Deleuze reserves for the artist as schizophrenic. As Mitchell (2000) points out, "there is too much of the 'other' in the empty body of hysteria" (230).

The normalizing procedures of clinical psychiatry in India are not singular or uniform, nor entirely disciplinary. Indeed, learning to live with the "good" and "bad" object, or seeing that they coexist and can be literally swallowed, as in the "buccal ethics" (Guyer 2007) of ingesting both the warmth and poison of the world, is recognized clearly in the Indian cultural context through its oral myths of Krishna, Shiva, and the Goddess, whereby the universe, with all its poison and beneficence, is contained within the mouth, to be ingested, and, of course, sometimes to be spit out (Doniger 2009). Literalism, serial forms of identification, and the erasure of this permeable and protean possibility of identity is, however, both the symptom and the cause. That is, monocultural fantasies and ideologies emergent today represent an archive fever, but are constitutive of fevered rationalizations. Destabilizing and deconstructing absolutes, a feature of Indian speculative and mythical thought for millennia (e.g., Smith 2006; Shulman 1985), is mirrored in psychiatric discourses around the term "hysteria," indexing indeterminacy, though the risk of a biomedical archive fever also lurks in the shadows of clinical care (Lacan 1997; Schechter 2014; Rose 2018; Kleinman 2009). As suggested above, however, I also take hysteria as an analytic in diagnosing matters of violence in the social, whereas the clinicians I observed gestured in this direction without the psychoanalytic language I elaborate upon in my readings of these cases. Therefore, the centrality of hysteria throughout this study occurs in two registers: one as analytic; and second, of a destabilizing of diagnostic certainty. Both are critical, I argue, as the second destabilizes psychoanalytic overreach, pointing to a paradox at the heart of Freud's legacy. That is, that Freud's insights around the indeterminacy of the sign, given its inexhaustible connotations, displacements, and condensations, rebelled against the diagnostic readings of case histories that purported a stable diagnosis. Or in Derrida's (1995) terms, the deconstructability inherent to the archive is already implicit within Freudian analysis, despite the latter's quest for scientific certainty.

In making this argument, through the cases and commentary that follow, I depart to some extent from the normative formulations of sociocentric theories of Indian (South Asian) selfhood, arguing that these formulations obviate the violence of the social by naturalizing hierarchy in gendered, caste, and communal forms. And, as Nabokov (2000) has shown, curing in the name of the sociocentric ideal can be extraordinarily coercive and violent, as well as psychologically traumatizing. Moreover, alterity and dissonance within Indian thought have a long been a force within the force of possession and dissociation (Smith 2006). And the modern provocations of these ancient idioms continue to destabilize sociocentric hierarchies and normativities (Ram 2013; Pinto 2014; Trawick 2017). The moral "good" objects of family harmony, filial piety, and ethnoreligious identity, while having possessive force, are also increasingly ossifying, alienating, and generative of inescapable failures and contradictions (Pinto 2014; Cohen 1998; Chua 2014; Varma 2020; Marrow 2012). Cultural idioms certainly have sway and power, and are interpolated within the self, but are increasingly deployed as anti-political and normalizing gestures, part and parcel of nationalism and its own version of archive fever, which in turn effaces its arbitrary orderings of power and privilege and the kinds of malevolence this unleashes.

While "schizoanalysis" (Deleuze and Guattari 1972) calls for a freedom of the unconscious to pursue its "own constituted machines," this in turn repeats, ironically, the duality of conscious and unconscious, inside and outside, which Derrida (1981) critiqued in his powerful essay "The Pharmakon." "Oedipus," like any writing or archive, is never singularly constitutive of consciousness, though it does, as any outside, permeate, whatever inside subjectivity might exist (Zizek 2003). Consciousness, as Hegel, Freud, Marx, and Lacan have shown, is *always already* mediated and exterior. But this exteriority is never singular, as it bears multiple traces, effaced and ostensible. The "anti" of Oedipus, though affording a timely and necessary, as well as an invigorating, critique of psychoanalytic hegemony when it was written, in short, negates too much, making singular and vitalistic what should be multiple and fractal, revealing a monadic libidinalization of the entire social field (Zizek 2003; Morris 2017). Derrida, more precisely, I would argue, reveals that each moment, each thought, and each utterance is divided within itself, an insight that Freud helped to decipher, but oftentimes effaced within his own scientific work (Derrida 1995). Learning to live with the ambiguities of Oedipus, or any filial/normative order, with its contradictions and injustices, is what hysteria or any "conversion disorder" arguably paralyzes, oftentimes with tragic results.

Living with good and bad objects, both being ingested and introjected through life's betrayals and intimacies, inoculates the subject against literalism, serialized forms of totalizing thought, and the need to negate alterity and difference with punitive vengeance. This is similar to what Obeyesekere (1981; 1985) has called "progression" through culture and symbolic elaboration and semantic openness, versus "regression" and symbolic closure. In the latter, the bad object becomes fixated upon, leading to obsessive and compulsive forms of self-harm. Progression through symbols, however, leads to greater self-understanding, as well as social integration and the spinning of cultural webs of meaning that have relevance to others. It is the difference between, in the more neurological language used by Malabou (2012), catastrophic injury versus adaptive plasticity. Whatever the organic versus psychological etiology of the wound, the self's capacity for healing and insight depends upon a language of expression that can speak to the wounds that mark the violence of the social, but also points to an ethic that goes beyond literalism, betrayal, and absolutes. That said, we wish to avoid the dichotomy of progression versus regression, as both can operate simultaneously through symptomatic and somatic distress coupled with symbolic elaboration. The scale may tip between functionality and paralysis, but absolute measures unnecessarily pathologize or romanticize what is more complex in the experience of mental illness (Pinto 2014).

While reciprocity and the desire to induce it animates hysteria and its demand against the Other, even its refusal can be transformative in either positive or harmful ways. Absolutism and judgement and the violence that ensues from this against the hysteric, or through the hysteric to the social field, can be one type of refused reciprocity that is harmful and immobilizing (Grosz 2005; Mitchell 2000; Pinto 2014; Willford 2014). A more positive type of withdrawal is another possibility, as Corin (2007) suggests for South Asia, in particular. The ascetic ideal is another road for progression, in Obeyesekere's sense, whereby the rejection of hierarchy and reciprocity is explicit, but not necessarily harmful. Here, contemplation and insights into the iniquities and relativities of social obligations and the identities they engender is given the relative freedom of a "becoming" other, and ultimately "imperceptible" in the mystical quest for a dissolution of self. Here, Deleuze's artist and philosopher, perhaps, meets India's mystic (Corin 2007; Kapur 2004; Corin, Thara, and Padmavati 2004). But in the everyday violence of the social, the psychiatric clinic is an increasingly important venue where the "crisis" of modernity's malevolence is enacted.

It has been argued that hysteria, and its modern replacement in various psychosomatic idioms of distress (Nichter 1982), is an attempt to control and master death through its enactment (Mitchell 2000). This is a virtual death, as opposed to the only absolute negation of the Other that is actual death, as Hegel most famously argued in his account of a possible refused recognition of the Other's mastery. Like Gregor in Kafka's *Metamorphosis,* the virtual death is, indeed, a becoming other in the sense that Deleuze suggests, but in the case of a hysteric conversion disorder, the refusal is not complete; it both speaks to a broken reciprocity, or the other's failure, a betrayal of intimacy bound up in familial politics, as well as a refusal to completely negate this other, bound, as it were, to a desire to have restitution and justice served. Such complexity is seen, for example, in Varma's (2020) and Cohen's (1998) discussions of *kamzori,* a fatigue-like symptom in North India that marks moral failures in the social in ambivalent ways, belying a singular external cause. As Derrida suggests, it is a resistance to resistance, an ambivalent attachment to a binding of self and other, where the hysteric's desire is bound and sustained in the Other's desire. Unlike the game of "fort-da" that, to Freud and Lacan, marked the subject's entry into language as substitution and sublimation, this becoming is more like simply "da" without the "fort." That is, a virtual death of the subject and marked by a drive to a death-like state to rouse the other's sympathy (Mitchell 2000). This, then, is the incapacitation of ambivalence and division to subsist, as in the "buccal ethics" (Guyer 2007), following Klein, that allows for the good and bad object to be consolidated within a grey zone or ambivalence that is tolerable and livable.

In my conclusion, I ask if we can better understand the pragmatic consequences of structural violence through a rethinking of hysteria's analytics (Kleinman 2009; Patel and Kleinman 2003). Aside from theoretical understandings, what are the practical implications of this rethinking in terms of a care-delivery model, and whether it is scalable or efficacious in relieving human suffering? Or, conversely, in sympathetically critiquing the global health movement and scalable models for community health systems through ethnography, do we potentially see the crisis of mental health as an excuse for medicalizing and pathologizing forms of alterity and difference that might not be pathological, unless when categorized as such through biomedicine? Finally, what are the potential racialized assumptions behind the resurgence of "native minds" (Sarin and Jain 2018) formulations in the light of indigenous studies and cosmo-centrism, ontological turns, and perspectivism? Is there a colonial phantom trace hidden within such "pharmakons" and archives of difference (Cohen 2012; Pinto 2020a)? Is a "pill for every ill" (Murthy 2018; Rose 2018) the inevitable psychiatrization of neuro- and experiential diversity? What might a psychiatric (and psychoanalytic) future look like in view of these questions (Rose 2018; Derrida 2007) that involve turning the gaze inwards upon a checkered history in which the violence of the social has been enabled by the normalizing violence of the clinic? Questions surrounding indeterminacy and determinacy prove critical, as "inside" and "outside" causation is figured in psychiatry and local cosmology. The question surrounding radical uncertainty and a failure of reason has, in the closed systems of magic and cosmology, and, arguably, psychiatry, found its solution through self-referential systems of coherence (Lévi-Strauss 1973; Mauss 1902). An ethical commitment to uncertainty and the unknown, on the other hand, opens that which is foreclosed in the hardened dichotomy of inside and outside causation, when the symptom is always indicative of an underlying determinant cause. Understanding the relentless and fevered drive to diagnostic determinism, in both cosmology and urban psychiatry, I suggest, opens up an alternative and radical psychiatry of the future.

Chapter 1

Shame, Stigma, and the Normalizing Impulse

The sense of crisis surrounding the question of mental health care in India has focused attention upon expanding coverage, educating the public, and combatting the stigma associated with mental illness. The key debates in the media and the academy have taken as given the preponderance of mental illness as statistically underreported, as well as a need for the expanded reach of biomedical psychiatric care. At the same time, there has been increasing recognition that the efficacy of traditional methods—faith healing and local health systems, such as Ayurveda, Unani, Siddha, and Yoga—deserves more research, given the acute needs within such a large and growing population coupled with the inadequacy of psychiatric resources in the country (Sebastia 2009a; 2009b; Fabrega 2009; Sujatha and Abraham 2012; Kakar 1982; Halliburton 2009; Lang 2018).

While this general awakening to the importance of mental health has been occurring globally, and is certainly important, the question of just how stigma produces its pathological object, the mentally ill patient, requires an opening up of the cultural and social forces that, in the name of normalizing and harmonizing relationships, enact regimes of power, oftentimes gendered, and quell creative and rebellious resistances to these hierarchy-enacting forces. How modern psychiatric clinical practice fits into, or resists, the violence of the social in producing the "normal" moral subject is the question this chapter examines.

The ranges of stigma, rebellion, and pathology versus normalcy within the NIMHANS clinical context are vast and varied, given its status as a major tertiary center. Indeed, NIMHANS is the main venue in all of Southern India for psychiatric and neurologic care, the training of future clinicians, and general research. AIIMS in New Delhi is the only institution of equivalent status and recognition, arguably, within the country. But NIMHANS, as mentioned, draws patients from all over the country due to its reputation, affordability, and relatively well-connected location within Bangalore.[1] Hundreds of patients pass through the Outpatient Department (OPD) each day, with a myriad of illness presentations. This chapter examines the parameters of shame, stigma, rebellion, and social abandonment, identifying certain recurring patterns out of this multiplicity. These patterns are a function of the cultural and social shaping of illness within families and communities, as well as of clinical modalities shaped by the physicians at NIMHANS, who struggle, oftentimes valiantly, against the pressures of high patient loads, coupled with a need to mitigate symptoms, and indeed, normalize and harmonize patients with their families and communities.

Though the myriad of case particularities suggests patterns of social causation, to some extent, it is also important to note that underlying biological vulnerabilities vary substantially from case to case. Therefore, it is impossible to separate thematics in a tidy lexicon, or to separate normalization pressures from agentive dissent or forms of resistance and rebellion that escape conscious intention. In that sense, we will see thematic overlaps across sections and chapters that would, in theory, allow us to restructure cases in alternative ways. That is, the thematic polymers that are my analytical rubrics can easily be reformed in alternate re-combinatory forms, given the questions asked. Moreover, these cases are exemplary to some extent, meaning that I cannot discuss all the cases that had, perhaps, similar resonances and dynamics. Finally, my aim, as stated earlier, is not to add another layer of diagnosis to the patients' diagnosed psychopathology. Rather, my intervention is to observe how the violence of the social is manifested in particular psychosocial etiologies (Pinto 2014; Cohen 1998), rather than determine individual etiologies which are, of course, quite complex and would require a manner of depth interviewing I was not able to undertake given the velocity of treatment within the OPD.[2] This, however, is where psychodynamic dimensions matter, as these point precisely to the social, where the ethnographic eye is most salient.

Shame and Stigma

Shame and stigma surrounding mental illness are pervasive and one of the key challenges facing professionals at NIMHANS. Even those patients and families that turn to psychiatry and, furthermore, make it to the leading center for psychiatric care are oftentimes uneasy about the care and advice they receive in the clinical context. The following cases address, in broad brush strokes, the manner in which stigma and shame impact family dynamics, revealing tensions that lie at the heart of the social. The intervention of psychiatry can powerfully reveal these tensions, providing not only a medical intervention but also, oftentimes indirectly, a social one, as well. On the other side of the coin, the pragmatics of the clinical encounter can also, conversely, serve to occlude or soften the sharp dichotomies of desire and tension within the family, offering a salve but not a direct psychosocial intervention.

Smita, a young woman from West Bengal, came to the OPD suffering from an inability to concentrate on her studies. She had also been vomiting for years after eating a full meal, particularly rice and curds. Her mother was very strict with her and did not let her mix with boys. But Smita's friends in school accused her of "stealing their boyfriends," though she was the "most shy with boys." Her teachers were "turned against her," she said, by these same friends. As a result of these tensions with friends and teachers she had to change schools a few times. Smita's father also suffered from panic and anxiety about the thoughts of others. It was unclear, however, if his relationship with his daughter was fraught, though I imagined the teachers as a possible figure of paternal transference, given how they were "turned against her." Prior to her treatment at NIMHANS, she had been prescribed lithium (for depression) by another psychiatrist. This was prescribed, she said, at the urging of her family, so that she could "get through her exams and study medicine." Of "all her friends," she said, her professional "ambitions are the highest."

It was unclear to the treating physician how much of her behavior was "normal teenage rebellion and anxiety." But Smita, we heard, had been teased for her being somewhat "plump" in school. As a possible victim of bullying, the doctor queried whether her vomiting was related to anything her mother might have said, in addition to the taunts of classmates? The doctor mentioned a Bengali proverb to the effect that "life is revolting" and must be vomited from the "bottom of the stomach." This was, perhaps, a culture-bound response to the vileness of human nature, he was suggesting, albeit, privately to me, after the patient had left the room. Of course, the question of anorexia/bulimia was also present in my mind as it indexed her "plump" appearance and apparent teasing for it. While her main symptoms were an inability to concentrate and vomiting, she also apparently lashed out at others within the home in ways that troubled her parents.

Her most recent exam scores in school were very good. Therefore, the doctor probed quite carefully about the source of her worries regarding her abilities to concentrate. He also asked if her parents had put excessive pressure on her to perform well academically. The doctor also queried whether the parents were very strict about not fraternizing with boys. To both questions, Smita answered affirmatively. These were not, of course, uncommon pressures faced by young women living with parents at home, and under the strictures of suppressing individual desires.

Clinical questioning turned to Smita's physical and social life. She enjoyed dancing but had no other physical exercise. It was not clear whether dancing was ever a social rather than an individual activity. Of some concern was her withdrawal from festive life within the family and community. In particular, she withdrew from celebrating Durga Puja, the most important Hindu holiday in Bengal. And though she claimed to have a few "good friends," it was apparent that Smita was socially awkward and anxious. Moreover, she harbored suspicions about what her peers and teachers thought of her, especially regarding "boys," which suggested an unease with her own desires, if read in psychodynamic terms.

The major psychiatric concern seemed to be her frequent and, apparently, volitional vomiting. Her doctor was of the opinion that she did not require a psychiatric diagnosis, though counseling was necessary. As the family had traveled from West Bengal, they were not in a position to stay at NIMHANS and to receive several sessions of psychotherapy. Moreover, without a more serious diagnosis, the doctor felt admitting her to the ward was unnecessary. The family, in turn, hoped for a "tablet" (medication), or quick repair, so that she could "work hard" for her upcoming critical exams, which would determine whether she could study medicine or not. "Counseling is a bit off the radar for most," the doctor explained to me. The time investment was greater, as was the potential for social stigma, given that the treatment would be potentially more visible if longer in duration. A "tablet" cure could be seen as general medical treatment by the wider community, and not necessarily treatment for mental illness (Lang 2018; Ecks 2013).

The doctor also felt it was not "proper" to have the patient counseled in the hospital environment of NIMHANS, in this case; but rather, it would be more efficacious if done within the "normal social environment" in which she lived. An effort to locate a couple of NIMHANS-trained psychotherapists in Calcutta who could provide services was initiated. It became apparent that there was, however, a crisis-level shortage of psychotherapists in the country, and especially in Calcutta, as I was told that the few there who practiced counseling were overloaded with clients. This seemed to contradict the idea that resistance to counseling is pervasive due to the stigma associated with mental illness. On the other hand, the sheer scope of the problem was, perhaps, enormous, in that even the minority of patients that were willing to seek counseling were sometimes at a loss in accessing adequate care. In this case, based upon her appearance and cognitive function, the doctor determined that Smita might have normal teenage anxieties, but exacerbated by abnormal "neurotic compulsions," as evidenced by the vomiting and social anxieties. Aside from her suspicions about her friends, she suffered no serious delusions or hallucinations at this point, though a follow-up appointment was suggested after some counseling had occurred.

Many cases were like Smita's, where a psychiatric diagnosis was not yet required, or was "borderline," or left undetermined. In cases like this, the pharmaceutical treatment at NIMHANS might be minimal. But, of course, there were many more cases where the comorbidity between psychological and neurological symptoms required a more aggressive intervention. For instance, there was a man who came frequently to the OPD. He suffered a speech and movement disorder that was caused by lithium, which he had taken while having a bad fever and depression; but this, apparently, was incorrectly prescribed by a local doctor untrained in psychiatry. This produced neurotoxicity within his system that affected his cerebellum. His speech and muscle control were permanently damaged. His cognition was still generally fine, though he was thought to have Bipolar Affective Disorder (BPAD), a very common diagnosis. He had been treated with medications for years at NIMHANS and returned regularly for follow-ups. Sadly, however, his children, whom he had raised well despite his condition, and both of whom were now lecturers in local technical colleges, no longer looked after him, finding him an embarrassment due to his movement and speech impediments. His doctor lamented their "cruelty," noting that for years he had asked the patient's children to accompany their father to the OPD, but he had always come alone. Yes, stigma and shame led to callousness and, even, as we will see, abandonment.

Stigma and shame also led to forms of social concealment to mitigate their effects. This could occur by isolating a family member from wider society or, conversely, sometimes hoping that marriage would cure disruptive symptoms. Indeed, marriage was thought to "cure" certain symptoms that, much like a Freudian analyst might argue, present themselves due to sexual inhibition or frustration. One day a cognitively impaired Kannadiga-speaking male in his mid-twenties presented with concerns raised by his family about self-care and behavior with others. There were questions as to whether he acted "properly with children" of various ages. His sister-in-law came with him to the clinic. She was asked about his ability to dress, recognize whether he was "neat or not," had certain food preferences, and knew how to "handle money," in addition to whether he exhibited "socially appropriate" behavior.

Ten years earlier, he had suffered seizures and during that time had some "behavioral issues." But with medication, he had improved a great deal. A motor skills assessment was ordered. Interestingly, the family, perhaps sincerely, wanted to marry him off as they believed that it "might improve his condition." His parents were now no longer alive, and he was cared for by an aunt and sister-in-law. Therefore, part of their reasoning behind marriage could have been influenced by financial considerations, though that is only speculation. This belief, as it came up in other cases as well, both in Bangalore and in the Nilgiris, is commonly held. The belief that marriage can offer an antidote for "seizures" (potentially nonepileptic)[3] or mental illness was fairly widespread among, particularly, the working class. This idea may be a culturally sanctioned way of talking about the relationship between various psychological symptoms and sexual frustration, suggestive of a Freudian analogue. But this was never explicitly explained as such. Marriage was said, however, to "stabilize" unstable people, and the sensitivities behind instability remained unsaid, as Freud would also maintain.

This case was also suggestive of the thorny issue of family quarrels concerning the assets that belong to the mentally ill. Doctors pointed out to me that declaring mental incompetency for one of their patients could have implications about the family's and patient's financial independence. In such cases, the potential for abuse of mentally ill relatives was great, as they could be cheated out of their inheritance, pensions, and/or savings by unscrupulous family members, though this was the exception, not the norm.

In another case, a man in his mid-forties with significant global developmental delay had been having "aggressive" episodes. He was deaf and mute. As he entered the examination room he smiled and signaled to the doctor by pointing to his mouth and ears that he was deaf and mute. The man was accompanied by his eighty-year-old father. He had two sisters but could not stay with them, and thus lived in an ashram-like orphanage for the disabled. While living in the orphanage, he learned a significant amount of language. He began to read and enjoyed writing things, though these were simple sentences. While it is certainly plausible that this man's occasional frustrations led to "aggressive" behavior, the doctor felt that his sisters were, perhaps, using this as an excuse to "abandon" him. The doctor mentioned that though there are "laws against desertion," in truth, nobody enforced them. Evidently, the sisters refused to come to the OPD sessions to meet with the doctor and had refused "family therapy." The doctor urged the father that the "family must get involved with the care." But how binding his evaluation and suggestions would be was a question that he seemed resigned to. A drug in the benzodiazepine family was prescribed for his "restless movements."

Conflict and abuse, of course, can take many forms. In one case, a middle-aged and highly educated man named Sarosh, perhaps in his late fifties or early sixties, came alone to the OPD. His regular doctor knew the man very well as he was a long-term patient from back when he was a resident at NIMHANS, over twenty-five years earlier. The patient was lucid but occasional unusual facial expressions betrayed a mental disturbance. When asked how he was, Sarosh answered, "She is trying to kill me." It turned out the man's wife had beaten him repeatedly and had told him that he "destroyed her life." One daughter had run away from the fraught situation at home, turning to a kind of charismatic Christianity (away from Hinduism) as a refuge. Another daughter lived at home but was working. She "doesn't talk to me," Sarosh said. The doctor asked what he enjoyed at present in his life. The man mentioned his dog. The dog, which it was his job to walk, is "my only joy in life," he replied. When pressed by the doctor, he admitted to emailing a few friends. His life appeared tragically lonely. Sarosh, at one point, evidently had many friends in the UK from his days as a PhD student at Oxford.

Sarosh admitted to some "florid states" when asked. He said, "I'm not allowed to do what I like. The voices I don't like . . . If I go on the internet, voices threaten and complain."

He complained further that he had no control over his finances. His wife had taken over managing these, and had, due to his "incompetence," made all financial matters opaque to him. For a while, he was lucid enough to give financial support to his daughter, as well as to help her land a good job. But eventually, he lost control over this aspect of his life.

On small details, Sarosh appeared to be quite sharp. He recalled precisely his medications and dosages, and had a "technical background" demanding precision, he himself noted. At one point, however, he said to the doctor that he "should end it all" before he "dies as a destitute." His wife, he complained, was spending all his money and "has vengeance." When I asked the doctor if the wife, in fact, did abuse him, or if this was part of his paranoid schizophrenia, the doctor said he believed "she did," but added that she found him to be an "evil man." Some background information proved useful: Sarosh, as mentioned above, was a brilliant PhD student at an elite school in the UK, and was from a wealthy family. His own mother was a doctor who cornered the market on abortions in her district. Evidently, the son had misgivings about her line of work, which involved some unsavory practices of illegal sex selection, impacting him emotionally. He developed his symptoms of schizophrenia while in graduate school, and due to his illness had to return to India. When he returned, his mother wanted him to marry. He met a woman who was counseled at NIMHANS about his condition and what marriage to him might entail (in this case there was no deception). Together, they had two daughters and somehow managed to get along fine for some time. One daughter became a high-ranked corporate employee in one of India's largest companies through his graduate school connections. The other became a born-again Christian, as mentioned. The wife, however, was very unhappy and complained that her husband was an "animal" and had sexually abused her repeatedly. Sarosh was, according to the doctor, described as an "evil madman" by the wife. The wife stopped coming to therapy and OPD sessions and became abusive to the husband. The doctor implied that Sarosh may indeed have been abusive at one point in the marriage.

Much conflict ensued within the household, especially with regard to money. Sarosh's mother, when old and an added burden, was confined by his wife to a room where she developed sores and eventually "died of neglect." It seems that at the hospital they discovered maggots and bedsores on her skin. This man now feared the same fate awaited him and was terrified of his wife. The daughters, having experienced too much chaos and conflict in the home, stopped speaking to their father, suggesting that they, too, felt he bore some of the blame for the dysfunctional home life. It seemed, too, that the daughter who received some help finding the corporate job resented the father for not helping her more financially, or for refusing to pull strings for promotion within the company, after this initial help with placement. Sarosh felt, however, that she had to "work her own way up" in life, and that doing more for her was against her own interest.

The doctor spoke to me about the long-term care of this patient and the possible side effects from a lifetime of taking antipsychotic drugs. That the symptoms stubbornly persisted despite many years of medications did not bode well for the future. He noted his fears privately to me, but to Sarosh said that things were going "fairly well." As such, he said to him that he should not change course with his treatment now. The man said in response, "As you say so, but I will not say so." He left on friendly terms, but clearly was not convinced that things were going well at all. While in this case stigma and shame seemed, perhaps, secondary to abuse and familial conflict, it seemed plausible that some degree of shame and stigma had, even within a professional and middle-class family, worsened what was already a difficult situation.

The next case, on the tails of Sarosh's visit, was equally complicated. A young woman named Shanti came with her parents. She normally lived in Canada with her husband and child, who was thirteen. But her schizophrenia had recently worsened to the extent that Shanti was sent home by the husband to live with her parents and get treatment, as the husband, working full time, had "no other recourse." She had intense and vivid nightmares in which she saw "corpses" piled on the floor. These corpses sometimes talked to her, or another malevolent group of entities urged her to "eat the corpses."

Shanti had been hospitalized in Canada for panic attacks before. The doctor felt she might be "willful" in the sense that she reported experiencing hallucinations all the time, but it was not entirely certain that this was, indeed, what was occurring. Her doctor suspected a possible excuse not to do certain "kinds of work for herself," such as "facing her problems." In that sense, the hallucinations were a kind of resistance, whether consciously malingering or not. One possible clue came in the form of her own resistance to family therapy. Shanti's aversion to therapy suggested, perhaps, psychical resistance close to the sources of her internal tensions. Her psychotic visions called attention to distress, but when asked to go deeper and explore their cause, she resisted. This is not to suggest that she did not experience psychotic symptoms; but, rather, the question was of their provenance in organic psychosis or other forms of distress. Moreover, she claimed she could "fight to control" these terrifying visions when asked how she could go back to Canada in her present state, which was her stated wish.

Shanti insisted she was well enough for her to return to her husband and child in Canada. But the doctor feared that in her present state her husband would not be able to take care of her. The doctor strongly advised against her return until her symptoms were under better control. Indeed, even as the doctor spoke to her, Shanti said she saw "snakes and eyeballs." She said she saw these things in the very examination room we were sitting in within the OPD. There were, she claimed, also lots of worms crawling about. Furthermore, there were twenty-five monstrous people standing there tempting her to eat the creepy crawlies. These symptoms, she explained, got worse throughout the day, reaching a climax every evening. During the night she had vivid nightmares. Her parents indicated that this was, indeed, the case.

The doctor asked about "healthy distractions" to keep Shanti's mind off these hallucinations. Could she watch movies or television, he asked? She said that she saw herself "inside of the TV" and would become frightened. But she had tried to watch television, she insisted. Shanti was quite nervous and apprehensive during the interview, as if she saw and heard the things she had earlier described. She also complained about "severe cluster headaches." Shanti kept a journal that described in gory detail scenes of blood and dismembered bodies. The doctor glanced at it, but did not wish to read it.

Her desire to return to Canada notwithstanding, Shanti was still receiving risperidone injections (an antipsychotic) and was advised to "finish this course" and "to try and stabilize" while she had the support of her parents in Bangalore. Moreover, her husband, she was told, would not be able to devote "full-time attention" to her given his job. She was adamant, however, about going home. Her parents, who came with her to the OPD, were ambivalent, I felt. On the one hand, they agreed with the doctor that the best course for her would be to stay in Bangalore until the illness had stabilized. But I sensed some tension or fatigue, and a hope, as well, to return to some normalcy in their lives. The parents were relatively well off, as best I could discern from their fluent spoken English, attire, and the costs of the risperidone injections running into the tens of thousands of rupees. The costs would have been minimal had they been poor or subsisting on a low income.

Interestingly, and perhaps revealing their ambivalence towards keeping her away from her husband and child and having to assume all responsibility for her care, the parents said that she was "improving" and was "shouting less" and having fewer panic attacks. Evidently, one of her unpleasant symptoms involved her shouting at her parents and, more generally, fighting with them constantly. When they claimed she was improving, she flatly countered it by stating that "they don't know what I experience." Shanti further claimed that she was in a "bad state." Something was clearly problematic at home. Her simultaneous and contradictory statements about being able to "control" her events and her desire to go home versus her proclamation that she was not improving and was in a "bad" state seemed to suggest a kind of mental paralysis in which she cried out, perhaps, for familial understanding and comfort, whilst simultaneously recoiling from the form this parental care exhibited. Moreover, her parents seemed to echo a contradictory sentiment of their own, in that she was "improving" but continued to shout and quarrel with them. Theirs was not a simple desire to either care for their daughter at home or abandon their daughter overseas. As was oftentimes the case, emotional attachments were complicated and nuanced, and did not fall into a clear dichotomy between an ethics of care versus a pressure for abandonment (Pinto 2014). I imagined at the time that this was also a collision between generations and values, given that her new life in Canada was probably markedly different from that of her parents.

There were elements in her hallucinations that suggested cultural themes at play, even religious ones. Her rage and her visions of corpses, eyeballs, and snakes, and even her desire to consume these demonic figures, seemed to invoke elements of the Goddess as Durga or Kali, the destructive and cannibalistic manifestation of the divine feminine that emerged in myths to slay the Buffalo demon, Mahisha (Doniger 2018; Ramanujan 1997; Ram 2013; Shweder and Menon 2010). Wearing the skulls of her victims, this "tooth" goddess not only slayed the demonic male figures but also drank the blood of her victims. Skulls and snakes are a key part of her iconography. The dangerous or violent Goddess expresses, many have argued, an illustration of feminine rage against the patriarchal and Brahminical notion that male power and social order (*dharma*) is premised upon the control and harnessing of *shakti,* the primordial power to create, which is a feminine principle. The myths of the Goddess as dangerous and malevolent reveal an alternative hierarchy that can unsettle the vanities of the male-dominated world, and even its reflection of cosmic order among the gods, at the same time that this "disordering" feminine rage also calls attention to the need to control and constrain its wild impulses (Kinsley 1986; Hiltebeital 2000; Ramberg 2013). That Kali's or Durga's tongue dangles signifies both her bloodthirsty nature and her "shame" (*lajja*) at dancing upon the corpse of her husband, Lord Shiva, in one ubiquitous artistic representation (Shweder and Menon 2010).

Good and Bad Objects

Sarah Guyer (2009), in a provocative reading of Derrida and Deleuze, suggests that "buccality," or the oral act of eating, harkens to a different type of ethical subject than that of the face and voice. In this sense, consuming the dead corpses of others, rather than simply being a form of necrophiliac cannibalism, is communicating an object-relation that is a "body without organs," or not connected by the "organs" of symbols, relationality, and the figure of the Law, as in the Oedipal theory of subject formation in Freud and Lacan. Derrida, Guyer notes, speaks of "buccality" as a kind of pre-oral phase, in which the opening and closing of the mouth is the first ingestion of the Other, in this case, the mother's breast, and the mouth's cry for it. It is simultaneously an opening and closing of the pre-subject to the world, and as such, is as much about "being eaten" as it is about "eating." The breast, rather than being the "good object," as Melanie Klein suggests, becomes simultaneously the "bad object," collapsing this distinction into duality (Kakar 1981; Kurtz 1992). The negotiation of opening the lips and closing them, then, was the first act of difference, preceding the apocryphal game of "fort-da" child's play that Freud (1961) suggested was the subject's entry into culture, the marking of difference, and the entry into the field of language, or the symbolic substation out of the first trauma of the mother's absence. An ethics of buccality, Guyer provocatively suggests, following Derrida, would be an ability to subsist within duality, mastering ambiguity and ambivalence marked by the splitting of the Kleinian bad and good object. One might note, however, that eating and spitting out the bad or poison is a common theme in the stories of the gods and goddesses of Hinduism. And while mortals must learn to live with ambiguity, the figure of divine law can harness the bad object for world-making ends, as in the story of Shiva as "Neelakantha," who removes the poison from the ocean through ingestion. The figure of the breast as locus of destructive power and restorer of divine law, against the failure of human (patriarchal) law, is perhaps best seen in the story of Kannagi in the great Tamil epic *Silappatikaram*, razing the city of Madurai to the ground with her breast, which she tore off and hurled at the city after the unjust execution of her husband by the king. In that sense, the "bad object" has been culturally objectified in Hindu thought, allowing for symbolic elaboration and progression out of an unconscious ambivalence, if read in psychodynamic terms (Obeyesekere 1981).

Read another way, however, the figuring of things bad and good, or the splitting up of that which is tinged with both simultaneously, as in the figure of the breast that one eats and is devoured by, in Klein's sense, can take on a pathological form, when it becomes literal or overly objectified. As Juliet Mitchell explains the Kleinian insight, "The ego can stop the bad part of the object contaminating the good part, by dividing it, or it can split off and disown a part of itself. In fact, each kind of splitting entails the other. . . . In self-protection it splits itself and the object into a good part and a bad part and projects all its badness into the outside world so that the hated breast becomes the hateful and hating breast. Klein describes this as the paranoid-schizoid position" (Mitchell 1986, 20). On the other hand, the bad can exist together in the same person, but rather than projecting and raging against a hostile world suffused with bad objects, the subject can feel guilt and anxiety, or what Klein calls the "depressive position."

This modification of Freud's theory of neurosis and psychosis notwithstanding, this object-relations approach not only resonates with the orality of Indian mythical imagery (Kakar 1981; Kurtz 1992; Obeyesekere 1981) as a correlate of unconscious fantasy, but it also suggests that literalism takes hold within a world of objectified relationships taken to excess. Buccal ethics, in Derrida's sense, would be an ability to subsist within a world that is permeable, fluid, and persisting neither wholly good or bad, but grey, ambiguous, and ambivalent. Being unreservedly open to the other, specifically, is a kind of hospitality and a disposition against literalism, archived legalism with its feverish rush to judgement (Derrida 1995), and a rigid boundary between self and other. Indeed, this relentless splitting of the good and bad, we will see, was a fundamental concern of some of my NIMHANS colleagues, where psychiatric patients suffered delusions and hallucinations that seemed to be worsened by the singularities being demanded of them in modern life, be they occupational or around questions of identity. That is to say that the "serialized" imaginary of modernity, as Benedict Anderson (1998) has argued, was productive, and exacerbated the ossification and literalization of good and bad objects within the social imagination. In short, the psychosocial causative factors deserved greater scrutiny than biomedical psychiatry's recent trends towards a pharmaceuticalization of treatment allowed for.

To return to Shanti's case: Noting that there was tension in the household, the doctor suggested family therapy. The family agreed to go for weekly therapy sessions together. The parents, however, also said that no decision would be made without the husband's consultation. Shanti was not satisfied with this resolution, having set her heart on a return to Canada. At the same time, there was, I felt, in the doctor's careful discussion of the case, a skilled navigation of the psychosocial dimensions of care that seemed to shadow the proclamations of hallucinatory visions. If our suspicions were correct, her hallucinations were not without meaning. There was a message within these florid and horrible scenes. Shanti felt it important, herself, to describe these nightmarish scenes verbally and in her diary's archive, as if to cry out for interpretation. That the doctor suspected "willful" dimensions within her asserted florid psychosis seemed to call forth the complexity of familial and marital relations, which, in turn, suggested that family therapy was needed, in addition to the pharmaceutical treatment of Shanti's psychosis. The psychosocial intervention was not always given this much emphasis in cases of florid psychosis. Perhaps the parents' class position, education, and openness to psychiatric care also influenced the decision to invest time and effort into psychotherapy. As Sudhir Kakar (e.g., 1982) has often noted in his many books, psychotherapy is generally more effective among the educated middle class, given the financial and time commitments it entails, along with a more secular understanding of mental distress.

The specter of death's presence in corpses or ghostly apparitions is often theorized in psychoanalytic studies as a haunting, indexing unresolved relations with the dead. But as the previous and following case show, the dead, and death more generally, might index an excess of meaning beyond that which is captured by psychodynamic approaches. For example, Devi, a woman in her fifties, came to the OPD and presented with a "generalized anxiety disorder." She spoke Telugu and came to the OPD with her husband. Devi was preoccupied with "family conflicts" and ruminated continuously about the wellbeing of her family. She suffered recurring panic that harm would come to her family members. Moreover, this harm was not random or accidental but would be caused by others with bad intentions. The doctor was not sure whether this was a "delusion of reference," the notion that her ideas about various random events have great personal significance or are directed at her, or a kind of paranoia, or both.

Devi told the doctor that she thought about her dead relatives all the time; and when she did so, she heard their voices in her head. But she had the insight that this was "impossible," and thus found the experiences confusing. The voices were very troubling because they spoke of her daughter being hurt by others. It was not clear whether she believed the dead relatives were themselves malevolent or whether they were warning her about other malevolent agents. In either event, there was a sense of contagion from death—that the dead will bring death—that was troubling her.

Devi explained that she was not happy at first with the antipsychotic drug she had been taking. She claimed to feel better, rather, with antidepressants. Evidently, she had stopped her antipsychotics as a result of this sense. But now, with the confirmation of her son, who came to the OPD with her, she said that she realized that she "got better" on the antipsychotic medication, because when it was stopped, the paranoia and panic became a lot worse. The doctor put her back on antipsychotic medication and requested a follow-up with the patient within two weeks to monitor the paranoia and side effects from the medication.

My impression was that Devi was not floridly psychotic, as she was able to function most of the time without hallucinations or delusions. It remained unclear to the doctor whether the voices of the dead relatives were experiences that audibly intruded upon her consciousness, or whether they came only during ruminations. If the latter, Devi might be able to "control it better," her doctor suggested. That she had insights into what is possible and impossible suggested an unclear diagnostic designation to her doctor. That she responded to antipsychotic meds to the extent that their termination exacerbated her paranoia was relevant, however, suggesting some psychotic tendencies. But this appeared to be a case where understanding the particular family dynamics would be important. That she spoke about and feared family conflicts and the harm that might befall her family, especially her daughter, indeed, that these were her preoccupations and ruminations, suggested that family tension was simmering under the surface.

I imagined that therapy might tease out the voices that haunted Devi. If these were dead relatives, did they speak "truths" that had been suppressed? Were there unresolved issues only verbalized by the dead, and not by the living, as psychodynamic models of hauntologies might suggest? These seemed to me key questions. The medical intervention, in this case, focused upon the question of more or less psychosis, and how best to manage paranoia and fear. Whereas the psychodynamic approach to hauntology explored the possible etiology for neurosis derived from suppressed, and ultimately repressed, traumas, desires, fears, and guilt, psychosis was given short shrift in these models, with some exceptions in Lacanian and Kleinian variants. In short, the psychodynamic approach would have the dead ventriloquize the patient, speaking on her behalf, or as her proxy. But the contagion and transformative powers of death upon the living was also relevant.

Death, as Deleuze has argued, is an expression of life, as a becoming and potentiality that made life possible. Death is a contagion in so far as it connects to life as a power of transformation (Deleuze and Guattari 1987). Devi, perhaps like Heidegger, thought of the "impossible" connection of death to life, an ability to coexist with death, though not without a daily cost. Thereby, her symptoms were, precisely and in actuality, not the Heideggerian being simultaneously haunted and liberated by death, but rather to deny death's possibility. This "impossible" exclusion being itself impossible, she was claimed by that impossibility in the form of a haunting or malevolent presence that pointed to the existential condition or immanent presence of death in order to imagine life. These complications of the psychoanalytic reduction of hauntology to unresolved interpersonal and familial dynamics notwithstanding, the pragmatic issue in Devi's case was to reduce her anxiety and fear by silencing these voices as much as possible. As the diagnosis suggested, "generalized anxiety disorder" is irreducible to the Oedipalized triangle of familial relations, though these factors are not irrelevant. Rather, as Heidegger (and Deleuze, in a different manner) would have it, it is a question of our existential relationship with the intimacy of death and life, as the one animates the other, driving the meaning-making engine of symbolic, indeed, cultural, reflection. Like Shanti, the corpse, or the dead's vocal presence, indexed the familial, but also to an excess in life, or connectivity to death, that exceeded and troubled human understanding, despite the efforts to better "control" or contain this fundamental contagion.

The Velocity of Care

While pointing to intractable existential dilemmas related to but exceeding familial relations, as suggested in the previous two cases, in many other instances the acute symptoms and their pragmatic significance to daily life did not arouse the kind of nuance and complexity that seemed to be called forth in the preceding cases. Part of this might have also been marked by the stage in which I observed the patient-doctor interaction. As in some cases, the patient was simply following up on a more detailed first interview that had occurred earlier, and hence, when I witnessed it, it was inherently less nuanced in the interests of time management, a very practical necessity within the OPD, given the patient load each day. In other cases, indeed, in the multitude of them, the acute nature of the illness and the social violence that might have been its primary symptom, and perhaps in some cases its traumatic cause, the ideal of patient insight was buried under the weight of urgency and the velocity of care within the OPD. Symptoms that led to abuse perpetrated by the patient, or its reverse, as caused by the social context in which the patient was traumatized, led to immediate and aggressive biomedical interventions. This, moreover, demonstrated to this anthropologist that the romantic constructivist view of mental illness as protest, or simply labeling, that is, the thinking of power (Foucault 2003), proved inadequate in addressing the acute and very palpable suffering patients and their families endured as a result of their illness (Kleinman 2012). For instance, "schizoanalysis," as formulated by Deleuze and Guattari (1972) as a creative and "deterritorializing" act against the reductionism of psychoanalysis to heteronormative familialism, worked fine for theory and innovation within the arts, or in analyzing the dissociative bliss of mystical quests; but, as an everyday ethics of psychiatric practice, was found wanting to the physicians and patients dealing with the very intractable and acute cases they had to deal with (in rapid fashion).

For example, a forty-two-year-old male, Murugan, presented in the OPD with a history of severe psychotic symptoms. He spoke Tamil, though he also understood English. His wife accompanied him to the OPD. His regular medication was chlorpromazine, though he had olanzapine on hand for emergency situations. According to the psychiatric resident who examined him before the consultation with the doctor, he was "clearly dysfunctional." Murugan had expressed "violent intentions" and exhibited violent behaviors to his wife in the past. The wife did not know of his condition when she married him, evidently. This was a fairly common occurrence, as mentioned earlier. There was much fear and stigma surrounding mental illness, and hiding its instance when marrying was, unfortunately, common (Pinto 2014).

Murugan had tried cognitive behavioral therapy (CBT) at NIMHANS when he was admitted some time back, but the wife, evidently, was unable to "sustain it" on her own. Murugan appeared to have a slight cognitive impairment when speaking. He also stuck his tongue out every few seconds, pointing it down. This was called TD (tardive dyskinesia), the involuntary movement of the lips, face, and other extremities resulting from long-term usage of neuroleptic medications, the doctor explained. Murugan appeared calm and let his wife speak for him until he was asked a direct question. To this he would answer in English.

The doctor spoke about the need for some disciplined training in self-care. She said he should be able to "care for himself, washing, cooking, shopping as much as possible." The wife tended to do everything for him, which was not good, the doctor said. She suggested that he learn "independence skills." She then spoke of giving him "tokens" and allowing him to shop for what he needs.

When asked what Murugan did at home, he replied, "Just resting." He was then asked about the kinds of chores he did at home. He claimed he would cut vegetables. The wife said he was able to fold clothes, wash himself, and other basic aspects of self-care. Murugan was previously able to work for his brother in a Lamborghini (luxury automobile) service center. New scripts were given by his doctor and a follow-up date was suggested. In this case, and many others like it that I witnessed, the pragmatic overrode any philosophical or even psychological considerations. While CBT had been tried, it proved impractical as a means of intervention for his primary caregiver, his wife. Treating his severe symptoms was most urgent, as the wife was the target of his violence. This, as a long-term case, and as indicated by the TD, suggested that coping with his disease and managing his care was the best they could hope for, given practical realities.

Another similarly acute case, and one with legal ramifications, was discussed in the OPD between various social workers, residents in the clinic, and the doctor on call. A man who was a regular patient at NIMHANS with "mild retardation" had killed a woman by throwing a stone at her. He was charged with murder (charge "302" in the Indian Penal Code). The victim was an elderly woman who had somehow enraged him. He had been admitted subsequently to NIMHANS where he was put on the antipsychotic risperidone. After a month or so he showed no abnormal behaviors. The question was whether he was competent to stand for trial. While he was not showing any abnormal behaviors, NIMHANS was of the opinion that he could not grasp the consequences of his action due to his "mild retardation." The magistrate wanted a letter of competency so that he could stand for trial. The opinion of his doctor was that he could, in principle, understand that he had hurt the woman, but did not seem able to grasp that she was dead. Therefore, he could never be fully competent. Moreover, this was a lifelong issue of retardation, not the sudden onset of psychosis. The *Of Mice and Men* quality of the case, whereby the actions of the patient mirror, to some extent, Lennie's fate in the famous novel by Steinbeck, demonstrates the legal, and thus very pragmatic, stakes that are grappled with within the clinic, particularly when cases were acute, long-term, and thoroughly interwoven with themes of violence. Stigma and shame, certainly as socially constructed, exacerbated the treatment of mental illness; however, the range of afflictions exceeded constructivist and power-determinative analyses. The next two cases point, in turn, to the complex entanglements over the long term between the mentally ill person and their caregivers, defying facile dichotomies such as care and abandonment (Pinto 2014).

One afternoon, during the hot season of April 2015, a forty-something male patient presented with a kind of incoherence and fidgetiness. He had been ill since the age of five! His brother, who took care of him, brought him to the OPD. As the man could not navigate traffic alone or take public transportation, he was very dependent on his family to function. The doctor asked the patient's brother if he had any social contacts or context for social life outside of the house. The answer was that the patient had no social life at all given his condition. Within the household he would only interact with those he "grew up" with and did not "welcome" or interact with those that had entered the household through marriage, such as his sister-in-law, the caretaker's wife.

The doctor mentioned that his social interactions had been severely affected by his illness, which, in turn, worsened his symptoms and prognosis. The brother then mentioned that his condition and ability to socialize was deeply affected by the death of his father some twenty years earlier. When the doctor asked the brother if the patient gave any emotional support or showed empathy for other family members, he was told that the patient would not show empathy or a desire to help others. But if specially requested to help, he would sometimes comply. While we spoke, the patient grabbed at his body with involuntary movements, which, as in the case above, looked like the TD effects of long-term treatment with neuroleptic medicines. The patient, we were told, had no empathy for others and was cognitively challenged. Between the ages of five and fifteen, he had been sent to various spiritual healers but was placed on antipsychotics at the age of fifteen.

While it was admirable that the patient's brother had not institutionalized him, it was apparent that the scope of his care had exacted a huge cost on his own wellbeing. Moreover, the care was tempered by the stigma and shame that led the patient to isolate and cut off the social contacts that could enrich his life. Doing so had, the doctor suggested, hastened the decline in his impaired brother's cognitive and social skills. It was also unclear whether his mild psychopathy worsened over time due to his isolation from others, or was its primary cause. In a case such as this, there were no heroes or villains, just the messiness and cruelty of life on full display.

At this point, after the patient had left the room, the conversation among the residents veered towards another case whereby, evidently, a patient refused to leave her father for any amount of time. But in this case, the father suffered from delusions of persecution and was schizophrenic. The daughter now shared his delusions as well as his diagnosis. The doctor, a very reflective and intellectual man, made the elliptical comment about family "intimacies" being "entangling," with regard to mental health. He cited a work by Sartre called "Intimacy,"[4] which deals with the impact that mental illness has on a family. The woman in this case felt that if she left her father alone, he would, in turn, be harmed by her mother. But in such a case as this, one first step towards recovery for both the father and daughter would, in fact, be to have them separate for a time. In her fear and psychotic panic, she refused.

Heat, Fans, and High Functioning

The hot season (April–May) had NIMHANS slowing down a bit, though hundreds of patients continued to flow into the OPD each day. The bodies, however, seemed to move in a more languid fashion now, with the full heat of May having arrived. One could see patients and their families huddling in the shade of the verdant campus. Cobra infestations on the grounds did not dissuade people from making use of every patch of green. The examination rooms and halls of the OPD did not have air-conditioning, though the normally swooshing ceiling fans moved now at their fastest setting, requiring all paperwork to be held down by paperweights. The sound of the fans drowned out voices, making it a bit harder to hear within the echoey examination rooms, though it also had the effect of drowning out noises from the hallways and waiting rooms, which was welcome. Doctors and patients had to speak a bit louder. But there were many instances when hearing proved difficult, and fans would be turned off. Many of the faculty were on vacation this time of year as medical student exams were recently completed. But there were doctors in rotation within the OPD and wards at all times, given that the patient load did not slow down, despite the heat.

One morning, Anita, a young professional in her thirties, presented with schizophrenia that was largely under control with medications. She had been seen at NIMHANS before and responded well to treatment. At this point, she was teaching mechanical engineering at a small college. She complained of troubles concentrating at work. Anita said that some parents of students had complained about her after she had disciplined certain "rowdy boys" for their misbehavior in the classroom. Though Anita's mother was the head of the department where she taught, the principal, evidently bowing to PTA pressures, sided with the students and asked Anita to resign her position at the college.

The doctor queried at some length as to why Anita's concentration levels were down. He kept asking her what "the issue really" was. With various teaching aids, such as "notes and PowerPoint," was she "getting bored," he asked? Or with these aids, was it "really that hard" for her to concentrate on the "task at hand?" That is, why, with all these devices and aids, should mental recall be a problem?

The doctor, who liked to provoke his patients with challenging questions, in this case seemed to directly challenge the patient's own statement about a "lack of concentration." He seemed to be asking if there was another underlying issue relating to Anita's apparent depression. His inquiry seemed to force the patient to articulate something that had changed, but remained unspoken, that, in turn, had produced this symptom, which, it appeared, was

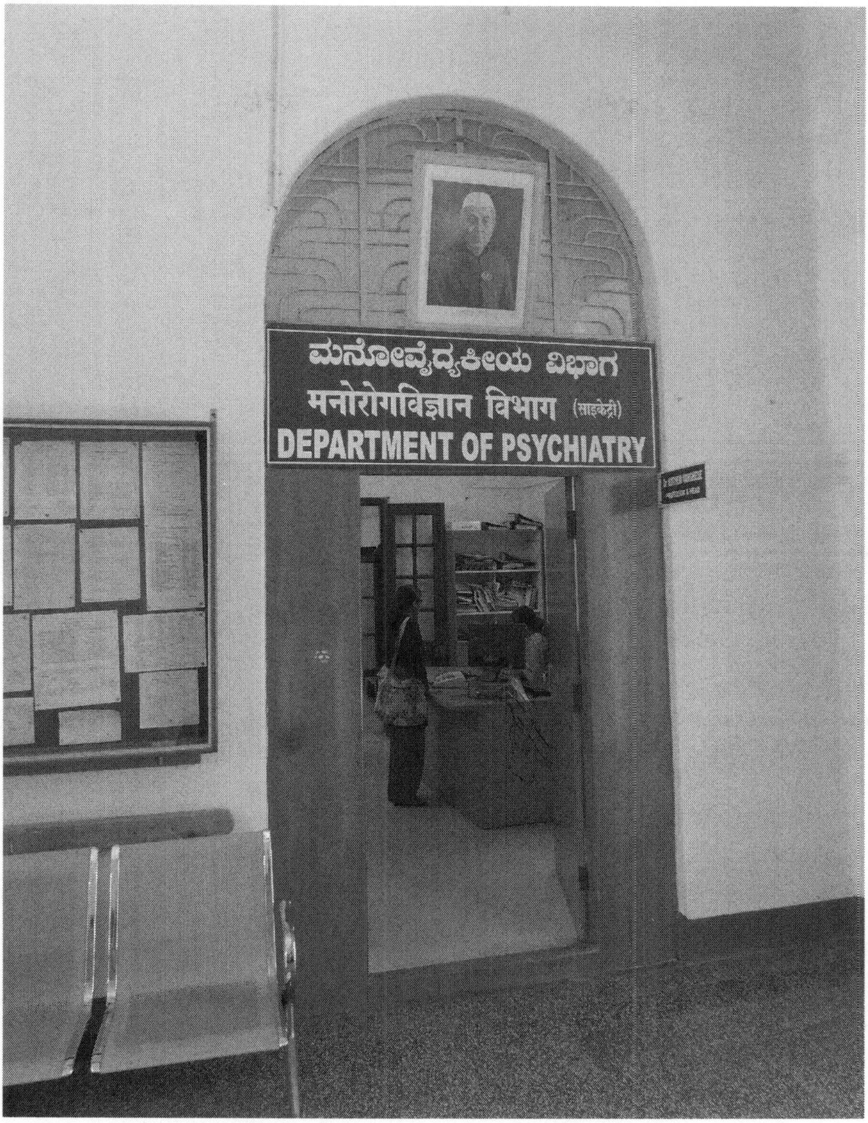

Administrative Office and Office of the Head of the Department of Psychiatry. (Photograph by author.)

separate but not unrelated to her schizophrenia diagnosis. After all, she had professed control of her schizophrenic symptoms. Her lack of concentration seemed tied up with the trauma of what had happened at work, and that her condition, in turn, might be discovered.

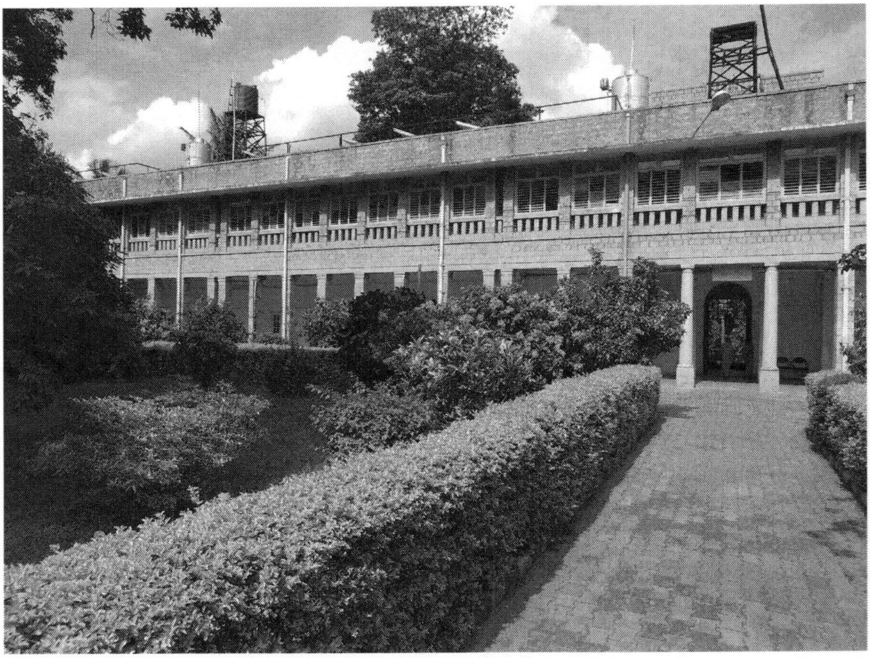

The Department of Psychiatry building seen from inside the NIMHANS campus. (Photograph by author.)

The doctor pushed on, asking whether the principal of the college had been kept apprised of her medical condition. A resident handling the case had advised a meeting with the principal to discuss just this issue. But there were concerns that, as this was a private college, disclosing this condition could, in itself, be grounds for termination. In public institutions legal protections existed against the discrimination of the disabled. But the patient's mother felt that as a private institution, this college could do as it wished. The doctor, in turn, thought the law applied to both private and public institutions, but was not entirely sure about this. Anita had more implicit worries about the stigma and embarrassment that such a disclosure would entail, particularly if it became known somehow to a wider group through a lawsuit. This could then affect not only Anita's present relationships within the college, but her employability in other colleges in the future.

Anita's mother and father felt, understandably, that she should have a "decent job." Anita, now depressed and lacking concentration, said she would like to "leave the job and stay home," looking after the house. The doctor, however, advised against this, saying it was tantamount to running away from her problem. The mother, for her part, wanted her daughter to quit the job, but also to take up an offer from her sister to work in an IT company. But the doctor pointed out that her training was as an engineering teacher, and that this change would be a "demotion" and non-utilization of her training. Rather, he counseled Anita to send her curriculum vitae to some other colleges whilst also considering staying put at the present job by appealing to the principal. He suggested a meeting with the principal. But Anita and her mother looked a bit apprehensive at the prospects of disclosing her mental illness, given the general stigma and shame that kept many diagnoses secret.

Secrecy, however, was not always ideal. As it turned out, Anita, now thirty-six, had not married on account of her honesty. When being introduced to possible grooms in the past, the family quite honorably explained the nature of her illness. This was enough, sadly, to frighten any prospective groom's family away, if not the grooms themselves. The rejections may have weighed on her depression and feelings of fatigue, disinterest, and ultimately, her lack of concentration in the classroom. Moreover, her fears of coming forward with further disclosures were likely founded in this experience.

In this case, we see not only the impetus to secrecy that must have weighed on many families with psychiatric diagnoses within them, but also the workings of college dynamics and implicit hierarchies that probably impacted upon women professionals more than men. That the parents of the undisciplined boys in the class sought her dismissal rather than question their sons' behavior speaks, perhaps, to the sense of gender and status entitlement that men might enjoy in the context of educational institutions. This violence within the social surely was an everyday reality, and one that might have also weighed on Anita as she pondered the difficult choices being urged upon her by the doctor. The easy choice would be retreat. But the doctor felt retreating in this case would only hasten more social withdrawal as she left work to "stay at home," to the detriment of her sense of self-worth and wellbeing. Here, stigma and shame were not directly expressed within the family, but rather were implicated within the professional life and legal rights of patients who were otherwise high-functioning individuals (Martin 2009).

High-functioning patients at NIMHANS, however, were not immune to a sense of betrayal, both within their families and in dealing with a wider society that still harbored prejudices. The attenuated social life that marked a person with mental illness could be witnessed across age and class divides, affecting family dynamics in profound ways, as the next case suggests. Harish, a young man around twenty years of age, presented in the OPD with a "borderline personality," depression, and marked social conflicts, particularly with parents. He also suffered from debilitating anxiety about public speaking and making friends.

Harish came with his parents to the OPD on a breezy afternoon during the start of the monsoon season in June. His father was a well-placed government worker who had been forced to move his family a few times. This had hurt the son emotionally, we were told. Moreover, Harish had been left feeling abandoned in boarding schools when growing up, leaving him very insecure about his parents' affection. Harish, the parents said, needed constant validation and certainty of affection from them. At the same time, however, he expressed great hostility towards his parents, saying they had "betrayed" him and were "not true to their words." Harish spoke fluent English and appeared alert and bright. He was now in a college in Bangalore, and despite his feelings of inadequacy and inability to concentrate, had scored right at the top of his class in his exams.

The parents seemed proud of his success in college, especially the father, who underscored just how smart his son was. Harish, however, said he had "not learned anything" and that his success was just "on paper." In his words, school "felt like" it was not going well. Part of his problem, he said, was that he only had two or three friends in school, despite being elected as a class representative. Though he had to communicate to the administration and staff on behalf of his fellow students, he complained of a problem with public speaking and of "social anxiety." He also said he suffered some "mental barriers." This, he said, was making it "hard to cope."

The doctor, unsurprisingly, reassured the boy of his abilities as "objectively measured." But at the same time, this objective measurement was something the boy distrusted at one level, but evinced slight pride in at another level, perhaps. Indeed, it seemed as though, despite all of his anxieties and troubles, he was, in fact, expressing his satisfaction that he was doing well, which was a matter of pride. But he did not trust in these objective measures and wanted validation and recognition from his parents and doctor, where I sensed some transference. He seemed eager to hear the doctor's validation of his success, as if his self-deprecating and self-psychologizing assessments were addressed to the doctor in demanding a response.

Harish explained that since the autumn of 2014 (the clinical interview was in 2015) his depression had worsened gradually. He said he always felt "restless" and "emotionally unstable." Moreover, this sense of unease peaked during the school exams. During this period, he could not focus, concentrate, or even stay awake. He complained that he slept up to twelve hours a day. He repeated the phrase twice that he was "emotionally unstable" and "restless." The doctor asked him to describe these experiences. The explanation veered a bit off point, as Harish said, "I used to get happy and then, sad, depending upon what I was doing. But now, I rarely feel happy, just [he paused], sorrow." The doctor interjected, asking, "Why?" at the exact moment he said the last word. Harish could not answer, and an awkward silence filled the examination room where the five of us were sitting. After a couple of minutes of this uneasy quiet, he said, "I think because I'm lonely and have very few friends. It is difficult to make new friends . . . and I always feel dazed."

I thought that he was pointing to his medications, as he had been treated by this doctor for several months already. But he never directly questioned whether his medications were the cause of his feeling sleepy and dazed; and the doctor did not suggest it, either. After a few minutes of probing and repetition by the doctor, the young man suddenly said, "I'm irritated often with my parents . . . only with them." He then said, "I have not been able to let go of the past. I get angry when I think about it." At this point he did not elaborate on this past, but would do so a bit later.

Harish returned to the theme of his alienation from others and the difficulty he had making new friends. "I have communication problems with other friends . . . communications are difficult. I find it hard to respond to their questions [pause], and I don't make much sense to other people." He reiterated again how sleepy he was, even pointing out that he felt sleepy talking right now and had a hard time understanding whatever the doctor was asking. When asked about his appetite, Harish pointed out that he "cannot be sure whether he is hungry or full." But he said he tries to remember to eat as, evidently, his weight had fluctuated in recent months, as had been pointed out by the doctor.

The doctor asked him about his plans for the future. Harish said he wanted to take the Civil Service exam and to follow in his father's footsteps. But he found it hard to study for this exam. Something was blocking him, he said. Confirming the connection with the medications, he said he had started a new medicine in March (a few months earlier) and said that during the past couple of months he had felt "very sleepy." Here he seemed to draw a line of connection between the drugs and his sleepiness. His self-described "dazed" state, however, lifted briefly as he went on to describe with animated expression a particular event that left him angry and "betrayed" by his parents. The doctor, however, noted that there was, despite his reporting of being dazed, a disjuncture between what he said he subjectively experienced and his actual communicative ability. Indeed, he seemed to be quite insightful and expressive about his own subjective states. But he had a decidedly lower opinion of his present functioning than that which was observed by the doctor, unless we take into account the transferential dynamic I suspected was taking root between his statements and the contradictory validation of his talents as expressed by the doctor. His self-deprecating comments were, indeed, countered by his doctor, perhaps to Harish's satisfaction.

Turning more concretely to his grouse with his parents, he described a period following his exams when his parents became "curt" and "rude" to him, whilst in earlier times they were more "warm and supporting." This had confused and hurt him. He wondered aloud what had changed with the exams being done, especially as he had "done quite well" in them, again evincing a certain pride. Here again, I heard Harish to be hurt that his parents were not more openly and lavishly praising his achievement. He clearly wanted, indeed, demanded, their approval.

Harish then elaborated further on this period. He explained that he had wanted to get his "driving license all of his life." His father, while saying it was possible to do, advised him to wait until after his exams. Moreover, his mother, who evidently had promised to buy him a car, was not fulfilling this promise, but rather made "excuses about money problems that the family had." As a result of the family's financial pressures, he offered to cut his daily expenses to help the family. When the family remained "curt," he felt particularly hurt and betrayed.

After Harish and his parents had been asked to briefly leave the room, discussion ensued between the doctor and an attending psychotherapist regarding issues within the family. Evidently, there were "family issues" that were being worked out in family therapy at NIMHANS. Family dynamics were also affected by financial pressures. With financial stability less certain, the family had made the decision to stay in Bangalore for their son's sake, rather than moving far away from him to accept a job opportunity. As a result, promotions and transfers for the father were on hold, as Harish had expressed a strong desire for certainty regarding their possible moves. His mother had evidently promised the son that they would not move, no matter what. But this was only a partial truth, as the father would eventually be forced to go wherever he was stationed as a government employee. While softening the blow in the short term, the deception had left Harish feeling that his parents "could not be trusted at their word."

Rejoining the clinical interview with his parents, Harish felt particularly incensed that he had not been able to obtain his driving license after his school exams, as "promised" by the parents. "All sorts of excuses were given," he said. He felt this was a particularly keen betrayal—so much so that it left him "very sad on his birthday." He complained that his father was "not a man of his word," before us all.

The father faced an imminent relocation that would separate the parents from the son, despite the promise that they would stay in Bangalore. The doctor chided the parents for making "promises" they "could not keep" in order to placate the son. He advised them to be consistent and honest with him.

Harish, for his part, admitted then that he had become violent with his parents in the past. Nothing about this, however, was elaborated, but he had reached the conclusion that his "violence" was inappropriate and he decided to become "passive," even when angry with them. The parents, however, were fearful of his violence and "caved" to his demands, even if they could not fulfill them. This had led to a pernicious cycle of false promises that could not be kept, spiraling their son's anger and sense of betrayal.

The doctor later told me that the police had been called once to their home to quell the violence directed towards his parents. Moreover, he said, the anger against the parents extended beyond the example of the driver's license, having its origins in feeling abandoned in various boarding schools while growing up. Therefore, as a result of his inability to trust, he sought constant confirmation and reassurance, and became a somewhat literalistic and legalistic child, wanting everything in predictable and certain contract-binding terms. Ambiguity and ethical grey zones made him uneasy. This theme of legalism and literalism, and its concomitant demands for certainty and singularity, is a theme we will often witness elsewhere in this study, particularly in response to the stresses, uncertainties, and demands placed upon identity and occupation in modern India (Appadurai 2000; Singh 2015; Hansen 2001; Willford 2018).

Harish had received sessions in psychotherapy from a younger doctor who was also present in this interview. But he said he had no recall of what he had learned in the sessions. Later the psychotherapist, who was a psychiatrist as well, confirmed that Harish would be given an exercise to practice but never "followed through" with the psychotherapy treatments. The doctor, while noting this, explained to Harish and his parents that psychotherapy and resolving his "issues" with his parents were essential to his recovery. For his relentless sleepiness, he recommended a reduction of one of his medications and the adding of another. The doctor also spoke of the need for more psychotherapy and made the psychotherapist arrange an appointment then and there for a date, with the parents also joining. He said that in order to become "in charge of your thoughts and life" he needed the introspection that only psychotherapy provided. He then asked Harish to keep a "diary" as a "personal reflection." The diary, the doctor explained, could be brought to the therapy sessions for the psychotherapist to review with him.

I was struck by the neediness in Harish's demands from his parents. He clearly wanted affirmation, material signifiers of this in the form of praise from others, including parents and, perhaps, friends who might have found this trait hard to satisfy, making it harder for him to forge close friendships. As for the suggested diary, there was perhaps a bit of risk, I thought, that such a self-oriented person might utilize a diary in mirroring an imaginary self that would contribute to a kind of solipsism. I had learned of this risk from doctors at NIMHANS who, noting the risk of hardening delusions, oftentimes ignored patient diaries when presented to them. I even verbalized to the two doctors, after Harish had left, that such an archive posed a risk as it could conceivably harden and objectify his grandiose sense of self as a victim of betrayal. After all, the material object—the diary—would serve as a kind of supplement, occluding destabilizing or unsettling insights from coming into being. This would solidify his narrative of self, perhaps, and exacerbate an already grandiose imaginary. A personal reference, too, like any archive, could become the filter through which he apprehended the world (Derrida 1995).[5] The doctors agreed, to my surprise, that this warning was merited, but felt it might still prove useful to have the diary around as a means to "take charge of his life."

My suspicions about the diary were seen as more relevant after his mother mentioned that he was suggestable to diagnoses. He evidently had done internet research on the medications he had been taking, particularly the side effects literature on these medications. Finding that he suffered the same symptoms as people with Bipolar Affective Disorder and Borderline Personality Disorder, he imagined, the mother said, he had these illnesses. Would he now pattern his response in accordance with known symptoms and presentation? He clearly used categories and models in a manner that had psychosomatic implications. Here his self-diagnosis seemed to align with the medical diagnoses he was receiving from the doctors.

On the other hand, the utilization or dismissal of diaries and other written thoughts by patients at NIMHANS seemed to vary from doctor to doctor but, more generally, was also influenced by the suspected psychiatric condition the patient was suffering from. In this case, mental illness did not include psychotic symptoms with florid delusions and hallucinations. Rather, Harish had to reckon, it appeared to the doctors, with his childhood traumas as the source of his distrust and literalism and a need for unrealistic and constant affirmation. His wounds were, in a sense, psychological, but not necessarily organic. The diary as a projection screen could, in the psychodynamic sense, allow him to express and project his thoughts and feelings onto the page, outside of the unhealthy dynamics that marked his family and school life, perhaps allowing for insights, via symbolic mediation, to emerge within the patient. In the cases of psychosis, doctors seemed more fearful that writings and diaries could make delusions and hallucinations more objectively real. Therefore, shattering the illusory self and not validating it through its self-produced archive was more appropriate. In this sense, biomedical psychiatry seemed congruent with certain aspects of Lacanian psychoanalytic therapy, despite their different ontologies.

Organic Causation, Cognitive Disability, and Family Dynamics

Family dynamics, particularly the tension and stress of modern Indian life, was, as has been already witnessed, a prevalent theme in psychiatric practice. Some doctors were more oriented towards family therapy and counseling than others. In general, I was told that the older doctors (by the older doctors, I might add) were trained more broadly, and taught to think holistically about the "person" rather than just the "brain." This, of course, is a sentiment expressed in psychiatry around the world, and not just in India. But in India, as has already been discussed, psychiatry had not developed within the psychodynamic tradition that marked both European and North American traditions in the twentieth century (Luhrmann 2000; Murthy and Jain 2009). Still, there were doctors very interested in "hysteria" and other conversion disorders at NIMHANS. In the treatment of these disorders, doctors explored psychosocial dynamics and stress factors without reservation. One such doctor was a young, thirty-something physician from the northeastern part of the country. I had collaborated with him on a case conference session focusing upon "hysteric" conversion disorders in early 2015, and thus had a sense that his interests were broadly inclusive of psychotherapy, psychosocial stress factors, and culture as well as the biomedical psychiatry that was the cutting edge at NIMHANS, with its focus upon organic and genetic causation behind the more debilitating neuropsychiatric conditions, particularly schizophrenia and degenerative movement disorders. The following two cases combine a focus upon family tensions and shame, as well as a focus upon organic disabilities that impacted both the care and family dynamics that affected this care, or lack thereof.

This young doctor's clinical approach was markedly inquisitive and time-intensive, detailing as much of the family and social background as the symptomatology and clinical presentation that was usually given precedent in the OPD. The first patient I saw him treat was a young man, Ravindran, whose mother was concerned about his poor performance in school, as well as irritability and anger outbursts that he directed at her. He was the second child of a family in the Coorg area, a few hours' drive from Bangalore, and part of the Western Ghat mountain range. The family had suffered much tragedy, with the father dying at an early age, as well as Ravindran's older brother dying a few years prior. The mother complained that Ravindran refused instructions from others and had "poor motivation." She expressed worry for "his future" as a result.

Ravindran was recognized as cognitively "delayed" and a slow learner. But the hope that he could still work and be self-sufficient was reasonable, the doctor suggested. The doctor asked first if he was "delayed from youth" or had recently lost acquired milestones. The mother indicated that he was "slow from birth," picking up language later than usual and even walking a bit late. Ravindran appeared coherent but somehow distant, as if he was disinterested. As a social worker had already spoken to the family in Kannada, their language, and had taken down a lot of family history as well as details of the present concern, he participated in the OPD session as translator and facilitator of the clinical interview. The doctor would pose questions to him and ask him to relay in Kannada in a very "sensitive" manner, as he did not want to upset the already distressed mother.

The doctor wanted to know about at what level the patient's mental functioning was, and after the translation to English, it was discovered that he was functioning more like a ten-year-old than an eighteen-year-old. This translated, the doctor said, to an IQ of about 50, well below average. He said that the patient would have to be directed towards employment in areas where he could succeed, and not be expected to handle responsibilities that would be beyond his abilities.

The doctor showed concern about the family history, particularly the death of the older brother a couple of years before, and that he died apparently of a jaundice-related illness. He first inquired, tactfully, through the translator, if the brother had had a drinking problem. The mother insisted that his jaundice was not related to drinking and had begun at the age of ten. The father had also died young, causing more concern. It turned out, however, that while jaundice had afflicted the brother, he had also fallen ill a few days before his death. The details surrounding his death were somewhat vague, but suggested a fairly sudden and acute crisis. But before this he had suffered an overall decline in his health. The doctor became concerned, though expressed this concern only in English to myself and the social worker, about the possibility of a genetic disorder within the family that was causing the jaundice and cognitive deficit. But rather than immediately mentioning this, he again asked if there was any progressive decline in mental or physical function with Ravindran.

As Ravindran had a fairly "flat affect" and a glassy-eyed appearance, the doctor asked the mother how he responded to his brother's death, and more generally, if he had normal emotional responses, such as "joy and grief." The mother said he was always "quiet," except when agitated, but did not show a lot of emotion openly. But he was "devastated," albeit silently, by his brother's death, she said. The doctor was keenly interested in his general "sensitivity" to others. He then turned again to whether the anger outbursts were getting progressively worse in the last six months, and thus, that is why she had brought him to Bangalore. The mother, however, said the symptoms were not really worsening, but she implied that her worries were now increasing for his future. His anger outbursts, it seems, were situational and followed some sort of "scolding" that he might receive for his "poor motivation" and performance in school.

The doctor asked the mother if she could afford to do some laboratory testing to rule out certain diseases. He told the social worker that he hoped he was wrong but had a fear that Hunter's Disease ran in the family. This is a progressive neurological disorder that invariably shortens life spans. The doctor ordered the laboratory test for this disease. This would cost the family roughly INR 5,000–6,000 (Indian rupees), he thought (about USD 100 at the time). The mother agreed to the test and said the money "would be available." The larger issue, however, was that the treatment for this disease, if diagnosed, was very costly, and could run into the thousands of rupees each month. And even then, this only prolonged the quality of life for a while, but did not cure the disease. He was unsure whether NIMHANS could help with the costs of treatment.

One of the indicators of Hunter's Disease, apparently, is a morphologically distinct look. Ravindran did not resemble his mother all that much. Therefore, the doctor asked the mother whom he most resembled. The mother answered that he looked "like the father and uncle a bit." He asked the social worker to ask this in a very sensitive way so as to not appear to be accusing her of anything uncouth, as in illegitimacy. The fact that he resembled the father was not a good sign, given his early death. But what was striking in this case was the equal attention the doctor gave to psychosocial factors within the family that were causing conflict, and the need to explore organic causation. This was also true of the next case.

A man in his mid-fifties presented with significant depression. This was his third bout of serious depression within the last decade. During the first instance, his depression had lasted for four to five months. It returned in 2008 for two to three months and was again this year (2015) ongoing for over two months, after many years of absence. The patient had a progressive neuromuscular disorder that affected his ability to move his arms. There was, as well, a family history of suicide. The key question, the doctor suggested, was whether the neuromuscular disorder was correlative or causative with regard to the depression. There were indicators that both could be at play, but sorting out the primary agent of causation would be important.

On the psychosocial side, there was the history of suicide and the recurrent bouts of depression. The doctor queried the resident who presented the case as to what he thought was going on. The resident replied that she thought it was "recurrent depressive disorder" or RDD. This was contrasted with "MD," she said, or major depression. The key question here was whether this was a case of lifelong depression with various peaks and valleys or episodic and acute instances of depression. The correct diagnosis was critical so that the appropriate medications and dosages could be administered. The training of the resident involved wanting to teach her whether acute treatment would call for a higher dose, whereas lifelong or recurrent depression would not require the continuous dosages of the same level for fear of lifelong side effects and a generalized decline in cognitive function.

In this instance, it was believed to be a recurrent depression perhaps correlated with the decline in neurological health. This, however, was also conjoined to constant worries about his son's poor performance in school. That this man's health was declining and his son was not performing particularly well could have triggered anxiety and depression as much as it being a direct comorbidity related to his neurological deficit. Here, again, the psychosocial and organic were both in play, receiving equal attention by the doctor. The doctor decided to taper his meds and asked him to return within a month for a follow-up. My admittedly brief impression, which seemed to be echoed by the doctor, was that the man was not suffering from acute depression, but suffered a degree of anxiety and worry, which exacerbated whatever baseline risks for depression he continued to possess. In any event, though the OPD was a place for rapid assessment and treatment interventions, the need for examining social context in many cases was equal to the need to document organic disease, despite the complaints by many doctors at NIMHANS that the general trend in psychiatry was towards narrow specialization, with pharmaceutical treatment far outpacing psychotherapeutic alternatives, given patient demands and societal attitudes. At the very least, the doctors were acutely aware of the tensions and contradictions they faced when treating patients. Some openly complained about the palliative and "Band-Aid" approaches they had to employ within the OPD, while others struggled valiantly to balance competing demands.

During a short break between patients, the doctor from the previous two cases spoke to me about aspects of the health care system in India that were of concern, touching on the tensions just addressed. On the one hand, he cited the presumption that the prognosis for severe mental illness in India might be generally better than in the US due to the support provided through the joint family structure,[6] though it was declining, he claimed. He also pointed out that there was a growing acceptance of mental health discourse in the public sphere, though it was not without challenges. A stigma surrounding mental illness still existed, and there was a severe shortage of mental health workers, particularly psychiatrists, within the country, as had been earlier noted.

But this doctor also suggested that a proliferating "industry of psychotherapists" posed its own challenge to providing sound mental health care. At NIMHANS, he said, one hundred hours of psychotherapy was required in order to received certification as a psychiatrist. But this was not, regrettably, a "high priority within NIMHANS" nowadays, with many doctors-in-training (students, residents, and fellows) viewing the psychotherapy training as just another "course requirement" rather than an essential part of their training as psychiatrists. He described a generational shift in biomedical psychiatry and how in previous times, doctors were much more "holistic in their approach" to diagnoses and treatment. Here and now, on the other hand, the doctors were increasingly specialized but, ironically, tolerated a large amount of concurrent care within Ayurvedic medicine and other forms of traditional/spiritual/faith healing.

Part of the problem with psychotherapy, and a chief reason why serious doctors at AIIMS and NIMHANS were wary of being identified as psychotherapists, had to do with the large percentage of fraudulent degrees that were being purchased, according to this doctor. To emphasize this point, he showed me a patient's file in which the psychotherapist's report from somewhere in Tamil Nadu was included. The "doctor" had, in addition to his MBBS, degrees or certifications featuring numerous acronyms that the doctor said were unknown to him, and most certainly to the patients. He suggested these "certifications" were largely purchased or based on fraudulent claims. Still, numerous doctors padded their "CVs and business cards" with these inexplicable "degrees." As if "buying degrees" was not enough of a concern, he went on further to explain that these poorly trained and fraudulent doctors routinely over-prescribed medicines in hopes that something would produce an effect. It was, I suggested, a "scattershot" method of throwing everything at the wall and hoping something would stick. He said, in response to my suggestion, that this was "exactly" what was happening.

A consequence of this trend was that it was very difficult to discern, once the patient arrived at NIMHANS, what exactly had worked and what had not. The variables were hard if not impossible to isolate. Therefore, doctors at NIMHANS were often left to interpret the results reported in the file but had to, in turn, reduce medicines in an attempt to isolate causal variables. A general trend, the doctor remarked, was "away from psychotherapy." Beyond NIMHANS, at AIIMS, the major medical school of the country, it went further. It was "patently antipsychotherapy," he claimed. We turned conversation to the "neurologization" of psychiatry and the desire of biomedical psychiatry to ground itself in organic biology rather than in the murky and hard to quantify theories of the mind or "psyche," or even more diffuse and vague, the "personality" (Luhrmann 2000; Schecter 2014; Rose 2018). There was nothing particularly Indian about this trend, other than the fact that in most Indian philosophical thought the mind is material, rather than in dualistic and Cartesian splits between psyche and soma, or mind and body (Fabrega 2009; Roland 1988). Indian psychiatry, as pointed out, never evolved a robust Freudian tradition, despite a few brilliant Freudian analysts that stood out over time (Pinto 2020a).

I asked how often psychotherapy was utilized at NIMHANS. The doctor said that most warded patients undergo "some sort" of psychotherapy. Indeed, when it is recommended that a person receive psychotherapy, they are often warded, given the intensity and frequency of sessions required. I asked whether forms of psychotherapy were utilized in the OPD. He answered that with time limitations and caseloads, "even the most basic psychotherapies" could not be utilized in such a short time span.

While this doctor was largely correct in his assessment of psychotherapy in the OPD, my own observations were a bit more nuanced on this point. In most sessions, not involving simply writing a new script during a follow-up visit, the doctor would ask several questions relating to wellbeing, happiness, functionality, sociality, and specific delusions—their content and presentation—in addition to writing out scripts for medications. While this may not qualify as the kind of depth psychotherapy that might have been warranted in some cases, it did suggest to me that even where there is some slight aversion or distaste for the complexity and thickness of the psychosocial world among doctors and patients, which was not always the case, by any means, it came in through the back door quite routinely. There would, indeed, be little substance to the OPD session if some psychotherapeutic techniques were not employed. On the other hand, there was often a quick resolution and return to biochemistry, symptomatology, and pharmaceutical treatment after whatever detours into the experiential aspects of mental illness had been explored. I rarely, for instance, witnessed a provocative question posed that was unanswerable in the moment but suggested as "homework" for future contemplation. Usually, rather, advice was immediate and didactic, and geared towards behavioral modifications that were thought to be healthy for the patient, given their particular distress. For example, a person who was thought to spend too much time on the computer or TV would be advised to keep themselves occupied with other activities, rather than probed for the cause of this addictive symptom. Or a person prone to depression or schizophrenia might be advised to have a structured daily schedule, leaving less room for rumination, and apparently, delusions to harden and take hold of the mind. Family issues might be explored, but provocation and probing in great depth, as in psychoanalytic technique, rarely occurred in the OPD, in my experience. Sometimes, however, the doctors would ruminate and speculate further on the psychosocial and cultural dimensions of the patients they were treating, once the patients had left the room. Perhaps it was considered good clinical practice to not speculate or delve into a line of questioning that the patients themselves had not brought to the table. And given heavy patient loads, insufficient time disallowed for extended interviews, though again, if patients were in acute distress and warded, this would be possible.

After several months I came to realize, too, that patients at NIMHANS often put on a very brave display when they saw a doctor. Rarely did patients cry or emote in any measure of force before their doctors. It seemed, almost, that it would be slightly unbecoming and inappropriate, if not disrespectful, in this cultural context where doctors commanded respect and authority from patients, at least, more so than I have witnessed in the United States. This was in accord with the observations by several NIMHANS doctors who told me that they have nearly never felt threatened by patients in all the years they have worked there. Ideas of "lockdown," bodily or verbal threatening, and panic are anathema, these NIMHANS doctors suggested, to the Indian ethos of respect for the doctor and a certain imposition of cultural and personal control mutually reinforcing one another. In this sense, the sociocentric theories of Indian selfhood discussed earlier were relevant insofar as outward behavior and normativity was concerned.

Conversation eventually turned to the absence of quality special needs education and issues of accessibility within India. With all the new income apparent within the middle class, absent was a reciprocal change in attitudes regarding supporting the disabled or mentally challenged, the doctor claimed. Therefore, just as there was still a stigma attached to mental illness, there was similarly a stigma, more generally, about disabilities. In both cases, particularly among Hindus, he claimed, there was an attitude that disabilities and madness signified past faults, sins, or "bad acts" now materialized by the forces of karma as punishments (Fabrega 2009).

Eventually we landed on the topic of weddings where one partner is mentally ill or an epileptic. The doctor described a law that allowed people to annul weddings when full disclosure of a mental health condition was not given prior to the marriage. In such cases, "dowry reclamation" for "wedding fraud" was available. On the one hand, this empowered women, in particular, who had been duped into marriage to fight back, after the fact. In theory, though not always in fact, this act meant the dowry could be recovered and the marriage annulled. On the other hand, some people abused this legislation in order to exact "revenge" on another family, which, in turn, could contribute to the abandonment and stress of those mentally ill or epileptic. While the intentions were to empower women, it had also become a source of abuse and conflict (Pinto 2014).

Returning to the scene of the OPD on another day, and a different, more senior doctor on service, we can see how cognitive disability becomes a psychiatric burden for families. The family's struggle to make sense of it, and finding the means of coping while facing a precarious future, was a fairly common occurrence. Ravi, a young man in his twenties, presented with cognitive difficulties from an early age. His developmental milestones were delayed, but after a "fever" at the age of seven, he began to "regress" cognitively. His memory, in particular, had worsened since this illness. Ravi's mother was asked why he had never been treated for his condition before this visit to NIMHANS, over a decade later. The mother could not answer, but did say that she "thought he would improve." The family had no prior history of genetic problems or disabilities.

When asked whether he recognized and interacted with people in their village (they came from a coffee-growing area within the mountainous Coorg region in Karnataka), the mother and brother who accompanied Ravi said he "recognized people" but would not interact with them. The doctor then asked if he knew "how to get help when injured." The mother and brother said he would not know what to do and would simply wait for others to help him. The doctor then asked about food preferences, and whether Ravi had any favorite foods or preferences (e.g., spicy, salty, and/or sweet). The mother and brother answered that he showed no preferences with food and would "simply eat whatever was placed before him." When asked about his social life and play habits, the mother said he used to play with other kids until the fever struck. After this, he withdrew and became "dull." He even stopped "going outside of the house." The doctor asked if he interacted with others in the house or tried to initiate conversations. He did not initiate but would respond to others in the house.

The doctor then directed his questions directly to Ravi. He could not answer all of them, but when asked to open and close his hands, or to hold his arms out, he could follow instructions. Ravi did not utter any words, but his comprehension of simple words and sentences was evident. The doctor, after this brief interview, explained that there was still significant hope that he could care for his own basic needs and even do simple repetitive work. This was meant to reassure the mother and brother, to some extent. The mother interjected, however, that he could not "handle money." The doctor then asked again, "Why, with these problems so severe, you never saw a doctor?" Once again, the mother could not offer a reason. And while neither she nor her other son were well off, financially speaking, based upon appearances, they were not living in poverty.

The doctor mentioned that with his "moderate to severe MR (mental retardation)," Ravi could get a "disability card" and receive a pension from it. The older brother then mentioned that an "uncle" in the family had already done this and the family did, in fact, receive some disability pension funds. Therefore, it became clear the family understood the mechanisms for state-sponsored entitlements, and as such, the doctor did not probe further in this direction. Rather, he then tacked in a different direction and asked if they took him "to the temple" and if so, if he could "do the correct things," or must he be "told each and every time what to do." The mother said he had to be guided each and every time. He did not, in other words, pick up on behavioral cues by observation and memory.

The doctor ultimately suggested that the best course would be to formally assess his cognitive capabilities, and thus suggested they stay for a while at NIMHANS. The family agreed to this. To the mother he emphasized that as she did "everything for him," such as washing, brushing his teeth, dressing, etc., Ravi needed to "learn how to do some basic skills on his own." Ravi was referred to a psychologist at NIMHANS who could work with him; and the mother was told that "psychosocial rehabilitation and training at NIMHANS would be good."

In this case the family was finally receptive towards psychosocial intervention but had previously been somewhat fatalistic, assuming his condition was just his and their lot in life and thus had to be endured stoically. Moreover, it became clear they did not have the financial resources that would have allowed them to seek aggressive medical treatment and associated occupational and speech therapies in the past. The mother was a widow, and supported, in part, by her other son and by the uncle who, himself, had a disability pension. The interview was conducted entirely in Kannada, with some translation done by a resident for the doctor, who spoke Kannada but not fluently. The need for some translation was often the case within a national institute like NIMHANS, as mentioned, but in this context it was also another indicator that the family was not from the middle class and by extension, English-speaking.[7]

It was also possible that stigma and shame played a role in the family's nonaggressive approach to Ravi's disability. It was not uncommon to hear about cases where cognitive and/or other disabilities would lead, due to stigma, to a family's desire to conceal or downplay this condition with others in the community. The reasons for this stigma were numerous, but included cultural beliefs about the moral status of a person born with a disability, and by extension, the family that he/she was born into. More pragmatically, but not unrelated, a disability within the family, as in the case of mental illness, might impact upon the marital possibilities for the disabled person and their siblings. In tragic cases, it could lead to literally hiding the disabled person from the community, sometimes resulting in horrific discoveries of neglect, abandonment, and early death due to malnourishment, bedsores, untreated infections, and other illnesses. In other cases, it was more benign, with the disabled person receiving adequate care in the home, but never brought outside of the home to participate in community events or social life. In Ravi's case, it was possibly the latter, and not the former.

The Violence of the Social

The OPD, as has been made clear through these cases thus far, is an arena where familial and social violence, structural contradictions, and tensions play out in a medicalized context. The next couple of cases illustrate the privileged role of the social in the presentation and treatment of mental illness, as opposed to the comorbid complications of neurological deficits as discussed above. In one case, a thirty-year-old woman from West Bengal came with her husband to the OPD. She had previously been diagnosed with BPAD (Bipolar Affective Disorder) as well as "dissociative disorder" and "borderline personality." She had been treated with the antianxiety medications chlorpromazine and clonazepam, as well as the antidepressant lithium.

This woman also suffered from severe anemia and had hypothyroidism, which may have been the cause of her anemia, we learned from the attending doctor. Additionally, she had "fits" (psychogenic seizures) often, which included thrashing and teeth clenching. There were also several suicide attempts in the past. She had also destroyed several cell phones in angry rages, and was, apparently, suspicious of her husband's fidelity. Moreover, for the past year she had been more "impulsive," spending money. The doctor thought, based upon her appearance, that she might be from a "tribal" (Adivasi) or very marginal Dalit community. He suggested she stop using the lithium and start sodium valproate, which can be used to regulate moods, but also is effective against epileptic seizures. I assumed the former was the doctor's line of reasoning, as he strongly suspected that the seizures or "fits" were very likely "pseudo seizures," as they were often coupled with acts of self-harm and thus were volitional. Thrashing and teeth clenching is also a fairly common symptom of a culturally shaped "hysteria," or conversion disorder, in North India (Kakar 1982; Marrow 2016).

The patient appeared to have the classic "hysteric's symptom" of trying to fulfill an imaginary wish by the Other for her demise and debasement, whilst simultaneously revealing the lack within the Other (the husband, and more broadly, patriarchy's grip, or the symbolic, as Lacan called it). The suicide attempts were an attempt to fulfill her husband's desire, as she perceived it, whilst simultaneously offering a form of punishment, which, as many scholars have noted, is a culturally pervasive pattern of protest in South Asia. I was curious if she had visitations by the wrathful Goddess, who oftentimes serves as the cultural template of protest (Nabokov 2000; Menon and Shweder 2010), and the ubiquitous correlate to this psychological and somatic presentation, but did not have the opportunity to ask. Nevertheless, her rages and "fits" seemed volitional and communicative, in response to her social predicament.

In contrast to the dramatic, and, arguably, culturally sanctioned and gendered behavior of the so-called "hysteric"—obviously a very loaded and problematic clinical term with a long and abusive history in psychoanalytic thought—passive self-neglect was another ubiquitous kind of social symptom we have also witnessed. One day a young man, Sam, came with his mother, father, and brother. He was said to "mutter to himself." Evidently, when he "studied excessively," suicidal thoughts would come to him. "What would happen if I were to die?" Sam would think to himself. He claimed he didn't really want to "do the act," but had thoughts about it.

Sam's family was based in Mumbai. But now he and his brother were both living and studying in Bangalore. Prior to this, he had been treated by a psychologist in Mumbai for seven years and had improved with medications. He then returned to school and stopped taking the medications. Sam then struggled in school, both academically and personally. The doctors told him to take his medications for two years without break. But he was noncompliant.

His thoughts of self-doubt had worsened over time. He managed to graduate, but after this he was unemployed, unlike his brother who scored better and had job offers right out of college. After his brother was "placed," he became more depressed. At this point, the family decided to see another doctor. The mother said Sam often blamed them for his failures at his studies. Sam did not speak as she told of this issue, however.

Now that he was on new medications, the parents complained that he slept excessively—sometimes the whole day. Moreover, he had no social life. His personal hygiene and self-care were poor, the brother and mother reiterated. He would lay around the house unwashed and unshaved unless prodded to "clean up." But when asked about food, the mother said he was a "foodie" and enjoyed eating out. Sam was then directly questioned by the doctor and asked if what the mother was saying was the "whole story" or if he would like to give his "version of the situation." Sam hesitated to speak but finally said that her account was "more or less correct." The doctor then repeated his question but said, "What is missing or still not entirely correct?" Sam did not respond to this question and looked uncomfortable in a moment of awkward silence.

Sam's brother and mother then described in more detail his poor personal habits of not shaving and wearing dirty clothes, as well as watching excessive amounts of TV or viewing the internet. He did not read books, however, in response when asked by the doctor. The brother said that Sam could engage in "reasonable conversation" with his brother about something they watched together. But these discussions only occurred with the brother and not with others outside of the house. Moreover, Sam was also often heard talking directly to the TV with nobody around. The brother had witnessed this behavior many times, he claimed. And in addition to oversleeping, he would sometimes have suspicions about other people's motives.

The doctor ordered a complete medical workup for Sam. When he repeated his request to Sam to say what was on his mind, the family members answered that Sam thought it was a "complete waste of time" for him to come to NIMHANS and that everything was, in Sam's mind, "fine with him." The doctor, however, suggested to Sam and his family that treatment was, indeed, necessary, based on their description of his behavior. That he could not answer questions directly or even indirectly suggested some a kind of paralysis of thought and speech that concerned him. The doctor was worried, moreover, whether Sam would come for psychotherapy and counseling, both of which seemed required. He had a history of noncompliance. And, as he lived in Bangalore, the mother and father, who lived in Mumbai, were worried he would not pursue his treatment and would again begin to neglect himself. The brother, however, as he reminded his parents, was there, so there was hope for reinforcement and encouragement. Sam, for his part, begrudgingly and reluctantly agreed to come for weekly treatment. The doctor appeared skeptical, however, that he would follow through.

Sam's case, as in other cases where counseling and getting the "whole story" was important, demonstrated an understanding that the social provenance of his symptoms of self-neglect was important. That Sam declined with his brother's success, and that he blamed his family for his academic failures, was indicative of an unhealthy dynamic within the household that contributed to his apparent depression and withdrawal from sociality. This dynamic appeared to be related to the pressures of academic and financial success, as well as approval from his parents and brother. His symptoms were, perhaps, a passive-aggressive response to these pressures by his becoming the very thing he was possibly blamed for, or in the terms of the case mentioned above, enacting the Other's desire in a hysteric refusal to act. In doing so he was simultaneously transformed into the abject figure of social failure, whilst also blaming his accusers of their culpability in his failures, thus also offering psychic resistance to this very discourse that pits brother against brother, and parents against their children. In this sense, while not discounting his suffering, Sam's symptoms could in some sense be called ethical resistance to the values of the age, which singularly herald a kind of achievement and success over and above all else.

While I have noted a legalistic or moralistic mindset in some cases as a form of patient symptom that is troubling, the larger cause of these symptoms is located in the singular and legalistic societal measures of success. We will further explore moralism and legalism in relation to the nuanced grey zone of ambiguity in later chapters dealing specifically with religious and professional identity. But even here in this chapter focusing on shame, stigma, and family conflict, the vicissitudes of singular and totalizing frames of reference can be observed with their concomitant manifestations of an affect of betrayal.

The Family Rains Down

June was a rainy month, with patients at NIMHANS taking more shelter in the covered halls near the faculty offices and lecture halls, as well as the canteens and coffee/tea stalls. The near-constant pitter-patter of rain and the dripping sounds of drainage pipes and gutters offered a nice rhythmic accompaniment to the day, softening the heavy traffic noise from the main roads that bordered the campus and bisected it. A nice chill in the air felt fresh, too, with some respite from Bangalore's horrific air pollution. Mosquitos were more plentiful as well, requiring the use of the fan and the electronic mosquito repellent that released its own toxic fumes within faculty offices. I was told to be careful when walking across the grass at NIMHANS, as snakes also liked to come out of their holes more frequently during the rainy season. Cobra nests were common, I was warned.

One rainy afternoon a middle-aged woman came to the OPD with her husband and son. She was in tears as the doctor tried to reason with her about her treatment plan. They spoke in Malayalam, which the doctor knew, and would translate to me every few minutes. A conflict between the husband and wife, with mutual recriminations, was being mediated by the doctor. The wife was animated and agitated, whereas the husband sat impassively. Their son, a grown man, said nothing during her angry speech to the doctor about her husband.

The doctor took a very active role in countering many of the things the mother was saying about the course of treatment needing to be followed, particularly about the medicines that "would take time" to help. I was struck by the authoritative tone the doctor used, as well as the possible use of suggestion and declarative truth having illocutionary power in the clinical context. After about twenty minutes of gentle argument between the mother and the doctor, the couple left, with the son indicating he wanted to talk privately with the doctor.

After the parents left the room, the son asked for a certificate from the doctor that would allow him to be posted to Bangalore. He was a medical doctor, himself, also working in a government hospital, and had to go where he was posted. He was arguing, politely, that he should be posted in Bangalore so he could be better positioned to help care for his parents, especially his mother. The doctor, however, refused to offer up any sort of certificate and asked him to leave in no uncertain terms. I was struck by his determined and adamant tone with the son.

After the son eventually left, albeit reluctantly, the doctor told me this man was "highly pathological." He explained that the family conflicts had "run deep" and a recommendation by him for family therapy was made awhile back. But the son had refused to come for the family therapy, out of shame or embarrassment, given his status as a doctor. But now he wanted "special dispensation to care for his mother" in Bangalore. The NIMHANS doctor said he had always been absent despite initially agreeing to come for the needed therapy that had been ordered. While I did not discover what the roots of the conflicts were in specificity, I was told they included both the father and son in relation to the mother. The mother was greatly saddened by the family conflicts, sending her into a tailspin of depression. My clinical takeaway was obviously limited, but socially stark. That is, even in a situation where there was a medical doctor in the household who would, in theory, be most receptive to expert care and therapy, the stigma and embarrassment, perhaps in front of colleagues or people he perceived to be colleagues, acted as a deterrent to participation in familial treatment. But this, of course, was ambivalent in that the son still wanted to care for his mother to the extent that he would privately ask for a special, and apparently inappropriate, dispensation from NIMHANS that due to hardship, he should not be transferred to another location.

The next case shows a more common pattern of family conflict, with the wife and mother-in-law forming the intractable line of tension between husband and wife. Like the previous case, this case also touched on the volatility and stress of relocation, as demanded by jobs within the public or government sector. The wife, Subhashini, a female in her mid-twenties, presented with the symptoms of "severe depression and death wishes." Subhashini also suffered from decreased sleep. The main social issue behind her symptoms, however, centered upon her relationship with her mother-in-law. When the husband, who was a policeman, was transferred to Bangalore, he did not obtain "family housing," being offered only "single housing" within the police housing complex. Like in the case of military bases, police in Indian cities have bases that include flats within housing complexes. Without a family unit, Subhashini had to stay with his mother and sister in their house about a two-hour drive from town. Therefore, most days, she was without her husband and left alone with her in-laws.

Subhashini had no psychotic symptoms, but experienced pain in the head and neck that was "too much" (Kannada: *ade jasti*) to endure, and suffered, as a result, a lack of concentration and could not sleep. Neurological testing done at NIMHANS had returned negative. Therefore, her symptoms appeared to be psychosomatic and related to her "severe depression" and stress at home. The doctor reasoned with Subhashini's husband for several minutes about a treatment plan. The husband asked a number of questions about the side effects of the medications being prescribed, as well as whether they were effective. The doctor tried to convince the husband to give it some time, as apparently Subhashini had been treated first a month earlier, and this was a follow-up. In this case, however, the doctor went further, advising the husband to rent a place in the city and to remove Subhashini from the "abusive" mother-in-law's house. The husband, it seems, continued to give his mother monthly financial support, which in theory could be used to rent an apartment. The doctor explained that the depression was caused by the "environmental factors" of living with the mother-in-law, who said abusive things to his wife, such as berating her as a "useless creature." The sister also joined in the abuse. When the husband asked his mother to stop "this sort of talk," she responded angrily with "Who gave birth to you?"

The guilt and hold of the mother on the son, however, was powerful (Kakar 1981; Addlakha 2008); and the son, moreover, was afraid to confront his mother, or dislodge his mother from the home, despite the problems it was causing to Subhashini's health and welfare. His hope was that through psychiatric medication, Subhashini's demeanor would "soften" and she would become a more compliant, dutiful, and, at the very least, a less agitated daughter-in-law to his mother. This was not an uncommon theme or symptom repertoire, as we have witnessed, due to the patriarchal values conjoined to patrilocal residence. The son felt caught between the rails of being a good son to his mother and wanting to remove his wife from an abusive situation. But the solution he sought was to normalize his wife through medication, rather than dealing directly with the social conflict that drove the symptoms and social pain felt by his wife. Economically, he had to make a choice whether to remove his wife through the payment of rent, or to remain filial through financial support to the mother. His salary, evidently, could not accomplish both aims simultaneously. But it is also important to note that while the doctor did, in fact, provide symptomatic relief for the symptoms of depression, sleeplessness, and tension, he was emphatic that a "cure" would require the husband's courage and initiative and a betrayal of his filial impulses, not to mention recognition of his own mother's flaws. Here, therefore, medicalization and normalization were mitigated by advocacy and the recognition that psychosocial intervention was needed. In this sense, psychiatry at NIMHANS was neither fully liberatory or disciplinary, as care and abandonment issues brought about by the strains of modern life anxieties and double binds regarding filial and conjugal duties were often impossible to resolve (Cohen 1998; Pinto 2014).

In another case, the filial bonds between mother and daughter were tested by the enduring stigma and shame associated with sexual propriety and marriage in an age when aspirations within a relationship as, perhaps, inspired by a conflicting set of values collided with older notions of decency and patriarchy within that order of hierarchy. Sita, an English-speaking woman in her late twenties from the Tamil middle class of Chennai who was currently residing in Bangalore with her fiancé, presented symptoms of depression. Sita complained about the "lies" that her fiancé and mother said about her to the doctor. Her mother, evidently, encouraged her to get married to the fiancé, as she had already been seen living with him and, by implication, would be seen as undesirable to other men. Sita, however, harbored strong reservations about her relationship.

She claimed that people were always "shouting" and wanted "softly speaking" communication in the house. The doctor advised her to continue "family therapy" as her relationship with the fiancé was the crux of her worries and indecision. Sita complained of "forgetfulness" for the past ten days. She explained further that finding herself in the kitchen, or having made a phone call, or just "being there" caused confusion, as she would not remember the moments that preceded her actions. The doctor asked with regard to the blackouts, "What caused this? What has changed in your situation?" Sita answered that "sometimes the fiancé shouts," so she would turn to her mother for support. The mother offered her emotional support and had come from Chennai to be with her daughter. But, Sita claimed, her mother had advised her to "weather the storm" with this fiancé given that "everyone knew" she was living with him before marriage. This issue came into focus as the conversation ensued.

Sita said she was suffering from lots of body aches and pains, as well as stomach ulcers. She had persistent gastritis and had lots of tests performed on her at various hospitals and clinics. Other than antacids, she had received "nothing helpful." And the tests had proven negative for organic illness, the doctor affirmed with her. But it was still not entirely clear whether these somatic symptoms were psychogenic. Sita also suffered severe constipation, which had become "very difficult" and caused frequent vomiting. She complained of "cramps in her muscles" and an inability to get out of bed. Overall, Sita believed she was physically unwell and had gone to great lengths to demonstrate this through medical testing, but she had only received antacids and antidepressants. The implication seemed to be that her symptoms all arose from her depression and were, therefore, psychosomatic.

Sita complained that her head and neck, in particular, were always "cramped and sore, making it difficult to get out of bed." The doctor commented that "the situation—the relationship problem with the fiancé has not changed." In response she admitted that she "is afraid" and that "people do not understand that I'm afraid." This must have been, I thought, aimed at both the doctor and mother, who encouraged her to make a decision regarding her relationship. Elaborating, Sita said she often did not fall asleep until 3:00 a.m. and often would wake up around 7:00 or 8:00 a.m. Moreover, she wanted to retreat "under the sheet" because she was not "getting support" and feared even her mother, who, apparently, had increasingly strong advice and was losing her patience with her. Though the mother had come from Chennai to care for her, she wanted resolution to the drama. The mother went so far as to tell her, "You are not a kid." This accusation of childish behavior was adding additional stress, Sita said.

The doctor asked, "What is the point you are trying to make?" Sita responded indirectly by asking a question of her own, "Am I confused?" She then proceeded to take out a notebook/diary in which she had been recording her daily thoughts and activities, as well as the things that people had been saying about her. She said, "I take notes so that I can see if people want to put blame on me." This prosthetic sense of self seemed to indicate that she was not confident in her ability to defend herself, or judge the guilt or non-guilt of the fiancé who she implied was abusive. Her supplemental archive, the diary, was a method of hers to construct the narrative of blame, whether it be hers or that of others, particularly her mother's or fiancé's. The doctor, indeed, later told me all indications pointed to her fiancé being abusive.

Sita's mother had at this point been staying with her for two months. She was increasingly telling Sita that she was "old already" and should stay with the fiancé despite her fears and reservations. The mother did not support her when Sita thought it best to end the relationship. It seemed clear that she had major reservations about continuing the relationship, but the pressures from her mother made her confused. Sita's condition deteriorated, and she had stopped working, explaining that this was because she was "confused and could not walk or pick up calls." Though this was lost income, an added stress, she felt it impossible to work until she improved or "until it is clear," suggesting an understanding of her situation and various symptoms. She underscored, "I cannot get up or do any daily activities."

Sita said she was trying to get back to work and to keep busy, following the advice given earlier by the doctor. The doctor also suggested couples therapy should continue, but the fiancé, evidently, frequently "forgot" to come or had a "bad attitude" about it. She said, "He complains if breakfast is late on the table," and also complained about other household work he expected her to do. He wanted his partner to be a "traditional housewife" with regard to cooking and cleaning and was angry with her for "failing in her duties."

Sita had seen another doctor at NIMHANS, a relationship counselor, who had advised her to focus on the relationship but at the same time to avoid placing blame on one person or the other. Her tendency, as noted above, was to try and locate blame through her daily written account, which would, as the word suggests, account in some quantitative sense for the objectivity of her situation, making her less confused. The "pharmakon" or supplement (Derrida 1981; 1995) that was her account would relieve her of the burden of uncertainty, but at the same time was threatening, as it could also invade her inner thoughts, as indicated by the doctors. Indeed, the current doctor had urged her to keep her "mind busy." By this he did not counsel contemplation, but rather, thoughts related to activities that would ward off too much "inward reflection," in the form of writing about her mother and fiancé, which, in turn, fueled her somatic complaints and confused thoughts. A different type of ledger or archive of selfhood was required, one that would supplant or efface these painful memory traces, more along the lines of cognitive behavioral therapy than psychoanalytic introspection. The former, one might speculate, would suppress what it effaced, rendering social violence invisible to an extent.

Sita, as the interview progressed, appeared increasingly sad and agitated, wiping away tears that were in her eyes. She said she was "thinking about running away." To this the doctor asked, "Will your mother and fiancé worry about you?" After a bit of back and forth with the doctor on whether running away was the answer, she agreed to take six more months to work on the relationship and decide whether to marry or separate.

The doctor clarified that the "job" he had suggested for her was not so much a command to sort out her feelings, but rather the more limited aim of managing her symptoms caused by the antidepressive medications, as well as helping her deal with the depression. Therefore, his intervention was in terms of a processual and behavioral modification to deal with daily symptoms that kept her immobile and "under the covers." In tears the patient cried out, "Either they are lying or I am lying." This was as direct as she had been about her mother siding with the fiancé. She added, "They confuse me. People have egos." It sounded like the "advice" she received caused her more anguish than clarity. But sounding slightly more confident, she added, "They just want to safeguard themselves. Mother just wants to marry me off." Sita had plenty of insight, I thought, of her social predicament and the values that undermined her own desires and agency for self-determination. But she still felt immobilized within her psychic resistance, turning this resistance inward upon her body, as a kind of resistance to resistance (Derrida 1998). If suffering is resistance, it is, while perhaps an ethical act, also life-negating and potentially suicidal, in the precise sense that Hegel articulated so long ago with his concept of the "unhappy consciousness." In this concept the slave's "freedom" in spirit was contradictory and split, as it called forth his corporeal reality in oscillation with his spiritual yearning, yielding increasing measures of guilt and self-negation. Or in Klein's terms discussed earlier in this chapter, the internalization of the bad object, the mother's ambivalent presence, produced the depressive position, culminating in hysteric paralysis.

At this point, the mother obviously had worries that Sita, having lived with this man, might be out of other options for suitors, and would be better off, reputation-wise, marrying. Reputation and stigma went hand in hand, even among the educated middle class. But Sita obviously harbored significant doubts that she could live happily with this man. At no point did she express her love or desire to be with him, noting only his apparent flaws. Her staying with him seemed to be driven by social pressures and a nagging doubt in her own health status, particularly in her confused and conflicted thoughts. If she was angry and confused, then how could she trust her feelings about the fiancé? That seemed to be the implication of her "confusion." As if to show a glimpse of her true feelings she said that the fiancé "pretends during therapy to be good and understanding." Under the therapist's gaze, she found it hard to complain about him. Moreover, the therapist had said that therapy will not change an individual per se, but rather only addresses issues that couples face together, which quite possibly inhibited her critique of her partner because she feared reprisals.

This doctor, who was also seen in the previous case, was slightly combative and provocative with patients, challenging them to take actions while not encouraging endless reflection and rumination, witnessing the paralysis and inward-directed stress this caused in somatic and emotional terms. At one point he asked what would happen if she were "to send the mother away?" He then asked more directly, "What will happen if the fiancé beats you after marriage?" This struck a nerve with Sita, putting the direct spotlight upon the unsaid elephant in the room. As he said this, Sita showed visible concern and discomfort. The doctor then abruptly stopped the conversation and said it was time to wrap things up. Sita said then that she did not want to do more therapy. The doctor, in turn, adjusted her medications to help with the depression. Sita left, I felt, seemingly unsatisfied, having wanted to talk more and receive some sort of clarity, which was elusive. The doctor, on the other hand, wanted to force a reckoning and movement past the status quo and paralysis on Sita's part, to make tough decisions on her own behalf. He wanted her to take some concrete actions, as her uncertainty was crippling.

After the patient left the doctor discussed with me what he termed the patient's "borderline personality." She was intelligent and lucid but clearly depressed, and had very ambivalent attitudes towards significant others, including, of course, the mother and fiancé. Part of her borderline personality involved misperceiving the other's motive, he suggested. This paranoid misreading of others' intentions would be self-defeating within any relationship, he suggested. But whether this relationship was healthy or not was equally important to determine. Therefore, some "action was required" to break the deadlock. Her ambivalence towards her mother and fiancé was part of her borderline personality, he pointed out. I wondered to myself if this was a subtle form of normalizing her for the most socially acceptable outcome, or whether a radical break was even conceivable given her ambivalences and depression. By what agency would ambivalence be overcome? The social and the individual were locked in an intractable struggle in which any victory would simultaneously be a defeat, as Hegel might put it. The full weight of filial and familial honor and reputation were clearly at odds with Sita's agency to choose her own fate. This doctor pushed for action, intentionality, and a decision as the only incision possible to cut this double bind that so paralyzed Sita, causing her many somatic complaints. The doctor mentioned to me that he had a background in "family therapy and systems approaches." Therefore, he saw psychiatry in a holistic way, putting the psychosocial on equal footing with the pharmaceutical or biochemical, but lamented that many younger psychiatrists today lacked this wider perspective and were becoming "linear in their thinking." By this he meant that they looked mainly at symptomatic relief, correlating symptom clusters with diagnostic categories found in the latest version of the ICD (International Classification of Diseases) and DSM (Diagnostic and Statistical Manual of Mental Disorders). Psychopharmacology was not systemic, in that nature, but only indexical, relying on symptom semiology and nosology alone, whilst ignoring the more open semiotic process of social life with its multidimensional impacts or "folding" experience upon local bodies (Cohen 2012; Pandian 2010).

Sexual Transgression

The final two cases of this chapter concern depression, compulsive behavior, family tension, and the sense of anxiety and guilt caused by sexual transgressions. In the first, a young man named Ajit presented with "anger outbursts" that were disruptive to his family. Ajit would also "harm himself" and was aggressive towards other family members. He had also attempted suicide twice. Medications had helped control the anger and aggression, but a depression remained. Ajit's father, mother, and sister-in-law, with whom he had some "sort of tension," accompanied him to the OPD.

Since the tenth standard (grade) in school, Ajit had begun cutting himself. He had slashes on his arms and expressed frequent death wishes. He had also hurt his schoolteacher once. He was, even prior to the cutting, a "problem since his childhood," his parents said. By the time I met him in the OPD, he was having crying spells and exhibited "excessive washing of hands" and a compulsion to do things a specific way. He also avoided certain tiles on the floor and expressed compulsive behavior more generally.

Ajit's father was a bank manager and his mother a teacher. His older brother was an IT entrepreneur and his sister-in-law stayed at home with the family. Ajit had been delivered as a cesarean baby prematurely and his mother had had two abortions prior to his birth. Asking questions about his birth weight and earliest childhood, the doctor wanted to know all the details of his early life. The parents said he was a bit hyperactive while in his early years. Ajit interjected that he experienced bullying in school. At one point, the sister-in-law, a woman in her twenties, was brought into the room and asked about her brother-in-law. The parents had noted that Ajit was "always watching her." The sister-in-law was slightly embarrassed when this was brought up in her presence. But she and Ajit's parents said that he harbored strong suspicions about the sister's fidelity to her husband, his older brother. His "suspicions" were excessive and caused friction between the two brothers and made the sister-in-law very uncomfortable within the household, especially enduring his stares.

The doctor prescribed new medications and predicted that there was a 50–70 percent chance of "improvement" with these drugs. He also advised them, and this was important, he emphasized, that they return for family therapy, and suggested a four-week stay at NIMHANS. This would not be easy for the family to arrange, as they were not from Bangalore, but they did not rule it out. The doctor also ordered an IQ test for Ajit. The parents, who displayed great worry for their son, expressed gratitude for the new medication scripts and offer of admission.

The obsessive-compulsive behavior (OCD), while a primary symptom, seemed subordinate, in this case, to the tension caused between the brothers over his inappropriate watching of his sister-in-law. The implication was clear: his obsessive suspicions of her fidelity masked his own inappropriate attraction to her.

While this was not the only sign of psychopathology, it was the most disruptive within the family. His aggression was better controlled with medications, as was his cutting and tendencies to self-harm. And while the doctor did not rule out that family dynamics might be contributing to his OCD and tendencies towards violence, the prescribed family therapy seemed more urgent given the tension that was mounting within the family over the triangle of relations between Ajit, his brother, and his wife. Harmonizing the family was paramount, as was normalizing Ajit's inappropriate behavior towards his "sister." While not threatening the sister-in-law, her discomfort at Ajit's compulsive stares threatened the fabric of sociality within the family. This was, therefore, not only about the structural problems of the patrilocal family structure that would likely be quite a common feature of family life, but, more centrally, about the disruptive force that mental illness brought, opening a breach into what should remain suppressed and contained. And, thus, while OCD is often linked to desires for control and power, particularly in response to sensing their lack in the traumas of early life, here it served as a harbinger of a disruptive and uncontrollable force—a violence that potentially destroys harmony and control, in short, a kind of "death drive" in Freudian terms, extinguishing spontaneity and life-affirming improvisations of daily life.

In a somewhat similar case, an eighteen-year-old male named Alok presented with "low mood and aggressiveness." This, apparently, had been acute for the past two weeks. Alok had an odd and compulsive habit of doing things in multiples of four. He said he did not "feel satisfied" if he had not done something four times, though this meant tasks took a lot longer for him to complete. Alok himself wanted relief from his compulsive behavior, noting the burden his obsessions caused him. Previously, when Alok went to college for two days and stayed in the hostel, he became so homesick that he quit school and returned home. This "dropping out" had been a constant regret, and perhaps a sense of guilt and anxiety. Later, he attended another school and performed well. But he felt very guilty about a sexual encounter he had there with his aunt. He was plagued by feelings of guilt and worthlessness. Alok explained further that "something weird I have [*sic*]. . . . It eats up all your time," referring to the compulsive need to do things in fours.

The doctor asked him why he felt "all this tension and worry." He could not give an answer, but he managed to say that medicines had not helped him. "They say I have Bipolar Affective Disorder (BPAD)—is this true?" he asked with a desperate curiosity, beseeching an answer from the doctor. The doctor answered, "We will see over time." The parents were then invited into the examination room. They expressed concern for their son "despite his doing well" in college. The doctor, as in the previous case, recommended admission to the "family ward" to get to the "bottom of things." The family said they would try, though being from the north, it was a bit of a hardship for them to stay in Bangalore.

After the family left, the doctor and I discussed the issue of guilt. He suggested that it had to be better understood in this case. Alok's OCD must have been related, in part, to a guilty conscience caused by the sexual encounter, he said. Alok possessed no psychotic symptoms, nor was he violent. He seemed, rather, a tormented soul. It was not clear he showed any signs of mania, so the BPAD diagnosis was questionable, according to the doctor. This BPAD diagnosis had come from outside of NIMHANS. In the older Freudian language, one could sense his OCD was a form of neurosis caused by a combination of trauma and subsequent guilt. Though this psychoanalytic language was not generally used in the OPD, the doctor's intuitive recommendation for "family therapy" suggested that Alok's symptoms were not reducible to the one traumatizing sexual encounter with the aunt. Rather, it was indicative of some familial dynamic that made Alok vulnerable to this transgressive act. Moreover, it was not clear (to me, at least) that the parents knew of this incident. Alok may have kept that secret with his doctor, alone. But given his unusually strong homesickness after leaving home for college, and his perhaps acute attachment to home, there was the possibility that intimacy within the home, or even the classic Oedipal attachments, were at play. The aunt, being the surrogate mother at the second college experience, had triggered these intimacies and had released their subsequent anxieties. These reflections notwithstanding, whatever the dynamics might have been at home, their affective power certainly exceeded the singular event of sexual trauma. Therefore, we can, as in the preceding case, note how the affective power of the familial, conjoined to sexual fantasy and/or intimacy, even when suppressed, caused compulsive and self-defeating forms of self-harm, be they behaviorally or psychically manifested.

* * *

Given the schematic nature and velocity of the OPD, there were, as is by now obvious, many facets of each case that could not be determined through a singular encounter. What I have attempted to illustrate, however, are modalities of familial conflict and, specifically, the styles of care and treatment that were provided by the doctors at NIMHANS. On both of the questions, there were themes and variations. Family conflict generated by mental illness was complicated by larger societal forces and iniquities in contemporary India, as would, of course, be the case everywhere. But in terms of Indian patternings of the social, shame and stigma influenced marital relations, and even the possibilities of marriage for patients and their siblings. Moreover, mental illness was, whatever its biological or neurological underpinnings and vulnerabilities within the patient, influenced by these same social patternings, bringing the violence of the social into the causative formation of symptoms. These oftentimes involved gendered norms that coerced a kind of normalization within the familial and social, inducing symptoms of protest or resistance, which, in turn, were then normalized within the clinical context through the desired "cure" offered by medications. But as we have also witnessed, the doctors, though varied in style, resisted patient desires for a kind of normalcy that suppressed symptoms but did not get to the violence within the social in which these symptoms found their provenance. As mentioned earlier, psychiatry was not wholly liberatory or disciplinary, but rather caught between these tensions (Pinto 2014; Lang 2018). While a sociocentric cultural ideology enacted embodied affects (and effects) of shame and stigma, with these registering at times as a resistance to resistance (Derrida 1998), or inward-directed and life-negating symptoms and compulsions, the "as if" (Sapir 2010) quality of this ideology was porous and contested by both doctors and patients.

Shame and stigma, coupled with the pressures of time, forced doctors to make rapid interventions. These interventions, however, as we have seen, are calibrated by their own deep understanding of the larger societal forces, which in turn determine the limits of care and certainty within any given diagnosis. The cases presented in this chapter, though wide and varied, and certainly not exhaustive, have attempted to illustrate the vicissitudes of shame and stigma as conjoined to some of the cultural themes that are resonant in Indian society. In each case, a level of indeterminacy was underscored in order to illustrate the skillful and difficult application of psychiatry in a primary center of care, where the skill sets of doctors are assumed to be of the highest caliber. And thus, though there is a trend in psychiatry away from the holistic focus on the person and towards organic causation (neurochemical imbalances, neurological biomarkers, genetics, etc.), there is still a great deal of psychosocial emphasis, given the provenance and presentation of symptoms being an expression of the social, in the broadest sense, with suffering clearly exacerbated by social violence and even experiences of social defeat (Luhrmann and Marrow 2016), particularly among those more vulnerable members of society (Kleinman 2012; Patel and Kleinman 2003).

The next chapter continues the exploration of stigma and shame, and the relationship between the social and the psychiatric. The focus, however, of this next chapter will be to examine forces of rebellion and resistance that are more intentional and agentive, and perhaps less passive, inward-directed, and somatic. This becomes most visible, not surprisingly, in a generational shift, where we might suspect to find instances of rebellion. Secondly, we turn to the themes of care and abandonment, as related to stigma and other social pressures impinging upon the social fabric. Rebellion, resistance, care, and abandonment are all inextricably linked to stigma and shame, and the sociocentric ideology of the "family" that is still hegemonic in South Asia, though increasingly incongruent with the social pressures of modernity (Cohen 1998).

Chapter 2

Rebellion and Abandonment

Excess and Antinomy

That shame and stigma impact upon individuals and their families in profound ways, exacerbating symptoms that in turn fuel attempts at normalization of these symptoms through psychiatry, is unsurprising. But we have seen the particular social and cultural pressures that modulate the presentation of illness and the psychiatric interventions within a particular Indian context. Factors such as the patrilocal joint family, the tensions caused by the increasingly competitive forces of education and labor, and the increasing legalism or literalism that are both symptomatic of a more bureaucratized society, as well as a causal force of today's demands upon identity and self-worth, have to some extent exacerbated the shame surrounding mental illness. The venue of the OPD, with its heavy patient loads and limited clinical durations, was also an arena where psychiatric focus magnified symptom alleviation, despite doctors harboring more complicated understandings of case histories and illness presentations than they were able to effectively treat at times.

However, in most cases shame and stigma did not lead families to reject the person possessing the illness. Rather, we witnessed conflicts that were difficult and strained familial relationships, but in most instances those conflicts did not lead families to the abandonment or institutionalizing of their kin. The lives of patients and their families were entangled in complicated ways, both in terms of the etiology of illness (the psychosocial causative factors) and their attempts at resolution (Pinto 2014). This chapter turns on a different foot. Here we continue to look at the pressures of normalization and the workings of shame, but also at the fissures that escape containment and normalcy. In the first part of the chapter we look at resistance and rebellion, particularly as arising out of the different aspirations of the young, and their rejection, at times, of the moral order that seeks to tame them. Secondly, we see in a few cases where rebellion and normalization meet their limit, leading to social abandonment, be it real or perceived by the person deemed mentally ill. Thus, while the previous chapter explored the entangled ground of everyday conflict as exacerbated by shame, stigma, and mental illness, this chapter looks to the more polarized ends of this entangled continuum, where an excess marks normalization efforts' limits. In the chapter's conclusion, we will return to the theoretical and philosophical implications of this notion of resistance, and its hypervigilant counter, a resistance to resistance, a double-negation that obscures the dormant yet lingering fantasy of the subject.

Resistance and Rebellion

Sometimes resistance to psychiatric treatment was quite routine, as in noncompliance with treatment that would occur quite frequently. What follows, however, moves beyond the kind of noncompliance that was experimental or careless. Rather, here we see social rebellion and resistance to psychiatry being linked in ways that demonstrate that fissures and tensions within society, and particularly between generations, are replicated in the clinical encounter.

Nalini was a divorced journalist who had been treated at NIMHANS for a few years. She appeared twice in the OPD while I was there, both times well-dressed and neat in appearance. Nalini complained of an inability to "meet deadlines" as well as not having any "structure in her life." Moreover, she found it hard to read, which was in her case a symptom to be taken seriously, given her profession.

Nalini had taken to freelance writing in recent months, as a "regular journalistic job" was proving too stressful for her. Even freelance writing, it seemed, caused her to experience some anxiety and she complained that as deadlines loomed she felt paralyzed and unable to work. When I met her first, she had complained of her relationship with her children. Due to her illness, and feelings of "strain" and tension, she found it hard to get out of bed on some days. Her ex-husband was a "hippie drifter" (the doctor's description) who had no money for alimony, nor was able to contribute much in terms of caregiving for the children. He lived in a different state in South India. Fortunately, however, she came from a middle-class family and had some help financially, which allowed her to have hired help at home.

Taking Oxetol, a mood stabilizer, for her depression, Nalini reported that she felt "normal" in her moods to some extent, though she still complained of mood swings within the day. Before, she explained, she would have "mood swings every few days." But now the oscillation was becoming more frequent, oftentimes within the same day. She also spoke of dizziness that occurred twice a day as well as having a "head that felt heavy."

Turning away from her life and its symptoms, Nalini then spoke of a two-month "vacation" from her children. They had been with her parents during this time. This time was "enjoyable," she said, as she could "go out and be free." But now with the children returning home and starting school again, she said she again felt very anxious. Moreover, she did not express happiness at the prospect of seeing her children, nor sadness at their absence.

The attending doctor suggested she add Tranxene, a benzodiazepine sedative for anxiety, to help regulate her sleep. She said she was sometimes sleepless at night or would sleep in very late in the morning. At the end of her OPD session, Nalini mentioned that she was writing an article on the mental health care performed at NIMHANS, in which she wanted to highlight how hard doctors worked for their patients. It was clearly intended to also impress upon the doctor her high regard for him. The doctor, for his part, suggested a foundation that might subsidize her article. The foundation, he noted, worked to lessen the stigma attached to mental health.

Nalini spoke fluent English and was clearly from the middle class, but she had been unable to hold a steady journalistic job for two years. She had come to NIMHANS in order to "restart" her therapy, expressing a strong desire to return to work. But she complained that she "cannot do anything nowadays" and would spend most of her time in bed. Sleep was a problem. Indeed, when she came to the OPD, Nalini said she had not slept in days. Moreover, she "had issues" with her mother and lived alone with her children, being divorced from her husband. Nalini complained that she "felt flat" when she was on medication, though it did, she admitted, lessen her anxiety and panic, as well as her anger outbursts. Her temper, in particular, had gotten her in trouble over the years as it manifested in the workplace, making it hard for her to hold a job. And her anger outbursts were often directed at her children. This led to a dynamic in which she complained of "not having quality time" with her children. Either she was angry at them for something or she slept all day in her bed, unable to function as a "normal mother." Nalini's daughter was "high strung," which proved too much for her mother. Furthermore, her ex-husband, it seems, had not "paid support for seven years." She had only recently been divorced, though they were estranged for many years. The ex-husband, Nalini said, saw the children every six weeks when he visited. He evidently refused to work and also refused to come for family therapy, which had been recommended at the outset of Nalini's treatment.

During the previous three months, the stress had been "just too much" and she was feeling overwhelmed by her desire to reclaim her life and work, whilst simultaneously feeling unable to function, exacerbating the stress. A well-educated woman with high professional aspirations, she clearly possessed a lot of insight into her condition and admitted that she could not handle stress well and needed psychotherapy to begin recovery. In her case, the desire for psychotherapy and understanding far outweighed her desire for medication. She said, "I was in bed all last week . . . and spent all day doing nothing." But as recalled earlier, she also said she had not slept for days. Her non-restful inactivity was compounding her stress, it appeared.

Being an educated and "progressive woman," Nalini sent her kids to a private school, which was based on the esoteric teaching of a German philosopher and educator. This, the doctor queried, must have been expensive, but she said that it was "normal" cost, though she also admitted to having missed several payments and being worried that the school might expel her children. She was asked by the doctor whether she received help from her parents, given her present non–income-earning status. She said it was "too much pressure" to ask her parents. And she added that she "should be able to take care of her children." The doctor reassured her that it was fine to seek temporary help from one's parents, as this would likely be returned in some form later on. This reassuring talk by the doctor went on for some time, as Nalini was clearly a bit embarrassed to be in a situation where she had no support from the father of her children, nor any regular income of her own.

At the end of the session, she was asked to keep a diary to see if meds were helping. The doctor urged Nalini to go back on her meds to stabilize her mood and sleep, as it was fairly clear that she had resisted the effects of the drugs, and perhaps had been noncompliant at times. As mentioned, however, she demanded psychotherapy and found it "insightful" in the past. The doctor, after she had left the room, said her "bipolar" diagnosis was not conclusive, and suggested that she basically suffered from a "borderline personality" making it difficult for her to get along with others. She had no delusions but did have, it seems, some manic and depressive symptoms, though not severe or pronounced enough for her to necessarily receive the BPAD diagnosis. Her rebellion was less against psychiatry per se than it was against the responsibilities that impinged on her freedoms. Deadlines that were professional in nature were stressful, as were the daily deadlines associated with childcare. Nalini rebelled against the structure and order of contemporary life, seeking a more creative freelance lifestyle, in which she would be able to craft her own narratives, rather than being subject to those of the people around her. But in this freedom, she also felt a sense of being "flat" and uninspired. Though a "progressive" person who wanted a more liberal and creative education for her children, she ran up against the structural reality of her aspirations for freedom, for herself, and for her children, and the hard reality of dependency. She resented that dependency, not wanting to take financial help from her parents. Even the "good object," in Klein's (1986) sense, had to be abandoned, rejected, and to some extent expunged from her sense of autonomy, as this would impinge on her self-image of "freedom" that she could only sustain while on her "vacation."

In Nalini's case, it was unclear what had triggered her symptoms, be it tensions at work, at home, or stemming from issues with her parents. She sought approval from the doctor, perhaps, in her desire to turn her journalistic eye to mental health treatment. On the other hand, her journalistic distance and analysis of psychiatric care seemed to also inhabit a critical disposition caused by a loss of control she had experienced while taking medications. There was certainly a rebellious side to Nalini's relationship to others, be they her parents, especially her mother, her co-workers, and even her children, with whom she failed to enjoy "quality time" due to her anger at their behavior. Clearly, the advice to keep a diary and to return to a normal schedule with work were intended to regulate the mood swings and unstable sleep cycles, with the concomitant stress this either signified or exacerbated. Some semblance of self-control and regulation seemed the antidote proposed by the doctor to Nalini's self-defeating rebellions against family, colleagues, and even the doctor. Psychotherapy seemed a promising terrain, in Nalini's eyes, though I could not help wondering how she might rebel, via transference, against whatever interpretative insights might emerge from the psychotherapist.

Case Conference

One Saturday afternoon in early January of 2015, I participated in the "case conference" that the Department of Psychiatry held routinely. These case conferences were largely exploratory for the patient's diagnosis and treatment, but also pedagogical for the residents and fellows. The theme this day was "hysteria"—a rather old diagnosis but one that still had some traction in India, as we have discussed (Pinto 2014; Marrow 2016). I was the guest "analyst," so to speak, being asked to comment on the cases from an anthropological perspective. This was not my usual modus operandi as a "shadow" within the OPD or wards, but I managed to say something for each case. What I said, I feared, could have either been obvious to residents, fellows, and others who attended, or conversely, was so alien as to be somewhat impractical. I was assured that part of the training for students and residents was, in fact, to see symptoms within their wider social context. Without offering specific diagnostic insights, or directions for treatment, my observations about the relationship between social stress and cultural beliefs might have seemed inconsequential, I feared. But the chair of the Psychiatry Department had also asked me to give some seminars on the key ideas in psychological anthropology, which I later did.[1] Therefore, I somewhat reluctantly agreed to lead conversation in this case conference, with the caveat that I was not a psychiatrist and would not speak to biomedical considerations. As the cases were selectively chosen on the theme of "hysteria," with its explicit psychosocial dimensions, it was decided that this was the appropriate session for me to moderate. The session lasted about two hours, and what follows are two of the cases that were presented.

We met in a lecture hall within the Psychiatry Department. There were perhaps fifteen to twenty in attendance, including a few of the doctors, clinical psychologists, and several students and residents. The cases were presented first by the fellows or residents. I was struck that the majority in attendance were female, suggesting either an imbalance among the students, or a bias towards attending this event (or not). It seemed that two of the doctors had instructed particular students to attend, given their own interests in having this broader training in anthropological thinking. As "hysteria" is already conceived as a kind of somatic rebellion or resistance to the normative order and, within it, a gendered dimension, these cases also fall under this section that focuses on psychosocial resistance.

The first case presented was of Manju, a woman in her late thirties who suffered from "regressions to childlike behavior" in which she spoke her mother tongue (though no longer living in her own state) and acted cheerful but decidedly "childish." This behavior had been going on for ten years or more. It was precipitated by her sister's suicide at the age of eighteen under mysterious circumstances. Prior to the presentation of this symptom, Manju used to fall down and remained unconscious for short periods. Seizures were suspected as well as syncope (fainting). After these events occurred, she would regain "normal functioning with some amnesia." Each time these "fits" occurred, they were precipitated by arguments, suggesting a possible psychogenic causation. Both epileptic seizures and syncope were eventually ruled out after neurological testing.

There was an incident in Manju's youth in which she almost had a bad motorcycle accident. This near-accident haunted her, we were told, contributing, perhaps, to her fainting spells. To what extent her "panic attacks" were different than her regressive and seemingly guilt-laden symptoms was murky, though there were hints of traumas in earlier life. She would also engage in acts of self-harm.

Manju married young and had one son. But neighbors had complained that she was not doing a good job as a mother and were "critical" of her. These critical neighbors drove her to depression and "extreme guilt" over her son. The content, however, of her purported "bad care" was not disclosed. I wondered: did she neglect her son and go out to enjoy herself? Or, conversely, was she sad that her illness-related condition inhibited a richer mother and son bond, or at the very least made it hard to provide daily care for him? If the latter, we might assume that the critical neighbors were blaming the victim, exacerbating her condition, with its somewhat classic hysteria-like symptoms of seizing or fainting. On the other hand, the implication that the neighbors were speaking ill of her, perhaps, seemed to suggest a paranoid response, which is, of course, typical of certain kinds of psychosis such as paranoid schizophrenia, or a tangible consternation over the young woman's morality.

For years, after precipitating factors and "fits" of unconsciousness, Manju would regain some semblance of "normalcy." But in recent years she had regressed to a cheerful but extremely childlike disposition. These episodes were tolerated given the patient's amiable state of mind, from her family's perspective, who were already used to her "fits" and unconscious spells. But Manju was admitted to NIMHANS after the "incidents became more depressive and dissociative in nature," and in which the woman did not resume normalcy as she had before. The guilt, fear, and shame from the neighbors' comments were worsening as well, contributing to a depressed and increasingly paranoid state.

Manju was medicated for depression and psychotic symptoms but it was concluded that she would need psychotherapy in order to learn "better coping mechanisms" than those she was using. Regression to childhood would certainly mobilize the support factors in her life (family, son, community) in a palpable way (Kakar 1982), though not without further embarrassment for the family, or for Manju herself. Moreover, the stressors that triggered her regression into childhood would remain opaque without further exploration.

My impression was that something must have happened with her sister and her suicide that prompted a guilt response. Fits and falling unconscious were a kind of simulated death, I speculated. Manju married very young, and may have assumed, in a strange sort of way, her older sister's identity in the process. It would be important, I suggested, that we know more about the sister's suicide as well as her romantic life, beginning with the feelings she may have harbored for her sister's partner (see Nabokov 2000; Obeyesekere 1981). It sounded to me as if the sister's suicide might have occurred over some unrequited love or sense of betrayal. This may have been a blind alley, but the son's purported "neglect" as well as the neighbors assuming the role of the "conscience" suggested something deeper may be at play with regard to this triangle with her sister and son.

I inquired about religious interventions as well as Manju's intimate life. Nothing was known about either, though it was said by the presenting resident that no religious cures had been sought. My impression was hardly innovative or insightful, given the missing pieces of the case. What I could muster was a question as to why these areas were not probed much more deeply in the intake interview, to which the resident, students, and faculty seemed to nod collectively in assent. That is, if hysteria, in the classic Freudian or Lacanian sense, is the language of the unconscious speaking somatically in resistance to an intolerable lack in the Other, coupled with an intolerable moral dilemma within the self that simultaneously attacks the good object, attempting to destroy it, as in the Kleinian sense (1986) of sibling "envy," the necessity of contextualizing this resistance and rebellion to the normalcy demanded by society is met with an aggressive gesture of inward-directed aggression. This simultaneously indexes the Other's wrong, and requires, in turn, a more rigorous catalogue of familial and conjugal intimacies, or their lack thereof. This was a case for a deeper psychodynamic probing of the issues of youth. What we can say with some confidence is that Manju's seizures and bouts of unconsciousness were psychogenic, as a way to control the uncontrollable, which was the near-accident, and the very real tragedy of her sister's death, for which, we might speculate, she felt some responsibility, real or imagined.

A simulated death-like state in this manner is a kind of self-mastering of death, though one that is hardly without consequence. The refractory nature of the illness was interfering, apparently, with the care of her son, which was noted by neighbors, or was imagined to be so in a paranoid fashion by Manju. More likely, it seemed to me, there was a synergy of symptom and comorbid feelings of guilt, whether the original symptom of "fits" was a response to some sort of guilt, such as something surrounding her relationship to her sister, and perhaps the sister's lover. In any event, her more recent retreat into childlike behavior, invoking the comforting mother tongue of youth, could have signified Manju's resistance to both parental responsibility and the pains of the previous twenty or so years, taking her to a time when life was less fraught with judgement. But even this rebellion had its limits, as it seemed to increasingly oscillate with depression and dissociation, so much so that she was brought to NIMHANS. Normalcy was retreating further from view, frightening Manju's family to take some action. Even forcing this action, one might imagine, was a form of passive aggression directed towards her family. Here, Manju's resistance was now assuming the face of a resistance to the resistance, and a retreat into a fantasy that guarded a more troubling yet obscured phantasm. There was an excess that exceeded meaning in her inexplicable, discomfiting retreat into a childlike disposition within her adult body. This was not cute or adorable in the sense that the Hello Kitty phenomenon in Japan might have marked a retreat from the reality of adult womanhood in Japan. Rather, Manju's childlike behavior, though initially tolerated, became the pathological site of an intervention, its repetition creating new strands of suffering for both Manju and her family.

Psychodynamic interpretations and interventions were less trodden paths at NIMHANS, as it was, historically speaking, driven by Kraepelinian organic psychiatry. In that sense, my psychodynamic speculation was different from the functional and symptomatic relief sought in most cases by patients and their doctors. That said, it had been clear that the older psychiatrists, who had a strong sense of psychosocial causation and found currency in the diagnosis of "hysteria," wanted students to be exposed to a kind of analysis that was not hegemonic within psychiatric practice in India. But, as Pinto (2014; 2022) demonstrates, the centrality of "hysteria" in Indian psychiatry also, and paradoxically, illustrates a preoccupation with the particular pressures produced by the sociocultural, and specifically sociocentric, forces in India, particularly in its gendered politics.

The next case we discussed concerned Anu, a woman in her mid-twenties who was unmarried and educated to the tenth standard in school. She came from a middle-class family and was somewhat of a child prodigy in South Indian classical dance (Bharata Natyam). She had been dancing seriously from the age of four and had won a dance competition at the age of eight. Anu's success on the stage of classical dance continued for another four years or so. But at the age of fourteen, she had an illness and missed school. During this time of illness she could not dance. Moreover, she stopped writing, another of her passions, and began to suffer leg pain and tremors. She was treated for forty-one days by a *vaidya* (Ayurvedic doctor) but felt badly about her "failures." Around a year later, at the age of fifteen, she was at school and noticed her name was absent from a roster of students that was posted on the wall (presumably those who scored high on exams). After this "insult" and its hurt, she began to have "episodes" of "falling down." Following these incidents she had trouble standing up again. Another *vaidya* referred her to allopathy (biomedicine) at this time. During her consultation she overheard the doctor say, "She may never walk again" to her anxious family. Overhearing this seemed to have worsened her symptoms.

For the next five years Anu lived at home and grew weaker, unable to walk unassisted, or on some occasions, not at all. By the age of twenty she was admitted into the neurology ward at NIMHANS. Anu had significant depressive symptoms for about forty-five days when she was warded, as well as exhibiting a "poor effort" in physical therapy. Depression became her primary diagnosis when no neurological findings were discovered after extensive testing. She did eventually learn to walk again with a "hand stick" (cane). But Anu remained convinced that her disability was organic, and not a "hysteric conversion disorder" as had been suggested while at NIMHANS.

After Anu's hospitalization she gradually and eventually emerged from her depression when she became an activist-advocate for the disabled, working mainly from home. With her social work on behalf of the disabled, she found some satisfaction and renewed purpose in life. But at the age of twenty-five, and while watching a youth dance festival on television, she began crying, sobbing in an uncontrollable manner. Thereafter, Anu's ability to walk quickly declined further. Anu was admitted again at NIMHANS, now for psychiatric treatment. After fourteen months of living in the ward and having psychotherapy, she had gained a considerable amount of insight that her symptoms of paralysis were indeed psychological. But her condition had yet to improve. She continued to receive psychical and psychological therapies at NIMHANS.

Upon hearing about Anu's case, I was reminded of the "Humpty Dumpty" syndrome among males in North America that neurologists had told me about when shadowing them in upstate New York. This syndrome in North America occurred when the ideology of self-reliance and toughness was shattered by a catastrophic neurological or psychological event, making the male patient question his self-worth when requiring the care and support of others. Due to the ideological resonance of self-reliance and the purported cult of individual capacity that permeates American male identity, in particular, when a situation arose that went beyond the control of the person, his imaginary sense of self was completely shattered in a manner that made putting the pieces of that image back together characteristically difficult, as it would require an acceptance of dependency and symbiosis that was anathema to these ideological notions of self-worth.

In Anu's case, she was an accomplished dancer, and even an award-winning prodigy. And like child actors who cannot cope with post-stardom and decline into depression and substance abuse, she seemed to have, after some traumatic events at school, become the very thing she feared the most. That is, her symptoms were the exact opposite embodiment of her earlier self-image as a finely skilled dancer. Moreover, her identity now as a disability advocate was predicated on her disability, and to that end, she had a negative incentive to overcome her disability. Furthermore, it had allowed her to resume writing, her second passion. Here we witness a resistance to resistance, and an inexplicable attachment to a symptom that is both negative and positive to Anu. In a positive sense, she could reject the identity of her prodigy-youth, becoming other than what the other desired of her (i.e., her parents). And in so doing, she received compassion and care from family and caregivers. In some sense, this is similar, then, to what Manju might have accomplished with her retreat into childlike behavior. In other words, it was a retreat into her pre-dancer life, as well as marking her post-dancer transformation into something that was other to and resistant from what was demanded of her as a prodigy. But faced with this transformation being based upon a hidden conflict, as well as a positive identification that gradually emerged out of her symptoms, she had a hard time convincing her body to know what her psyche had come to realize through over one year of psychiatric treatment at NIMHANS.

I wondered aloud if Anu's early years as a dancer were happy ones, or if her symptom was also a calling of attention to the potential hypercriticism and overly vigilant scrutiny that a child dancer might be subjected to, which I had witnessed in another context (Willford 2006). In that sense, her disability could be, in its inception, a form of passive aggression against her parents. Like the case of "Sundar" that Kakar (1982) writes about, open expressions of ambivalence, much less hostility, to one's self-sacrificing parents are unthinkable. In Sundar's case, partial paralysis was psychogenic, protecting him from striking his father in anger, a great filial sin. Becoming disabled might have had a similar function for Anu in negating her parents' desire without open conflict; and moreover, this certainly brought some measure of concern and attention to her at a very different level than would have been the case as the perfect idealized child artist.

This, in turn, would also explain Anu's sensitivity to even the slightest insult that could not be managed by her without a complete collapse of self-image. Could the school incident have simply been a recurrence of the same slight she might have endured from her dance teachers and parents? Or alternatively, was her inflated and grandiose sense of self, cultivated by success in public, simply shattered by real-world experiences that could never repeat indefinitely the illusion of perfection? Was this, in other words, akin to an Indian female version of the Humpty Dumpty syndrome, whereby idealized self-images were shattered by reality?

A third possibility, of course, would have been that there still was an undiagnosed neurologic condition causing her paralysis, and that Anu's depression and anxiety was comorbid from that unrecognized illness, as well as a sense of frustration that she was being treated for a "hysteric conversion disorder," even after a long and mentally laborious admission in the hospital. That is, was Anu now facing tremendous pressure that she heal herself, taking accountability for her disability through the insight of psychiatric diagnosis and psychological counseling? If an underlying neurological condition did exist, then her failures at recovery would be understandable, but not to the clinicians and family members perplexed by her "stubborn" attachment to a disabled persona. If this was the case, I imagined that, like a case of failed exorcism, Anu faced the double jeopardy of an illness coupled with the social pressure to have enough faith in expert knowledge to overcome it. This third scenario seemed the least likely to me, given her extensive neurological workup at NIMHANS, a leading center for neurological research. Had Anu's neurological testing been done at a less esteemed institution, as was the case in Biehl's (2005) now classic study, *Vita*, speculation and doubt would have arisen more to the psychiatrists and psychologists at NIMHANS who were now tasked with helping her.

In any event, the cases of Manju, Anu, and others also discussed in the case conference indicated a moment of reflexivity and expansive openness in what was otherwise a more rapid-fire OPD, where doctor-patient interactions were limited due to time constraints. As such, decisions about medications, admissions, and whether to suggest psychotherapy had to be made in relatively short sessions. In many instances, sessions, particularly follow-ups, could last as little as five minutes. In new and oftentimes complicated cases, thirty minutes would be the upward limit of a session in the OPD with the attending psychiatrist. Appointments with specific time slots were not offered. Patients and their families had to commit to spending the good part of the day waiting in the OPD for their consultation. In addition to meeting with the attending doctor, they would be examined and interviewed by the residents, who would then usually brief the doctors when the patients entered the doctor's office. Therefore, the case conference allowed for a more holistic discussion among faculty and students at NIMHANS, looking at each case from its psychosocial dimensions in addition to its biological determinants. In this case, where "hysteria," and specifically hysteric conversion disorders, was the theme of the conference, the psychosocial was given extended attention, especially because organic causation had already been determined to be secondary to the social provenance of symptom presentations. Moreover, it followed that even anthropological perspectives could be entertained in the nonclinical space of the teaching classroom. I was struck with the ambiguity that each case continued to contain. Meaning and signification was elusive and allusive. Something resisted facile interpretation by physician, psychologist, or anthropologist, though ideas were suspended within clouds of reflection, which, it was hoped, would enrich future psychotherapeutic explorations. Hysteria invited thinking, and left a productive indeterminacy within psychiatric diagnosis at NIMHANS against the pressures of biomedical determinism based upon symptom nosology.

Boredom and Rebellion

We have considered how psychic resistance might manifest in somatic symptoms, and in so doing, have speculated about the psychosocial and cultural tensions that might have contributed to these illness presentations. But sometimes, rebellion or resistance as an explanation was not countered, contradicted, or denied. Indeed, sometimes patients openly expressed their culpability and blame with regard to their self-destructive behavior yet found it challenging to stop it. There were many, many cases of addiction, particularly substance abuse of alcohol and marijuana (ganja) that passed through the halls of NIMHANS. Oftentimes, these were working-class males who used substances to cope with the pressures of making ends meet, working in arduous and physically demanding jobs, or even peer pressure. In the majority of these cases, however, addiction could lead to drug-induced forms of psychosis, which in turn became even more debilitating than the addiction itself. These cases would then require psychiatric evaluation and, at times, psychiatric medications coupled with detox counseling. But in other cases, particularly among the young and more affluent, addictive behaviors could mark a rebellion against the normative order, or even mark a boredom and fatigue with the increasingly alienating pace of life in the urban metropolis.

One afternoon, Abhirami, a young woman in her early twenties dressed in jeans and a t-shirt, came with her more conservative parents to the OPD. A long-time patient of one of the doctors at NIMHANS, Abhirami had lost weight and waged an ongoing battle with "boredom," alcohol, drugs, and more recently cocaine use. She spoke fluent English and obviously came from the Westernized youthful middle class of Bangalore. She lived currently with a friend in their own apartment, but also had "rendezvous with boys" that her parents did not know about. Though she said she had quit drinking and drug use, she complained of boredom and lethargy.

Abhirami's parents said that they saw some improvement in "her attitude" towards them. They were asked to leave the room for a few minutes while the doctor questioned her. She said to the doctor she was bored with her friends, her life, and felt very "detached from everything." Abhirami got along with a sister, she pointed out, but "basically" wanted to "work and come home and sleep." She had no stable relationships in her life, but said she "fools around sometimes." Her work habits were, she claimed, "demotivated," and "average to below average" in performance. Due to Abhirami's proficiency in English, she worked as a proofreader for a local publisher. She had plans for journalism school but said that she "feels very lost these days." Abhirami said she lived "day to day," and had "no direction in life." She added that she "gets sick of everything: food, conversations, and people." Sometimes in the middle of a conversation, she would "lose patience," and would stop talking or listening. Moreover, her sleep was disturbed. "But if I take a pill to help me sleep, I'm like a log," she said.

Abhirami's parents, who had been called back to the room, complained of her long work hours. She was waking late in the morning and working very late at night, when she returned home. But this, apparently, might have been Abhirami's excuse for staying out late. She had battled her conservative and "orthodox" Hindu parents for many years about her lifestyle. Her doctor told me that the parents "did not know the extent of her self-destructive behavior," only seeing her moodiness, lethargy, and late sleeping, but not knowing, evidently, of her drug, alcohol, or sexual life. Abhirami already had experienced a couple of abortions, and quite recently had been convinced to take cocaine with a "boy." But as with everything else, the drug bored her, she claimed.

Abhirami's parents wanted her to move back home and to quit her job. But she had no interest in moving back home, though she herself claimed that her life was aimless. Moreover, this "aimless life" had depressed her. Her presently undisciplined life was a rejection of her parents' values, embodying everything her parents feared, and then some.

Abhirami was seemingly quite intelligent but had not found anything that could hold her attention long enough to pursue with any zeal or passion. She got by on her wits, but just barely, as she stumbled from one form of intoxication to another. But these distractions, or retreats into rebellion, only left her ever more bored and empty. Her compulsions, in other words, were self-defeating and aggressive, not only to the goodness of her parents, but to herself. That is, while she clearly was, in Klein's sense, disillusioned by the flaws and/or lack in her parents' world, despite their care and apparent uprightness, and sought to attack that "goodness" by becoming its opposite, her compulsions and addictions were a resistance to resistance, as Derrida (1998) would say, in that her explorations of the "dark" world of sex and drugs were empty, boring, and without the potential for creative transformation. Progression was blocked, and regression to the "bad" object of her desire to negate the "good" became self-defeating, redoubling the contempt she must have perceived at some level from her parents, as she embodied that which they feared the most.

Bangalore, with its large middle class, has a fairly robust and hedonistic youth scene, rife with clubs, drugs, alcohol, and opportunities for casual liaisons. But we might imagine that in this case, Abhirami was dissatisfied with her own rebellion, having to some extent internalized her parents' disapproval, which now punished her, albeit indirectly, with the compulsions that led to automatism, boredom, and emptiness. Her resistance to resistance, then, was to occlude her deeper issues with her parents, which might have driven her initial rebellious rejections of their values.

These psychodynamic thoughts notwithstanding, the doctor took a practical route, whatever he might have been thinking, and advised her to return to school and pursue something of interest. How to get her to take the initiative when Abhirami was in "this state of mind" was a difficult clinical question, the doctor admitted. Therefore, the management of symptoms seemed the best option for now. Perhaps Abhirami had bipolar symptoms or a more generalized depression, he wondered, that contributed to her self-defeating and self-destructive compulsions. Her apparent lack of a belief system, culturally speaking, was not only a problem to her parents but also caused her to have cynicism towards everything in her life, including, and perhaps, especially, towards psychiatry and psychotherapy. Indeed, when I asked if she had tried psychotherapy, the doctor said that the few times it had been tried, Abhirami, owing to her intelligence and education, would get "very bored and anticipate the questions" and the logic behind them. Therefore, the generalized angst of depression that, in turn, might have produced her primary symptom of boredom and rebellion, found no remedy that could easily penetrate the veneer of cynicism, her toughest armor of self-defense. This cynicism anchored her self-image within modernity's chief value of status and professional success, but at what cost, I wondered.

Siva, a young man around twenty, came to the OPD with his parents one morning. The parents complained that Siva did not "want to study," and expressed both concern that something might be "wrong with him" as well as exasperation with his frivolous and carefree attitude. Siva, we heard, had started taking cannabis a few months back and had stolen family money to buy drugs. He was out of control in many respects, disappearing with his friends for days at a time. While away, he would draw money from the ATM and stay in expensive hotels.

Siva was quite rebellious of his parents. He made demands on them for purchases that were beyond their means. The family appeared to be middle class and perhaps had not suffered materially. But the boy's demands could never be satisfied. Within the past couple of years he had become increasingly irresponsible, skipping school and taking drugs, as well as spending money in frivolous ways.

The doctor spoke with Siva in a very soft and gentle tone and said it was important to find out whether his behavior was just a "normal" rebellious stage, or whether something deeper with psychiatric significance was causing this behavior, which, in turn, exasperated his parents. Her interaction with Siva was, I thought, the exact opposite of what one might expect from his parents. She spoke softly and offered no judgement whatsoever, in order to, I thought at the time, get him to open up and trust her. That things had worsened significantly, from the family's point of view, was relevant, she explained. Siva listened politely but offered no opinion or insights. The doctor then recommended admission and family therapy within the family ward. The admission would be, she explained, for a limited period, in order to get at the root of the problem. I jotted down in my fieldnotes that "the patient was counseled in gentle and careful terms." The words "psychiatric condition" or diagnosis were never mentioned, nor were normative categories used to condemn him for his rebellious behavior.

After leaving the room, the doctor asked whether it was a "soft form of bipolar" or just "adolescent trouble," in Siva's case.[2] My impression at the time was that this was likely a combination of peer pressure and adolescent rebelliousness, and not a severe mental condition. It was not clear that Siva was depressed or manic, or even self-destructive in the way that Abhirami appeared to be. He did not open up within the OPD, making it hard to know whether he felt inhibited by his parents' presence or was dealing with significant depression. But upon reflection, it seemed that the doctor had, in her recommendation of family therapy, suspected that there might be more at stake than simple youthful rebellion and carelessness with money and drugs, resulting from peer pressure. This particular doctor was a known expert in dealing with addiction and substance abuse. The next few cases, albeit brief encounters, revealed a bit more about the comorbidities between substance abuse and psychiatric diagnoses. But even in this brief encounter, her suspicion of family drama suggested a keen psychosocial understanding of the cultural demands for a particular kind of morality, and most likely, filial or sociocentric pressures that remain quite strong in India. This was more ostensible in the following case.

Addiction

Arjun, a young man perhaps in his mid-twenties, presented with drug-induced BPAD (bipolar affective disorder) in the OPD. He was admitted at NIMHANS in 2014 for cannabis dependence and a severe episode of depression. He was put on lithium, baclofen, and clonazepam, a powerful combination of antidepressants and anti-anxiety medications, as well as an antipsychotic (risperidone). Arjun still suffered from anger outbursts but showed some improvement, though a side effect from the medications was slowness of speech.

He had been, according to his father, "withdrawing socially" and had "sexually inappropriate behavior" (staring at women), and was not interested in going to work. Arjun's father worried about his drug use, and had "cut him off from a gang" that he was in. Without his old friends, Arjun was angry, and perhaps lonely. But he was not taking drugs anymore, Arjun claimed. His speech, however, was slurred, perhaps due to the prescription drugs he was on.

When specifically asked about ganja use, he said he no longer used it. But his father, who came with him to the OPD, reported that he fought with his sister. The "manic symptoms" had subsided with the medications, but behavioral issues remained within the family. Arjun would only work, his father said, when compelled to do so; and he continued to "stare at women." The doctor mentioned, however, that now that there were no longer any BPAD symptoms, it was possible to say that this was, to a degree, "normal adolescent strife." His "lithium and risperidone must be reduced," she said. Arjun's medical condition, in other words, was drug-induced. His psychiatric condition was contingent upon his addiction. The addiction had induced his symptoms, and the treatment with prescribed drugs had, in turn, made him functional enough to reduce the medications that had been prescribed when he was admitted in a more acute state. Without current severe symptoms, the father's complaints about his behavior suggested that medicines were a tool for normalizing social compliance, to some extent. The doctor, in her experience, implied that replacing one chemical dependency with another was counter-productive. Indeed, it had left Arjun somewhat enervated and contributed to his lack of initiative with regard to work. His staring at women was not pathological, nor a psychiatric condition, she determined, but rather a part of adolescent strife. Arjun, though a few years older than adolescence, might simply have had a lingering period of awkwardness relating to women as a result of his dysfunctional period when he succumbed to cannabis addiction and depression.

I witnessed many cases like Arjun's, where addiction to alcohol or ganja was the primary symptom, and psychiatric symptoms were secondary. Sometimes these cases were tragic, in which family members, particularly wives, were victims of their husband's addictions, as in one case where a woman came to the OPD on behalf of her husband, who suffered from severe bipolar disorder and addiction. She was only thirty years old, and had a very tough time of it because her daughter had committed suicide, and her husband was abusive due to his alcoholism. The wife received no support from the father-in-law or the abusive and now mentally ill husband. In cases such as this, the doctors were invariably sympathetic, and indeed, compassionate in their care, but could do little beyond adjusting medications. When the patient suffering addiction would appear, almost always men in my experience, they were questioned a bit more rigorously to determine whether they had been "using" or not, and to what extent they had made progress. In addition to adjusting medications and making queries regarding patient progress, there were, in most cases, and especially when addiction was comorbid with other psychiatric diagnoses, directions given in a more didactic manner regarding regulated activities, such as exercise, work, and sleep-related rhythms.

For instance, an English-speaking middle-aged man presented with repetitious thoughts that were "troubling." He was diagnosed with schizophrenia and BPAD and had, in the past, been verbally aggressive with his doctor. He was fairly calm and lucid in the OPD, though appeared to be a bit depressed. He was now walking at night, following the doctor's suggestion that he exercise in order to regulate his moods and reduce his urges to consume alcohol. With this exercise there was an improvement to his condition. Prior to taking up walking, he said he suffered from a poor appetite. Now it had improved, and he could even work and "do things" that had eluded him before. In another case, a man in his thirties presented with "problems at work." He worked in a factory but had been admitted twice in the past year with complaints of "tension." During these episodes he would refuse to work, and would also be tempted to abuse alcohol and/or ganja (cannabis). The man complained of an acute sense of "burden" and decreased sleep, coupled with reduced social interactions. The doctor suggested that he be admitted to the ward. This would provide the "motivational support" to send him to work. He was told to go to his job daily, straight from the ward, and return afterwards so that he would get into the "rhythm of work." The motivational support in the form of cognitive behavioral therapy would establish a routine, thereby breaking his "tension" and sense of "burden" that led to addictive behavior. He was also given a small dose of chlorazepam to reduce his anxiety.

Though there were numerous cases of addiction that were treated similarly on a daily basis at NIMHANS, the cases dealing with rebellion and resistance were more complicated, and indexed familial, and by extension social, contradictions and tensions that elaborate on themes we have already touched upon, and will continue subsequently. To some extent, I was, as should be clear by now, trying to find thematic patterns in the cases that pointed to larger social tensions that were enacted in the arena of the clinic. On the other hand, as I was not producing the kind of biographical ethnographies of the person that would reveal, with specificity and nuance, the particular etiologies in each case, I was recreating the accelerated rhythms of clinical life in the rapidity, and even superficiality, of my case studies. Therefore, I was also doing an ethnography of the OPD itself, as a kind of social ritual, in which the doctors were the ritual specialists who operated by a unique set of exacting procedures, given the constraints of the ritual arena in which they operated. This said, there was with each doctor a unique style of interaction that, if I wanted to highlight these differences, would necessitate creating personas for each doctor, and abandoning my efforts of concealment and the attendant focus upon the social field from outside the ritual arena that produced the patterns of illness that appeared within it.[3] The final three cases of this section on resistance return us forcefully to the familial, with all its entangled murkiness.

"Hysteria"

A young man named Ajay came to the OPD with multiple issues. The main concern of his uncle, who accompanied him to the clinic, was with his studies and his "confusion" in dealing with certain problems and responsibilities. Ajay's father had committed suicide when he was still very young. His mother had quickly declined and died after the father's death. The boy was, in turn, raised by his uncle.

In 2009, Ajay had a serious accident that left him with a significant head injury. After this he began to suffer seizures. The uncle claimed that his communication skills had decreased since this time as well. And Ajay was increasingly "not responsible for his duties." Moreover, he had some difficulty recognizing letters of the alphabet since the accident. He had also suffered from erectile disfunction for the past fourteen years, though this had been treated with medicine. This latter problem persisted, despite the medicine and a steady girlfriend for several years.

The seizures were apparently fairly well controlled at this point, but Ajay complained of an unspecified anxiety. The uncle said that since the accident Ajay's communication skills had changed and he noticed some slurring of words. The doctor focused on what was different after the injury. The uncle answered for Ajay that it was his "speech and concentration" that was most affected. But just as he said this, I noticed a distinctive rolling of the eyes on Ajay's face, albeit briefly, in response to his uncle. The uncle had a slightly accusatory tone regarding Ajay, which was also mentioned by the resident presenting the case to the doctor. This left me also wondering if behavioral resistance to the uncle, albeit mainly passive, was also part of the equation.

Ajay also appeared slightly "nervous," the doctor noticed. This again suggested that perhaps the young man felt uncomfortable talking about his issues in front of his slightly overbearing uncle. According to the uncle, Ajay "never concentrates in work." Moreover, he was "not obeying orders" and "gives credit to customers," which was against the rules of the family business.

All this, coupled with rolling of his eyes, suggested that his behavioral issues were not directly caused by his earlier accident. These behavioral issues had to do with authority figures and following rules. The doctor, after I had mentioned this (without the patient present), also made brief note of this in Ajay's file. I suspected the uncle was the key player in his psychodrama. The key question that emerged was whether Ajay could handle his work and make basic transactions in a reliable fashion. Therefore, the doctor asked a series of questions aimed at deciphering his ability to think clearly and reliably. After hearing responses from the uncle, primarily, who spoke for Ajay, the doctor then suggested that Ajay's cognitive abilities had not been compromised by the accident. Indeed, the uncle even admitted that his nephew did not take responsibilities seriously even before the accident. This was not, in other words, a case of cognitive decline with associated behavior problems resulting from a head injury. Rather, his resistance had a social message, particularly to the uncle and other sources of authority.

Ajay was asked about his moods and whether he was depressed, to which he answered that he was not depressed and was generally fine. In this instance, both uncle and nephew concurred. But when the question concerned aggression, there was a difference of opinion between the two. It was said by the uncle that Ajay's aggression always occurred in response to being reminded about "his responsibilities." Once again, this suggested a social message or psychic resistance was at play. Eventually, the uncle was asked by the doctor why Ajay was brought to NIMHANS. What was his special area of concern? The uncle mentioned the issue of responsibility again, saying that he worried about his nephew "taking charge of his life." The uncle, it should be mentioned, was relatively senior in years, and was perhaps wary of getting old and needing to care for a slightly impaired dependent. The uncle also mentioned his concern again that the nephew was having trouble identifying certain letters. The latter, the doctor suggested, was nothing to worry about, as he had this problem from a young age, and was not declining as a result of the accident. The doctor seemed to be implying a degree of dyslexia, rather than a progressive decline in Ajay's function, as the uncle feared.

Ajay, who remained quiet throughout the interview, displayed mild displeasure at his uncle's assessment but did not speak out. The uncle was asked, however, if Ajay spent a lot of time on his laptop or television. The uncle said yes, indeed, Ajay did spend a great deal of time with these devices. Ajay was then advised to cut back on his usage of these mediums. As he was, at the time, taking three anticonvulsants and seemed to be relatively seizure free, the doctor wanted to eliminate one or more of the drugs in order to elevate the one that was "actually working." The doctor did not believe that all three were working together to control the seizures. The anticonvulsants, he felt, could also be causing cognitive impairment, resulting in Ajay's problems with work.

My impression, based upon the doctor's instructions, was that Ajay was suspected of having a mild disability caused by his accident. This was coupled with dyslexia that predated his accident. But as a result of the demanding uncle, Ajay had also created a shield of resistance to the authority figure in his life. This resistance, Bartleby-like, as in Melville's classic short story, and a refusal to do his work responsibly, was perhaps a good defense for Ajay, given that he did not seem to suffer any untoward depression or debilitating mental illness. That is, what the uncle took to be a worrisome lack of initiative related to his cognitive decline was also quite possibly an act of passive resistance that guarded Ajay from taking on greater responsibilities. But his relationship with his uncle was worsening over time and now, from the uncle's perspective, required some sort of clinical intervention. Ajay, however, remained mute and passive, though he did, as mentioned, roll his eyes when his uncle complained about him. With the death of his parents at an early age, it was also not clear what sort of traumatic impact that this had on him, or whether some elements of anger and/or blame were displaced onto this uncle. His refusals to "obey orders" clearly showed an ability, indeed, to refuse his uncle's demands. This, in turn, meant that normalizing him, from the uncle's perspective, was not just about preparing him to face life's difficulties when he was no longer there to protect him, but rather that the uncle increasingly demanded from Ajay compliance and labor. Ajay's resistance to this, while possibly influenced to some degree by his dyslexia and injury, exceeded biological causation, and had as its core an element of psychosocial determination. One might even suspect that his withdrawal from his duties was positive, a volitional reclaiming of his own agency against the stultifying demands of the Other (Deleuze and Guattari 1987). But this positive withdrawal or resistance was not without pain. Ajay, as we recall, admitted to feelings of anxiety, certainly related to earlier traumas that were unresolved, coupled with his awareness of his uncle's expectations, that, indeed, he may never realize. And given his history of seizures and his use of anticonvulsants, with their unfortunate side effects, it was reasonable to first assess his cognitive function before recommending more extended psychotherapy.

Therefore, a first step in treatment would be performing a complete neuropsychiatric and cognitive assessment. The doctor ordered this to get a "baseline," and requested a follow-up after it had been completed. The objective measures, in turn, would be useful in determining how much of a psychosocial intervention through psychotherapy might be useful.

Anxiety over familial expectations was, as we have seen, a common thread that tied discussions about normalization to the inherent vice grip and "everyday" (Das 2006) violence of the social as embedded within kinship. These often figured around gendered forms of hierarchy. Faridah, a woman from West Bengal, came to the OPD complaining of "heart" and "chest tightness," also describing a feeling of "heaviness" and loss of appetite. She worried a lot about her heart, in particular. Faridah had an anxious look upon her face as she described her concerns. Her husband, however, did most of the talking in the clinical interview with the doctor. They spoke Bengali with the doctor, who was also assisted by a translator to make sure he understood key details. The couple appeared to be working class, based upon the language they spoke and the clothes they wore.

Faridah had very difficult fights with her husband's family. She moved into her husband's family house after marriage, as per the custom, and for twenty years had faced escalating tension with her mother- and sisters-in-law. This, as many scholars of the patrilocal family in South Asia have noted, is oftentimes stressful and structurally fraught for the brides, as they become the most subordinate member of the household, and are expected to do the bulk of cooking and cleaning for the husband's family (Kakar 1981; Pinto 2014; Addlakha 2008). Her primary symptom was "morning anxiety" that was most acute when the day began. As the day progressed, the anxiety would lessen.

Faridah ruminated constantly about the quarrels she was having with her husband, who failed to "support" her when she was being criticized by her in-laws. Thus, she worried about her future excessively. The couple had one child. While the husband was talking, I noticed Faridah becoming progressively more anxious, though I could not say if his exact words were provoking her. Aside from her anxiety, which was causing her to have panic attacks, complete with palpitations and a loss of appetite, she had become very irritable, according to the husband. She also had, he said, occasional thoughts of suicide, or at the very least threatened it.

Though she had a history of anxiety symptoms, palpitations and fainting, she had no previously known psychiatric issues. Her son was now eighteen and showed no symptoms, himself, and was her only child. Faridah also had three sisters she remained close to. Due to the severe marital discord, she moved back into her natal home two months prior to her being seen at NIMHANS. This was an extreme step, the husband claimed, given that her family was not in a position to support her financially, not to mention the apparent stigma attached to moving back into the mother's house and out of a difficult marital context.

The doctor asked Faridah, "How did this go on for twenty years?" He then asked, "What has changed in the last two months that prompted you to move out?" This was followed with a question as to whether the brothers and sisters married after her. Here, I assumed he was talking about the sisters within the in-laws' family, where that dynamic would alter the in-house hierarchy between the daughters-in-law. In any event, answers were not forthcoming, but she did indicate that her panic symptoms were becoming much worse in recent times. Something, apparently, had become acute and unbearable.

One might wonder if the family conflict had made Faridah "mad" or "ill," or whether they labeled her as such, a diagnosis that marked deviance, as in Biehl's influential (2005) study of the life of Catarina in Brazil, who was deemed "mad" by her husband and his family when she resisted their will (also see Pinto 2014). Perhaps the doctor was also thinking this because his next question, in fact, was, "Were you able to handle the daughter-in-law duties?" But again, nothing was said in response to this question. A palpable tension between spouses seemed to inhibit Faridah's response.

The doctor noted that Faridah had a somewhat puffy facial appearance. He thought this could be due to malnutrition and proceeded to ask questions about her diet, which was apparently, and not uncommonly, rice based, but was not supplemented with adequate vegetables and proteins. She did not appear underweight, per se, but weighed, the doctor noted, only forty-five kilograms. Aside from her weight, the question of quality in her diet remained. Faridah pointed out some skin rashes on her arms and suggested that she had gotten these rashes in response to a medication she had been given. It was unclear to me what medications she was taking, as she had not yet been treated at NIMHANS.

The doctor suggested that family therapy was needed, given the relationship with the in-laws involved a core tension. But the feasibility of this treatment was thrown into doubt. The family, as expressed by the husband, was interested only in making Faridah compliant to her role in the family. This was to be obtained through medications, not in resolving underlying social dynamics. This was a characteristic case of the joint family in dysfunction with the daughter-in-law bearing the brunt of the tension, being the least powerful person in the household. Faridah's resistance, insofar as her symptoms of fainting and anxiety brought to attention her pain, was limited in its agency. Indeed, it was her refuge in her natal home that was intolerable and shameful, requiring the expertise at NIMHANS for a resolution. But having received the best advice for admission, it was apparent that understanding the provenance of Faridah's anxiety, irritability, and fainting were not considered as important as the disciplinary hope that drug-induced compliance promised.

As Faridah and her husband were not going to stay at NIMHANS much longer (they had stayed in the family housing for a couple of nights),[4] they were referred to a psychiatrist in West Bengal, near the town where they lived. For now, they were counseled by a Bengali-speaking resident and psychologist about the familial "crisis." But as a crisis intervention, it was doubtful that one or two sessions would produce much result, particularly given how silent Faridah remained, coupled with her husband's strong and patriarchal views.

When I witnessed cases like this, I wondered why patients and their families would travel vast distances to NIMHANS only to be sent back home with the referral to a local psychiatrist, who, through a connection to NIMHANS, was thought to be reliable. With wealthy patients, a short flight to Bangalore was, indeed, feasible. But many patients would make long multi-day journeys by train or bus, only to stay at NIMHANS for a day or two. The question I had, as exemplified by Faridah's case, was: What did they expect this visit to NIMHANS to accomplish? Without an extended stay and intensive family therapy, what could be accomplished in one session? Again, the implication was that the husband and in-laws were hoping for a quick and normalizing pharmaceutical fix. This was the "magic tablet" cure that we have encountered in many cases. In a sense, this was akin, in some respects, to the magic of an exorcism or faith healing, with NIMHANS becoming a sort of pilgrimage-ritual journey, efficacious by reputation and the magical properties of the tablet cure (Kakar 1982; Nabokov 2000; Ecks 2013). In this case, however, there was a palpable sense that Faridah wanted to express herself and explain her side of the story, but feared doing so in front of her husband. On the other hand, the husband just wanted to "repair" his wife so that he could bring her home. Sad cases like this would pass through the OPD each day, leaving the doctors exasperated at times, or at the very least, feeling resigned to the limits of care that were imposed upon them. And of course, even more than the limits the doctors were resigned to, Faridah's resistance was circumscribed within the everyday violence of the social, with its gendered normativities (Marrow 2016; Pinto 2014; Das 2006).

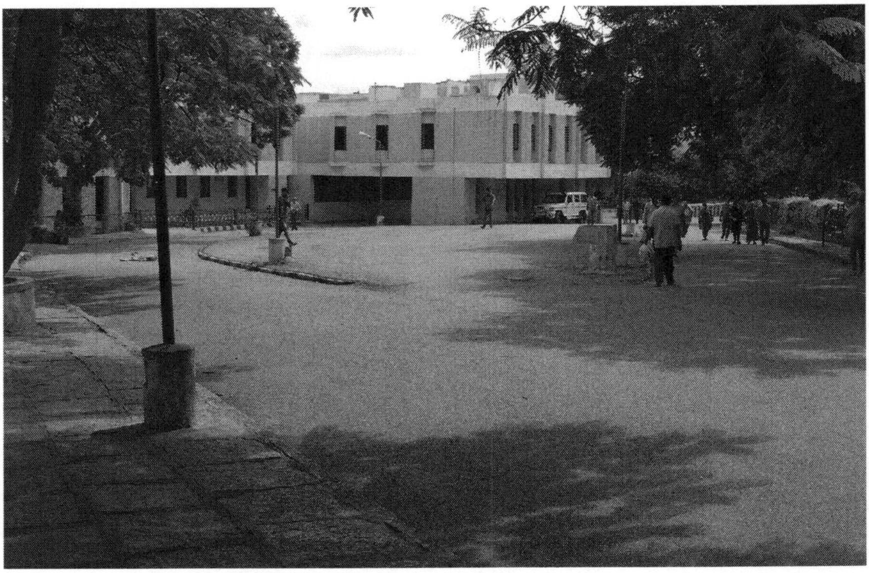

The NIMHANS Outpatient Department (OPD). (Photograph by author.)

Resistance, as we have seen, takes many forms. We have traversed a terrain where rebellion was youthful and agentive on one end of a spectrum, to the other end where the resistance is at the core of somatic pain and, to an extent, spoke its message of conflicted thought and compulsive behavior within a part of the self that was inaccessible to the patient, at least in conscious terms. Symptoms, however, redoubled the normalizing pressures that were the source of their provenance. This was labeled as "hysteria," an old diagnostic term no longer used in biomedical psychiatry but one that had continued disarticulating and deconstructive relevance in the OPD, marking an important uncertainty within diagnosis and treatment that, in turn, called for social analysis. But aside from its deconstructive potentials, a compulsion to resist, like the classic repetition compulsion, could be punitive to the self that expressed it, whatever masochistic pleasure, a secondary form of *jouissance*, in Lacan's (1977) language, was also derived in its act, as well as drawing punitive attention to the unfilial freedoms it exhibited against the moral order. We can witness this dual aspect of freedom within a "cage" (Willford 2006) in the case of Meera.

Meera, a woman in her mid-thirties, came to the OPD presenting symptoms of being "withdrawn and angry," according to her husband, who accompanied her to the clinic. She would compulsively move objects around the house, reordering them over and over, to the dismay of her husband. Arrangements of objects were never satisfactory and led to endless acts of reordering. Meera, we were told, did not have an "outgoing personality" and did not tend to make friends.

Meera's husband spoke for her in the clinic as she sat quietly. He was a helicopter pilot for the army and lived with her in military housing. After noticing her flat affect and strange obsessions with reordering objects, as well as some strange gesticulations while walking, he contacted her family and asked whether she was like this before marriage. The family tried to reassure him that this was "just her personality" and that she was fine, just a bit quiet and "different" in some respects. But due to her social withdrawal, strange behavior, and some "delusions and magical thinking," usually concerning the necessity to place objects in a certain way to, in Meera's mind, prevent disaster, she was seen by a local non-NIMHANS psychiatrist and put on a low dose of risperidone. She was diagnosed with schizophrenia by this local psychiatrist before arriving at NIMHANS.

The doctor in the OPD asked whether Meera interacted with her son. The husband said she did, and furthermore, was good at teaching him "reading, maths, and writing." At this moment, Meera mentioned that she had an abortion after the birth of the first child. It was not clear whether this precipitated any of her gesticulations or OCD behavior. Meera appeared flat and remote throughout most of the interview, but began to exhibit, too, a slight look of concern. She questioned her own behavior and said that after hearing her husband tell her that her behavior was "not normal," she "felt bad." It was then revealed by her that she, evidently, was not performing her "household duties properly" with regard to cooking and cleaning. She felt bad about this, she said, and asked the doctor if there was something wrong with her. We might call this her resistance to her resistance, where she ostensibly identifies her behavior as problematic, but in so doing, seems to demand a response, not only in answer to her symptoms of OCD but, more pointedly, to her character.

Her inability to have her own circle of friends was a symptom that caused her husband great concern, he said. The husband said her friends, to the extent that she had any, were his friends. She did not seek out any friendships on her own. Like the compulsion to order and reorder the material objects in their house, she had, evidently, reordered her social existence around her marital objects: her husband, his friends, and the military house in which they lived. It was as if she had renounced, in excess, her own self, taking upon herself the Other's demand of her. But in so doing with obsessive, self-negating ferocity, Meera was also signaling in this excess her resistance to the moral order by becoming its very perverse form: she revealed to her husband that she did not have any pleasures that were hers, and hers alone. The OCD was an automatism that called forth his concern, and demanded an answer to the question of what was normal.

We might speculate that pleasure can be derived in the compulsive reordering of objects, as this does provide a semblance of control to someone who has become reordered and made into an orderable object, perhaps, in post-married life, particularly into the regimented life of the military. But even in this pleasure of reordering, where agency is at least enacted, uncertainty and repetition tear down as much as they build up a semblance of order. We might then see this behavior, though in this case obsessive, compensatory in precisely the sense that Freud (1961) apocryphally wrote about in *Beyond the Pleasure Principle*, where he described the ordering of objects (fort-da), as the great cultural achievement of the toddler who has learned to make objects appear and disappear to compensate for the first and fundamental trauma of maternal absence. But, according to Freud, when an elaborate symbolic ordering of social reality was constructed as a chain of symbolic substitutions to fill the lack experienced out of this foundational trauma, there also emerged a desire to tear it town with aggressive zeal, as a kind of desire for nondifferentiation and return to the pre-symbolic. Meera may have, indeed, exhibited some OCD traits before marriage, as her family intimated to the husband, but we can probably assume that her symptoms required diagnoses only after marriage as a result of their worsening presentation, and when the symbolic order became more oppressive in its patriarchal demand, precipitating its automaton-like repetitive symptoms of OCD (Lacan 1977).

There was, apparently, a very tough period prior to diagnosis, when "an episode" of "flat behavior" with increased OCD lasted for six months, ending only after being prescribed risperidone. Meera's social withdrawal coupled with her compulsive behavior had come to a head, in her husband's mind, prompting him to bring her to the clinic. The doctor, upon hearing the husband describe her symptoms, recommended a monthly follow-up. Meera then suddenly asked with great alarm whether she had schizophrenia. She said she had read about it online and was "very worried" she had the disease. The doctor said he was not at all certain at this point whether she had it or not. Therefore, he said, further follow-ups and "investigations" would be needed to determine this earlier diagnosis by the outside psychiatrist.

After Meera left, the doctor expressed some doubt about the certainty of the earlier diagnosis. She, he said, could also suffer "severe depression" or some "schizoid value." I certainly wondered about depression, noting her affect exhibited in the OPD, as well as the husband's description of her "flat" disposition at home. The abortion seemed obviously significant, too. She had only spoken twice, once mentioning the abortion, and the other, addressing her diagnosis, and by extension, her status as a person. The details surrounding the abortion were yet to be discovered, though it appeared in conversation at the precise moment when her husband had turned his praise to her parenting of their son. As if to turn the tables on any positive evaluation of her person by her husband, she had to pivot to a profound reordering of objects, in this case, her fetus. Again, it was a kind of resistance to her resistance, a self-denial of worth. Was this reordering of self-object volitional and/or compelled by the husband? Herein might lie the clue to her depression and OCD, I thought. Moreover, having heard the husband, who obviously was sincerely concerned about his wife, one could not help being suspicious, too, that the husband was fairly dominating and expected the very model of a compliant military wife, an image she was finding difficult to maintain in front of his friends. His concern that she did not make friends on her own, I imagined, indicated the desire that she have her own social network within the military compound, already a limited social domain, in order to compensate for his regimented schedule, which, in some cases of military households I had encountered at NIMHANS, led to loneliness and feelings of neglect.

Along the lines I suspected, after Meera left his office, the doctor told me about a morning patient that he had seen who had heard "voices of the gods" for some time and had schizophrenia. She heard the voices of the great gods in Hinduism and would sometimes speak "abusively to the gods," for which she felt "extremely guilty." Vulgarizing the gods was somewhat uncommon, particularly the great gods, though it is fairly common for demigods in both myth and everyday language to be insulted (Doniger 2010). Scolding, but not vulgarizing, the gods is fairly common. Though this woman was schizophrenic, apparently, it is interesting to also think of her symptom through the lens of "hysteria," where the gods become a projected displacement for other law-giving figures, such as the husband and in-laws. While this was a more flamboyant symptom than was the OCD witnessed above, there is the common thread of transgressive behavior followed by guilt and a self-demand (or demand from the Other) for moral or clinical evaluation. In that sense, resistance against resistance short-circuited and contained great transgressive displays of resistance. Dialecticism and antinomy were operative even where resistance manifested itself. Therefore, a romantic reading of psychic resistance, one in which normalcy and pathology are mere constructs or byproducts of power, was clearly insufficient to the doctors who had to deal with the pain and suffering of their patients (Kleinman 2012).

Abandonment

Within the familial stress caused by shame and various types of trauma, the vicissitudes of care and abandonment were always in tension. We have seen that it is sometimes hard to define what care, abuse, and abandonment mean in the entangled lives of patients and their families. Shame and guilt sometimes caused withdrawal from more intimate and active social participation within families and communities. At the same time, abuse that either caused and/or exacerbated mental illness could occur in many forms. And abuse was not only directed at the mentally ill, but was sometimes a symptom of illness being directed at other family members. In cases where the refractory nature of the illness was likely organic and understood, as in the case of florid psychosis or paranoid schizophrenia, the impact of the illness upon family and marital discord was tragic, though not without explanation. On the other hand, there were "borderline personality" cases where a diagnosis was harder to reach, and the site of illness, be it dysfunctional relationships, tension and stress, or an undetermined organic cause, led to ambiguities, as we have seen around the term "hysteria," for instance, that impacted upon the spectrum of care and abandonment by family members. This section, however, explores the perception and experience of abandonment by patients and its subsequent impact upon the trajectory of an illness, as understood by doctors at NIMHANS.

Mohammad, a young man in his early twenties, presented with "low moods" and a "lack of initiative." He also heard voices and, specifically, heard the voice of a neighbor saying, "I will kill you." Mohammad had recently been at a kind of Islamic retreat and had been mistakenly accused of being a "thief," and was consequently sent home. This was significant, perhaps, because he had been raised by an uncle after his father was arrested for being a thief. After his father's arrest, his mother had deserted him for the father's younger brother. It was this uncle-father that had brought him to the OPD at NIMHANS.

The uncle complained that his "son" would "sleep excessively and refused to work." Moreover, Mohammad would "bang his head on the wall" and have anger outbursts. At times he "lost control" and would have thoughts about his own death, along with the auditory hallucinations he had regarding the neighbor's threat. As one might expect, given his traumatic childhood history, he already suffered symptoms as a child. But these, apparently, had worsened significantly in the past six months. One of his oddest symptoms involved a kind of involuntary sleepwalking in which he would go to the neighbor's terrace and speak incoherently, perhaps, at the threatening voice.

Mohammad, however, had no clinical history nor any significant "social problems" before the recent downturn. He had, however, failed most subjects in school, the uncle stated. At one point, the uncle-father sent him to a madrassa (Islamic school) for eight years. These were decidedly unhappy years for Mohammad. He performed poorly in school and, as a consequence, was often scolded by the teachers. The uncle said that Mohammad would react negatively to a "teacher's scolding." He was deemed "defiant" and unrepentant, the uncle said.

This "defiance" happened at home, as well, where now he was very short-tempered with his uncle. While Mohammad was not hearing voices anymore, now that he was on clonazepam, he still "felt low." Indeed, his affect was demonstrably flat during the entire interview. During the interview, most questions were directed at the uncle in Hindi. But the doctor also spoke to the young man directly. At one point the doctor asked Mohammad to solve a simple subtraction problem. Mohammad looked confused for some time, and only with prodding from the uncle, counted backwards using his hands. Solving this took around three minutes and produced visible nervousness on the young man's face.

The doctor suggested that Mohammad might have a "cognitive deficit" and ordered an IQ assessment. As it turned out he could read Arabic well, but not Kannada, suggesting, to the doctor, a kind of dyslexia, or SLD (specific learning disorder).[5] It was possible he had some form of ADHD (attention deficit hyperactivity disorder) as well, given his inability to focus and complete tasks at hand or study. Whether he had something more specific was yet to be determined, the doctor suggested.

Mohammad also suffered headaches and dizziness, as well as a loss of memory, the uncle explained. Given that he had these strange fugue-like states in which he would sleepwalk to the neighbor's balcony, it suggested a possible neurological problem, the doctor offered. Therefore, a referral to neurology at NIMHANS was ordered. I wondered whether these symptoms, particularly the directive sleepwalking, could be epileptic-induced fugue states. I had my doubts, as the behavior seemed purposive and meaningful, particularly given the auditory hallucinations regarding the neighbor's death-threats.

The initial psychiatric clinical interview ended without clarity as to whether Mohammad suffered a mild cognitive handicap, which, when negatively evaluated by teachers and his uncle, caused the depression, lethargy, and irritability that the uncle was exasperated by. Indeed, this was a common occurrence at NIMHANS—a family member would be exasperated at the failure of the patient to fulfill a role, be it work-related or household duties (see Luhrmann and Marrow 2016). In response, doctors would sometimes try to explain that cognitive deficits were a factor, and that families should temper their expectations so as to minimize experiences of failure or "social defeat" (Luhrmann and Marrow 2016), which, in turn, would worsen a patient's symptoms.

Mohammad had suffered a traumatic life event when his father was arrested and his mother ended up with his uncle. Moreover, he had suffered the repetition of this wound when he himself was accused of being a "thief" while in the Islamic retreat. That this happened recently seemed an obvious trigger for his rather sudden downward spiral in the previous six months. If his problems were neurological and predated the traumas he experienced, it would be perhaps surprising that his disposition had changed rapidly. But Mohammad also clearly possessed some cognitive deficit, as evidenced by the dyslexia and inability to subtract simple numbers.

Mohammad, his cognitive limits noted, was otherwise "functioning." He dressed neatly and piously, wearing a clean white skullcap and kurta, and appeared well groomed. But it was very obvious that tensions with the uncle manifested in his behavior and attitude towards him. The uncle, moreover, had otherwise blamed Mohammad for his attitude and failures, which, as the doctor was trying to suggest, might have been due to his disability and not intentional, as the uncle seemed to imply. The uncle's aggressive criticism, given Mohammad's possible learning disability, would be a source of tension and frustration, reinforcing a sense of failure, as Mohammad was unable to satisfy his expectations. I wondered whether there was intentionality in his night-time walks to the neighbor's terrace. If so, and if this is the same neighbor who would send him messages of his impending death, there might be something related to his past at play.

We might speculate, perhaps, that the neighbor who threatened him was, in fact, his uncle. Within the extended family in India, uncles are, in fact, neighbors, perhaps only separated by walls and rooms, but not in separate households. That Mohammad could sleepwalk to the neighbor's terrace suggested a kind of mobility within a building that would be characteristic of the extended family's household. Prior to his mother's abandoning his father, the neighbor could have been the uncle. Could the voices in his head be a reaction formation to his own parricidal wishes towards the uncle? While it seemed reasonable to ascertain his cognitive and neurological deficits, as these limits could lower his uncle's expectations, and therefore lessen his moralizing criticism of his "son," which I am certain the doctor was trying to achieve, it seemed there where psychodynamic issues at play that would be harder to evaluate without some sort of psychotherapy. In any event, in this case, while not of literal abandonment of Mohammad by his uncle, a sense of abandonment was felt by the patient. There was the abandonment by the father, first, with his arrest and disappearance from the family. Then there was the abandonment by the mother, who literally left the father for his brother, an undoubtedly confusing and traumatic event for the young boy. Moreover, there was the abandonment through neglect, arguably, of placing the young Mohammad in institutions like the madrassa where he was bound to struggle, given his cognitive limitations. Now, within the OPD, the uncle abandoned his culpability in Mohammad's symptomatology, blaming him for his irritability and "lack of initiative." Mohammad, for his part, was left to "bang his head" against the wall and to ruminate over his own death. In this light, abuse, neglect, and abandonment are part of a complex of actions and affects in which those who suffer mental illness and cognitive deficits face a myriad of social sanctions that contribute to and even worsen their cluster of symptoms. The psychosocial and neurological factors are thus oftentimes conjoined and comorbid with one another, as we have now seen in several cases.

Oftentimes the cases that pass through the OPD are devastating, poignant, and tragic. One patient, a woman in her thirties named Zareen, was adamant that she speak to her doctor. He had already spent upwards of twenty minutes with her within the OPD. Still, she kept interrupting him with other patients, requesting more time. He, like the other doctors, could not spend this much time with each and every patient, particularly on follow-up visits. This woman had originally come from Kerala. When her father died, her mother had married a Jordanian man (they were Muslims from Kerala) and moved the family to Jordan. After moving to Jordan with the new stepfather, Zareen developed extreme OCD coupled with paranoia. When she developed severe symptoms of mental illness as a teenager, the family put her on a plane and returned her to India without supervision, and without a destination "other than Bangalore." The family had literally abandoned Zareen so that the family (in Jordan) would not be burdened or face the stigma of mental illness, which, evidently, would impact negatively upon the marriage prospects of her sisters, all of whom were also there. They had put her on a plane with a one-way ticket. Moreover, as she was without Jordanian citizenship and had lost her Indian passport, she was essentially "stateless." Somehow, however, she was able to enter the country but ended up walking the streets of Bangalore for two years suffering all sorts of delusions along the way. In addition to her delusions, she had OCD and could not succeed with the placements within group homes that NIMHANS had tried to broker on her behalf.

Homeless and stateless, abandoned by family and unacceptable to any potential adoptee parents, Zareen wandered the streets until she was rescued by NIMHANS. After a long admission, her symptoms finally stabilized somewhat, though she still had delusions and difficulties working with others. Most noticeably, her sense of social etiquette was absent. Though the patient appeared lucid, she was obviously agitated and manic, and she felt a pressing need to command the doctor's attention. Perhaps a fear of abandonment, grounded in real life experiences, exacerbated her demand for personalized care from the doctor. If so, it would be completely understandable, given all that she had endured.

On another occasion, Zareen came into the OPD shouting at the doctor, asking that he let her "die in the streets." She claimed he was not her "real doctor" and accused him of not taking care of her "for one year," which was untrue. Zareen had lived in the ward for the past year plus, after being found wandering the streets, as mentioned above. She, being stateless and living in the NIMHANS ward, had no other family within India to look after her. Moreover, she was often unwilling to take her medicine (fluoxetine) and as a result, her psychotic symptoms were worsening. She kept loudly repeating that "there is a God" but spoke mostly in a nonsensical and disordered mode of delivery. To the extent she made sense, she accused the entire team of caregivers of not treating her, and particularly, "not speaking" with her. She was highly agitated. Zareen suggested that those around her were conspiring to "kill me off." She said she would rather "die in the street than in this shit NIMHANS." Zareen also said that there were only "bad people in India." She accused the social worker of "putting dirt" on her belongings, and kept repeating, too, that "I don't want you people treating me."

Zareen, evidently, had strong and florid delusions that people were hurting her in the ward, or "putting dirt" in her bed and clothing. She harbored a special hostility towards a social worker at NIMHANS who had worked more closely with her. One of the residents was singled out for additional scorn, claiming he had never spoken to her though he had been her doctor for many months. In the times I saw her in the OPD, Zareen would express disappointment, and oftentimes anger, at not having time to talk about the problems that she claimed actually caused her symptoms.

She wanted a kind of attention to her story that the doctors were not prepared to give, because of time constraints, which were obviously a factor, but also to not entertain her delusions. For instance, she wrote numerous notes to herself on sheets of paper in Arabic and kept presenting these to the doctor. In response, the doctor said he did not read Arabic. But he also told me that he did not want to "entertain her delusions."

Her shouts and screams became so disruptive that a guard was called to remove her from the OPD, but there was nobody around to help. Even in the hall, on her own, she cried, screamed, and cursed at the top of her lungs. Finally, somebody escorted her out of the OPD after over twenty minutes of shouting in a public space where other patients would hear her. Her doctor tried to calm her by telling her that nobody wanted to harm her and that she needed to take her medicine. This was to no avail. Later, when asking him about her, he said this was becoming "increasingly her baseline." She never took her meds, was noncompliant, and was increasingly delusional and suspicious of everyone at the hospital. Her situation looked bleak. Another doctor mentioned that Zareen came around the faculty offices, across the campus, and abused the staff and doctors whenever she was wandering the campus. She even shouted at the head of the Psychiatry Department from outside of his office. The doctors, for their part, tolerated this behavior because they knew that if Zareen was "on the streets" she would only get worse.

Zareen's case was the most direct and tragic case of abandonment that I recall witnessing at NIMHANS. What made her case so devastating was her complete rejection of the care she was receiving from her doctors and social workers. Her deep sense of betrayal and paranoia was fundamental, leaving little room for redemption. There "was a God" and cold judgement had been passed on the world, she implied. Zareen felt her abandonment continued within the institution. The refusal to engage with her delusions, however well-intentioned and clinically sound, also further enraged her, leading her to accuse her doctor of not treating her for over a year.[6] Her case was at an impasse with no light coming forthwith. Zareen's despair was matched by hopeless resignation on the part of her doctor. Sadly, when I spoke again to her doctor a couple of years later, I had learned that she had passed away. I never learned what the cause of death was.

The tragedy of Zareen's case is a reminder of the reality of mental illness, against either a romantic or constructivist view of power and resistance. While normativity is undoubtedly violent to those cast as abnormal within any society, producing exclusions and typologies of illness, as well the legal ramifications of these, what was true to Zareen was true of many other cases I witnessed. That is, Zareen, despite the extensive efforts of doctors, psychologists, and social workers, was unable to trust either the process of treatment or the individuals who were to carry it out. And while we might wonder whether her paranoia was caused by a genetic predisposition or by the traumas of early life in which she was uprooted from her home and lost a father, these early experiences coupled with her later abandonment overdetermined her perpetual unease and distrust of care providers. Her illness was intractable, and the tragedy of her case was that even institutionalization and prescribed medicines could not save her when she was noncompliant and hostile to those who wanted to help her, however understandable her mistrust in authority figures was. There was only one answer, "There is a God," and this answer, sadly, did not leave room for trust in other failed authority figures, if we imagine her caregivers at NIMHANS assuming the parental role for her.

The disturbance that Zareen caused in the OPD was somewhat unusual, which—unlike what I had seen in the Hollywood representation of psychiatric wards where disruptive and wild gesticulations were the stereotypical way in which the mentally ill were represented—was usually calm and orderly, despite the long waits in the waiting room and the serious cases that were being treated every day. A few of the doctors, on separate occasions, had told me about the formal protocols with "orderlies" that exist within the Western psychiatric clinic as compared to the atmosphere of the clinic in India. The lockdowns, panic buttons, and orderlies had not "yet arrived here," but there were some calls being made for more of these protocols to be put in place at NIMHANS. One doctor mentioned that in his thirty years or so of practice, he had only been attacked physically a couple of times, implying that the risk was higher in Western contexts. We spoke about the "cultural limits" that mark aggression in India versus the US within clinical contexts. This doctor suggested that norms of respect and even deference for doctors were very high in India, even within those who had serious mental illnesses. A patient would rarely challenge a doctor, observing general rules of hierarchy with regard to respecting those in a position of authority, such as educators, gurus, and doctors. In short, what has been called the sociocentric self in South Asia inhibited the behavioral repertoire, to an extent, towards observing deference to elders, doctors, etc. (Kakar 1982). The cultural repertoire for clinical practice did not include either verbally or physically assaulting the doctor, despite the everyday structural and symbolic, if not actual physical, violence that permeated the lives of patients and their families. This never failed to impress me. To draw an analogy from my previous fieldwork, I told the doctor about my experiences witnessing spirit possession. In these cases, the disorder and even violence (Willford 2006; 2014) within rituals were contained by the authority of the priest/healer and specific mantras they would utter, or other means employed to quell the unruly spirit's presence within the individual.[7]

Most cases of abandonment were more entangled within the vicissitudes of care than was in the case discussed above (Pinto 2014). For instance, on a hot April afternoon, when even the stray dogs at NIMHANS were lying under the campus's many shady trees, a pregnant woman in her mid-twenties came to the OPD with her mother, exhibiting "mild mental retardation," according to the resident's notes to the doctor. She laughed and spoke to herself while the doctor tried to address her. The doctor asked her a series of questions about her husband but the young woman seemed a bit oblivious to her surroundings and did not respond. Her husband, we learned from the patient's mother, was now estranged from her and denied fatherhood, adding to her woes. It was the mother who answered questions raised by the doctor. In this case, the doctor mentioned that this might have the makings of a "legal case of abandonment." Even the mother-in-law had renounced the young woman at this point. She was cared for alone by her mother now, which was a very large burden, emotionally and financially.

Her doctor mentioned that she had been treating this patient for nine months already, though improvement was hard to measure. The young mother-to-be was prescribed olanzapine for her psychosis. The doctor then mentioned to the resident that the files of this patient were incomplete, as some of her drug prescriptions were "not duly recorded" in the file. The patient, evidently, had begun on risperidone, but was switched to olanzapine more recently when it was determined that her psychosis was not improving all that much. Some confusion was expressed between the mother and daughter regarding what her medications should be, and when she was supposed to follow up with the doctor. The daughter responded to her mother, whereas she did not answer the doctor's questions. The mother, who was not wealthy, asked for free medications from the doctor, and had the proper BPL (Below Poverty Line) card to receive them from the NIMHANS dispensary.

In this case, though the husband and his family had abandoned her, perhaps due to her mental illness, and perhaps justified it by claiming that she carried an illegitimate child, she was cared for by her mother, who apparently had managed to devote several days to her daughter's care at NIMHANS over the nine-month period. Given her poverty, giving up a full day's wage to visit the OPD was, indeed, a hardship, requiring a heroic effort on the mother's part.

We might recall an earlier case of partial abandonment, where a male in his forties presented in the OPD with "significant global developmental delay," meaning he suffered a cognitive deficit. His aggressive episodes in recent years had been concerning, and he had been seen previously a few times at NIMHANS. He was deaf and mute, and as he came into the OPD he smiled and signaled to the doctor by pointing to his mouth and ears. This individual was accompanied by his eighty-year-old father to the OPD. Though he had two sisters, he lived in a facility, because the sisters were unwilling, apparently, to care for him. Somehow, while living in an orphanage run like an ashram, he had gained a degree of language proficiency. He liked to read and enjoyed writing out simple sentences as a mode of communication with others. While he had been occasionally "frustrated" and "aggressive," the doctor felt that the sisters were, perhaps, using this as a pretext to "abandon" him at the orphanage. The doctor, in frustration, had noted that "laws against desertion" existed. But, in practical terms, these were rarely enforced, an oft-repeated frustration voiced by the doctors at NIMHANS.

We can recall, too, that the sisters refused to come to the OPD sessions with their brother to speak with the doctor and had refused family therapy. While the doctor impressed upon the father the need for the family to get involved with the care, there seemed little hope this would occur, based upon his pessimistic tone of resignation as he spoke. A sedative was prescribed for the patient's "restless movements" and aggressive behavior, after which the patient was sent back to the dormitory where he lived—an unsatisfactory solution, the doctor reiterated.

As in the case above, we see the partial abandonment of a patient, whereby one parent takes upon her/himself all the caregiving responsibilities. In both cases, the doctors blamed abandonment on certain family members, suspecting that the burden and stigma of mental health influenced their actions. This pattern of abandonment within ongoing care was probably characteristic of the majority of cases I witnessed, and was a feature of cases discussed in other chapters as well. As Pinto (2014) has persuasively shown in her landmark study, care and abandonment are not opposites in practice, but rather are entangled realities within the ambivalent intimacies of kinship and the harsh realities of medicalized modernity.

There were thirty beds at NIMHANS reserved for those "abandoned." These patients were all under one doctor's care, who had taken it upon himself to advocate for this space. It was here that patients such as Zareen, discussed above, could be rescued from homelessness and receive specialist care. But I was told that the central administration of the institute was now pushing to "open up the space and discharge the patients." This was lamentable, I was told, and showed the pressures of resource limitations and the "logic of capital" making its way into a public and government-subsidized tertiary care center. We will have more to say about privatization, financial pressures, and the future of the public health care delivery system later.

To conclude this chapter, however, let us conjoin the question of abandonment with that of cosmology. In the next chapter, we will look at the prevalence and increasing manifestation of another "modern" symptom. This modern symptom, particularly relevant within excessive attachments to ethnicity, religion, and nation, was to divide the world into absolutes in which betrayal is a common theme, as is the dualistic, almost Manichean struggle between good and evil, and the concomitant inability to live within the grey zones of ambiguity where battle lines are not so starkly drawn between self and other, good and evil, and the sociocultural categories that, in their hypostatized, postcolonial, and serial form (Anderson 1998; Appadurai 2000; Hansen 2001; Willford 2006; 2018), pit communities and individuals against one another. In one sense, I will argue, these dualities and their pernicious othering tendencies are symptomatic of the modernist and serial imagination (Anderson 1998). But in another sense, I will also suggest that the instantiation of these bounded forms of identity is itself productive of the symptoms of othering. Moreover, the madness potentially unleashed by totalizing and ossified forms of identification, when conjoined to underlying symptoms, be they psychosocial or organic, intensifies the conditions of betrayal and cosmological suggestibility, providing for, and exacerbating the content of, the repertoire of symptoms that are compelled to speak in the name of the Law or archive (Derrida 1995) that supplements a deficient reality.

Thomas, a man in his forties, came to the OPD. He spoke in English, complaining of memory lapses. He appeared to be lucid and relatively high functioning but had recently failed to remember the word for "latch" in the bathroom. He also suffered from depression and was very "suspicious of other people." Previously, Thomas was involved with the Christian ministry, but complained that "Indian politics and the Church" were vicious. He meant that within the church there was political struggle. He said he had experienced a "very hard life" and spoke of his own "insecurity and low self-image" as a result of life's weathering experiences. With these blows in life, he was now easily provoked and had difficulty maintaining social relations.

Thomas was quite interested in my presence within the clinic and volunteered, looking at me, that he "first got depressed in England." He had worked for ten years within a software company in England. Evidently, there had been periods within his life when he had felt very good about himself and periods when he had been very low. It was unclear whether a clinical diagnosis of BPAD was warranted, however.

His struggle, aside from that within the church, was within his own family. Evidently, he has clashed with a brother about the inheritance of some land. Moreover, when he visited a sister recently, the same estranged brother threatened her not to have any contact with Thomas. The doctor suggested that sorting out the familial dynamics and conflicts would be the key to his recovery, and recommended psychotherapy. The doctor added, however, that it could not be "done overnight," but would involve a long-term commitment on his part, perhaps lasting six to eight months.

Thomas reported the odd symptom of not knowing sometimes whether he is sitting or sleeping. He doesn't believe he sleeps at certain times, but he was told he does, in fact, sleep. Thomas told the doctor that his sleep was poor, in any event, and that he felt quite depressed, particularly now that he was not within the ministry anymore. He claimed that someone "jealous" of his role in the church ruined his clerical career, which, in turn, brought him down. He said his depression had even extended to his religious convictions. Nowadays, he complained, he no longer felt the same inspiration reading biblical verses that he once did. His faith was rattled, and he alternated between feeling betrayed by a rival, but still committed to the faith, and being disenchanted by religion altogether.

The doctor suggested that there was an oscillation in his life story and self-understanding in which he, on the one hand, would meet great figures who help him, whereas there are also antagonists who destroy him. Therefore, his life became a dualistic struggle between good and evil in his mind, as figured by an idealized leader and a satanic one who betrayed his trust. Moreover, there was a narcissistic streak, despite the modest demeanor that Thomas ostensibly displayed. His grandiosity came in the belief that idealized figures favored him or negative figures persecuted him. In either case, he seemingly constructed a reality around himself, in which he was singularly important, suggesting a narcissistic and grandiose tendency (Kakar 1981; 1982). The grand drama that was his life led to his oscillation between the very high highs and the very low lows, as might be suggested by a bipolar diagnosis, which was suspected by the doctor. But it was also clear that something was seriously amiss within the family's intrigue and conflict between siblings. Whatever template for betrayal that existed within the cosmological realm might have been prefigured by familial tension between siblings and, of course, the parents that raised them.

We conclude this chapter with Thomas not to suggest he epitomized abandonment, though his being disavowed by a brother, and potentially a sister, surely constituted a sense of betrayal, if not abandonment. Rather, his case offers a segue to the connection between familial stress and cosmological tension. Moreover, the degree to which he participated in a grand drama of cosmological significance seemed to suggest a sliding of the personal struggle into the cosmic or collective struggle of categorical significance, the subject of the next chapter. We might then ask: What is it about modern life, and particularly in India, that compels this apparent sliding of significance into cosmic drama?

Chapter 3

Singularities and Their Discontents

As soon as there is the One, there is murder, wounding, traumatism. The one guards against/keeps some of the other. It protects itself from the other, but in the movement of this jealous violence, it comprises in itself, thus guarding it, the self-otherness or self-difference (the differing from within oneself) which makes it One . . . the One forgets to remember itself to itself, it keeps and erases the archive of this injustice that it is.

—*Jacques Derrida*

As was noted earlier, India's velocity of social and cultural change is producing discourses of "crisis" within the media about a potential mental health emergency. Most often these debates about modernity's discontents point to the kinds of anomie that are well established and associated with urbanization and a diminution of traditional familial and community sources of support and social connectivity. This simple causal model obscures much by discounting the cultural shaping of illness presentations, as well as the cultural forces of rationalization and serialization within modernity that are productive of ideological supplements and displacements. As Lang (2018) discusses in detail, "depression" is the form this discourse of crisis addresses, pointing to not only anomie, but a nexus of neoliberal economics and individual oriented self-care. She notes a shift in discourse to "mental health" as opposed to mental illness, and with it, an attendant shift towards de-institutionalized self-care through pharmaceutical interventions.[1] This form of biomedical malevolence, we have seen, has been resisted by doctors at NIMHANS with varying intensity, drawing focus upon the social, despite the gravitational force of pharmaceutical treatment.

In this chapter, I turn to forms of malevolent haunting that spiritualize mental illness presentations and their consequent treatment by patients and physicians alike. I draw out and examine three main themes of malevolence and social violence as perceived by physicians, to some extent. First, I describe the spiritual hauntings that are oftentimes associated with possession and sorcery in South Asia. Though the philological and anthropological literature on spiritual hauntings is vast for South Asia (e.g., Obeyesekere 1981; Smith 2006; Fabrega 2009; Kakar 1982; Taneja 2018; Nabokov 2000) and specifically for India, less attention has been focused upon the intersection of psychiatric diagnosis, treatment, and the wider cultural forces that are productive of these spiritual hauntings. Second, and related to the first, I discuss how "reforms" and reformist discourses within the modern, serialized, and rationalized religious life in South Asia are productive of frustrations and thwarted aspirations, ossifying a more porous, creative, and fluid field of identifications within the social and cultural fabric of religious life. This ossifying, or contracted social field, in turn, is productive of obsessions and delusions that shape an already existent symptomatology in new and more bounded forms. Third, and as a consequence of the latter, the prevalent themes of betrayal and categorical truth, as opposed to a toleration of ambiguity and uncertainty, take root in accusations and uncanny hauntings, as well as in a kind of legalist subjectivity that is supplemented through the fevered archives of the other's transgressions. These three and broadly malevolent poles come in bundles, and are inseparable, though the emphasis or presentation may vary substantially from case to case. Rather than artificially disentangle these thematics into discrete analytical categories, I will present the cases more organically in the rhythms of the OPD, as they might actually appear sequentially within the clinic. Moreover, these thematics are not isolable from the other patterns of illness I discuss in other chapters. These themes of malevolence resonate, to a greater or lesser degree, throughout this study. The recognition of patterns, or analysis, following the lead of the doctors I shadowed, is necessarily retrospective, and thus, synthetic, in the conclusions I draw.

Spiritual Hauntings

A thirty-year-old and slightly overweight Muslim woman named Salma came with her husband and young son to the Outpatient Department (OPD). The woman had a visible scab on her forehead caused by hitting her head against the wall. It seems that she was unaware at the time that she was doing this until the "blood would flow." Upon seeing blood, she would cease her head banging. She had been checked by a neurologist for epileptic seizures, having both an electroencephalogram (EEG) and magnetic resonance imaging (MRI) performed. But her neurological evaluations had been negative. As this was possibly a case of psychogenic seizures, she was referred to psychiatry. Salma came from a lower-middle-class background and used to be better presented in terms of her physical appearance, according to her husband. It was only after marriage and childbirth that she had depressive episodes and exhibited seizure-like behaviors.

The husband was a tailor of second-hand clothes who earned a modest wage. Salma had, in fact, moved downward, in terms of material wealth, after her marriage. The doctor treating her said to me privately (after the patient had left the room) that economic frustration could, indeed, be a factor in her illness. Prior to coming to NIMHANS she visited two *dargahs*. These are tomb-shrines for Muslim, and particularly Sufi, saints. One *dargah*, however, was for a Sufi saint, whereas the other was for a Wahhabi-influenced, or reformist, one.[2] While spiritual healers at both *dargahs* suggested that she was possessed by devils, their prescribed cures were different. With a Sufi healer she had been told, in the course of her treatment, that she was possessed by a *jinn* (a spiritual being, oftentimes malevolent in character) and drank a whole bottle of rum, which had been demanded by the *jinn* in the presence of the *Pir*, or spiritual healer, within the *dargah*. She had never tasted alcohol before, we were told by her husband. This did not appease the *jinn*, nor cure her of her madness.

The Wahhabi-influenced healer in the other *dargah* discouraged this behavior and wanted her to follow orthodox teachings to drive the devil out. This also did not work. When both failed, she decided to try neurology, and eventually was transferred to psychiatry at NIMHANS. The physicians examining her deduced her behavior to be volitional and communicative. If her seizures were epileptic they would not fall into a pattern of self-injury in the manner it presented. Moreover, she would not be able to stop her head banging upon seeing blood.

Salma appeared sluggish, depressed, and somewhat uninterested in the doctor's evaluation, while her husband showed visible concern. Her illness had caused marital stress and discord, as well, as will be made clear below. This notwithstanding, the family had upward aspirations and wished to send their son to an English medium institution, a path towards the middle class, they hoped. The son, in fact, spoke English to the doctor while accompanying his parents to the OPD.

The patient was described by the doctor as a "30-year-old mother of two who suffered from a compulsion to bang her head." She now experienced "economic distress as well as social marginality." Discord, especially with her in-laws, had worsened over time, making her very "sensitive" to their criticism. She, as mentioned, had been more autonomous prior to marriage, and

"South Asian" in her "liberal" practice of Islam, which, not uncommon in India, incorporated Hindu and Sufi elements (Flueckiger 2006; Taneja 2018). Moreover, as she had worked as a hairdresser prior to marriage, the in-law family saw her as a "bad" Muslim woman, having themselves embraced a "reformed" or purified Islam. Her father, a Sunni, had not been as strict as her in-laws and husband. Religious tensions were playing out in this family, indicative, as the doctor suggested to me, of a wider canvas of religious tension in the country in a worsening communal climate with the ascendency of Hindu nationalism (Hindutva) in recent years (Menon 2022; Jaffrelot 2021). Being caught between normative models of gendered religiosity was a cultural strain that worsened the symptoms of many female patients, as their freedoms and aspirations were increasingly frustrated after marriage (Marrow 2016; Pinto 2014).

Salma's primary symptom of head banging had, as pointed out, left a large scar on her forehead. While banging her head, she said she "feels alive" but this had, understandably, frightened her husband. Sometimes, her husband said, she suffered from hemi-paralysis, as well. Though neurological tests were done, nothing organic had been discovered. Her paralysis appeared to be psychogenic, according to the doctors who had examined her. Sometimes while banging her head during a seizure, she would speak in the voices of other people who were "not me." When she had earlier visited the Sufi-oriented *dargah* specializing in demonology and exorcism she was found to be possessed by an "evil *jinn.*" The *jinn* was originally thought to be the spirit of a sixteen-year-old girl who had purportedly committed suicide. But sometimes the *jinn* spoke as if he was the deceased brother of the woman, calling attention to a "murder" that had occurred. While somewhat ambiguous, the sixteen-year-old evidently had claimed to have been murdered, or someone else close to the brother had been murdered. The *jinn* spoke from beyond the grave to an injustice that had been done. This empowered the woman, making her "alive" as an arbiter of justice, or at least, its siren from beyond the walls of death. We might even speculate that the traces of death within her—a renounced self with its aspirations for life, an ambivalence towards the letter of the law as opposed to the "living" or organic flow of religious life, and the repetitive and seizure-like self-harm that marked her as alien and uncanny to her in-laws—were externalized and concretized through the figure of the *jinn*, leaving her inner being alive, if only for the moment of possession. In those moments, she commanded care and fear, not unlike the figure of the Goddess in much South Asian thought (e.g., Ram 2013; Doniger 2009; Ramberg 2014; Shulman 1980; Obeyesekere 1981; Trawick 2017). The "knots" of gendered normativity and religious discourse exacerbated by reformist modernity would not abate (Pandolfo 2018; Taneja 2018; Ramberg 2014) but appeared in the clinical symptoms and guise of what the doctors labeled as "hysteria."

Aside from frightening her family, she received attention and a degree of support, though it must have been also ambivalent, given the family's more orthodox orientation to Islam. Here the validation and continuity of a more fluid, syncretic, and demonological system of belief and healing was enacted by Salma, though her symptoms and their treatment called attention to the clashing cultural models of Islam at play (Taneja 2018; Pandolfo 2018). But beyond the cultural context, which was also marked by socioeconomic strain, why did the woman identify and find some degree of enlivening pleasure with the symptom of *jinn* possession, particularly given the familial disapproval of this, and therefore its invitation to create more discord within the family? And why the emphasis on murder? Why a sixteen-year-old girl? Was this woman around this age when she married? Was her injustice within the husband's family tantamount to a kind of murder? Might the knot of self-harm she was enmeshed within be both resistance to gendered hierarchy and yet also a resistance to resistance that was punitive and hysteric, in the Lacanian (1977; Fink 1995) sense?

These questions could not be answered with any certitude given the limitations of the psychiatric encounter I witnessed. Even the doctors often admitted that their speculations of psychosocial causation were, while tantalizing and possibly useful for determining the level of biomedical intervention prescribed, never resolved to their satisfaction. Most of them had possessed some insight and knowledge of local cultural psychologies themselves, so as to repeatedly question the boundary between psychosis, schizophrenia, conversion disorders, and transient or situational forms of mental illness (Young 2007). Moreover, they were often not in a position to convince patients that psychotherapy might be warranted, given patient preference for a magical "tablet" providing symptomatic relief (Ecks 2013). Still, this and many other similar cases of malevolent haunting, frustration, and thwarted aspirations seemed to suggest an emergent pattern of response to reformist pressures and the categorical (serialized) truths they purport, as well as the psychological consequences thereof (Kakar 1996; Hansen 2001; Menon 2022). The hemiparalysis and self-harm also suggested a kind of inward-directed aggression that could not find an external target, which might suggest that the failure of exorcism looms large, changing what is at stake in the encounter between traditional and biomedical healing within an ever-encroaching modernity—a point central to the second volume of this study set in rural India. Again, this accords with Kakar's (1982) model of paralysis and self-harm through malevolent spirit possession as a means to defend oneself against the greater horrors of being unfilial (Cohen 1998). There is certainly, too, a strong cultural model that the *jinn* must be exorcised through the banging of an iron nail utilizing the forehead (Halliburton 2009). This is powerful among both Hindus and Muslims, with *pey*, *bhut*, *preta*, and *jinn* possessions being quite common (e.g., Smith 2006; Kakar 1982; Ram 2013; Ramberg 2014; Halliburton 2009; Pinto 2014; Nabokov 2000). Following the psychoanalytic line of reasoning pursued, for example, by Obeyesekere and Kakar, it would be relevant to know whether this particular woman had harbored strong romantic feelings for anyone before her marriage had been arranged. In this light, the deceased brother could be a disguised and abandoned lover (Nabokov 2000). Could he have committed suicide? Or conversely, could she identify with the suicide of another vicariously? Could this be one of those transient mental illnesses that Allan Young (1995) writes provocatively of, whereby the ecological niche for a particular symptom presentation resonates to such an extent within public discourse that a public symbol becomes very personal, but not merely private fantasy, as Obeyesekere (1981) argues?

While a number of cases I observed surrounding thwarted aspirations and malevolent spirits were of Muslim women, the same pressures of reformist and modernist religiosity were felt by Hindus and Christians, as well. And men were not immunized against spiritual malevolence and symptom repertoires that were part of the social fabric of modern India. Indeed, identity, I argue, is a battleground that conjoins more or less benign forms of identification to cultural politics and serialized forms of nationalism, be it linguistic, religious, or regional (Anderson 1998; Willford 2018; Hansen 2001).

Susila was a Tamil-speaking Catholic woman who had been waging a war in her head between devils and angels for years. She was well known to the doctors at NIMHANS, as she had been seen and admitted several times. I observed her a few times within the OPD, as well as in the ward where she had been admitted. On one occasion she brought her mother to the OPD with her. The mother had a degenerative bone disease in her spine. Susila had suffered severe delusions and hallucinations for years, but she was urged to take care of her mother by the doctor examining her on a particular day in the OPD. She was, despite her illness, high functioning, cognitively speaking, and had masked her illness for years. Indeed, some years earlier she convinced a local parish priest to leave his flock and marry her after they had fallen in love. They had one son together. But upon learning of her mental illness, he had left her and taken the child. This trauma worsened her psychotic symptoms and feelings of haunting by malevolent spirits. Aside from the possible guilt she may have felt in turning a priest away from his vocation, her traumas revealed a new intensity after turning to a more demanding form of Christianity.

Susila's condition worsened over time. Eventually, she had to be admitted into the ward when she began to have symptoms of severe depression, fatigue, and weight loss. One afternoon, while I accompanied her doctor on his rounds of the ward, my heart sank upon seeing Susila. The rooms in the ward were monochrome, as was her mood. The distinct smell of Dettol antiseptic, used to mop the hospital floors, always stung my eyes and nose. But against the sterile smell of antiseptic, the distinct smell of natural body odor and used linens lingered. This was not a strong stench, but a lived-in smell. Clearly, Susila was being cared for and bathed, but not to the extent that her room had the smell of soaps or fresh linens. A few unwashed dishes and a pot for cooking sat next to the bed on a small table. Her food, mostly rice mixed with vegetables, appeared to be half-eaten. Plastic chairs were provided for family members to sit.

When we first entered, Susila was lying down. Seeing us, she tried to sit up. She was lethargic and said she felt very ill, had a fever, and was unhappy to be in the ward, and she begged the doctor to be released as she claimed that the hospital was making her sicker. She was not eating well, though her mother tried to feed her in front of us, and was there by her side. Her doctor tried engaging her in conversation, but she was unresponsive to most of his questions. I noted "excessive tiredness" in my notepad. Susila's mother told us that her daughter had also been vomiting after meals. The doctor said he understood her desire to leave the hospital, but could not release her "just yet" as there were still "too many symptoms." Aside from her psychosis, her physical condition appeared to be in decline from when I had first encountered her a few months earlier. Her coloration was different, probably from fever, vomiting, and being inside a hospital room for many days. More shocking, however, was her complete disinterest in our presence, and her extreme symptoms of fatigue. I did not think to ask what could be causing her fever and vomiting. Rather, it seemed that the doctor's main concern was her depression and psychosis, though I assumed her medical charts indicated whatever comorbid conditions she was presently suffering from.

Susila had been experiencing a proliferation of "demonic forces" in her life struggling with "angelic" ones. A cosmic struggle was being waged within her between these dualistic forces. As in the case of Salma, discussed above, a clue to her dyadic struggle, at least its cultural shaping, could be seen in her religious turn to a more "reformed" and demanding version of Christianity. She had been raised in a more syncretic and characteristically South Indian style of Catholicism (Mosse 2012), but turned to a more charismatic and Pentecostal kind of Christianity. In short, South Indian Catholicism, particularly in Tamil Nadu and Kerala, had over the centuries incorporated many elements of worship style from Hinduism, such as a particular style of *puja* (worship with flowers, incense, and fruit offerings, for instance) and saint veneration. Modes of oracular healing and notions of immanent sacred power within particular shrines were shared across religious divides (Mosse 2012). This was also true for Islam, as noted earlier. Sacred sites such as particular churches, *dargahs*, and temples draw devotees from all three religious traditions within the same spaces of worship (Halliburton 2009). Boundaries between devotional communities were generally fluid, though the processes of serialization and boundedness had taken root in modern life, demanding a suppression of the Other, as well as the heretical elements in the Other's faith-based traditions. True belief, therefore, increasingly involved a disavowal of a part of the self, now proscribed by the processes of becoming "reformed." The uncanny residue of these suppressions and repressions (Willford 2006) were, in turn, manifested in self-conscious assertions of difference, a more legalist mindset in which truth was determinate and fixed, and, in turn, was generative of archival tendencies, in Derrida's (1995) sense, utilized to buttress the shaky bed of conversion.

Susila's conversion had heightened a sense of cosmic struggle against demonic forces, and she increasingly saw and heard the presence of evil beings that caused her to doubt her own spiritual worthiness. And while her hauntings were not reducible to religious conversion, or the trauma of a failed marriage, given her long-term diagnosis of psychosis, the shape and intensity of her delusions and hallucinations were exacerbated by the volitional force of her conversion, and the impossible demands it placed upon her. The traces of her failures would instigate her guilt responses, perhaps, animating and emotively charging her psychic life with cosmic implications. At the same time, the disavowal and externalizing of these traces into the cosmic realm was also a defense and partial erasure of said traces.

What were these traces? We can, for one, speculate that she bore the traces of decisions she had made that violated her Catholic beliefs. The marriage to the priest would have, perhaps, been a transgression against faith and belief. The guilt of that transgression is evaded through the path opened up by Protestant and, more singularly, Pentecostal Christianity. This action of disavowal violently suppressed Catholicism from her self-identity, solving one problem of transgression. But it also opened up the palpable reality of experiencing God's presence in daily life, as the constant struggle to be waged with the devil becomes real and animate through not only the voice of God working within, but also in the daily "signs and wonders" that validate the life of charismatic Christianity (Luhrmann 2000). As her doctor seemed to suggest, her conversion was a key factor influencing the shaping of her psychosis, exacerbating its intensity. In addition to displacing the traces of guilt associated with transgression, the traces of Catholicism undoubtedly lingered within her, these in turn bearing the traces of filial and familial intimacy. These intimacies transgressed through the intensity of denunciation that a stricter and bounded Christianity demanded, producing the hauntings characteristic of the serialized form. That is, one must constantly reinvigorate the struggle against the "evil" that threatens to drag the self into intimacy with the traces that have been surmounted in the charismatic euphoria of the new.

The text that comprises the narrative of selfhood matters. The archive, in Derrida's (1995) sense, is supplementary, buttressing the law that has taken root, retroactively validated but incompletely, through the archive of, in this case, "devils" and "angels" waging their battle. Susila, in short, was caught between a rock and a spiritual hard place. Her rejection of her mother's Catholicism must have strained their relationship to some extent, animating and intensifying her spiritual drama. The father's role in her illness was not made clear, as I did not hear his name ever being mentioned. While this aroused my suspicions that his absence was, indeed, a large presence—a lack that was, in Lacanian terms, productive of the psychotic break with reality—it was not clear that he was truly absent. Her symptomatology seemed to inscribe the law and legalism into the core of her inner struggle.

In addition to Susila's religious visions and delusions, she was having symptoms of myoclonic (epileptic) seizures.[3] It was unclear if these were epileptic or psychogenic seizures, that is, behavioral or possibly a reaction to the clozapine medication she was on. Her lethargy and general sense of fatigue could have been, in part, a reaction to the medication. For present purposes, I wish to underscore how the bounding of identity through "reform," in this case religious identity, produces a particular kind of haunting and dualism that pits an already unbearable psychological ambiguity into the realm of certainty, as expressed through the idioms of faith-based assertions. An ambivalence and possessive force, however, betrays assertions of truth and certainty. Sadly, Susila did not survive her illnesses, passing away a month or so after we had visited her in the ward. The cause of death was never revealed to me, though my first thought, recalling the last time I saw her, was that she had lost the will to live, being haunted by devilish forces and desires, as well as the wrathful judgement of the "angelic" ones. The question that lingered in my mind, indeed, haunting it for days, was whether the sense of betrayal in her tragic story was of her own doing or, conversely, was powered by the ideas of a threatening betrayal that lie at the heart of the reformist creed with its impossible demand for singularity against the traces of the past. That is to say that the psychic archive we all inescapably possess has social predicates that can turn malevolent when singular, ossified, and "molar" (Derrida 1995; 1998; Deleuze and Guattari 1987).

Delusions and Hallucinations

The next case illustrates less a religious imaginary than a grandiose delusion of betrayal that shared some similar structural features. A forty-two-year-old man, Sanjay, appeared in the OPD with his two aged but highly educated parents who appeared to be from the middle class. He had been suffering with delusions for over ten years, and had been diagnosed with schizophrenia. His affect was, I noted in my notepad, "a bit flat and diffident," though his parents had a look of long-suffering patience upon their faces. His parents said that Sanjay had lost his jobs and his "ability to work outside" (the home). As a result of this, Sanjay had moved home where he relied on his parents for his care. He was articulate in English and told us that he had been a "reasonably successful person" at one point. But his disease, his parents said, had caused him to lose a good job at a major electronics brand from Germany that manufactured and distributed products in India. Now he complained that "nobody would hire him," though he could not attribute it to his illness, which he disputed with his parents. Indeed, he said he was fine, and that his parents were exaggerating his condition in order to get him out of the house. Rather, Sanjay proclaimed that "all were against him," a signal that his delusions were also paranoid, which is fairly common with schizophrenia. By implication, he seemed to be saying his parents were also against him, and that their bringing him to the OPD was an expression of their animus towards him.

This notwithstanding, he expressed a keen desire to "reclaim his life." He said that getting a job was the "key to his happiness." But, as his parents complained, he never left the house, and had a severe vitamin D deficiency according to his lab results, suggesting he did not receive enough sunlight. Regarding his termination from a good job, Sanjay explained his version of events. While working, he "learned that an actress [her name escaped me] was infatuated" with him. When probed by the doctor as to how he came to know this, he said the others in the office "told him everything." He said he was terrified to go outside because the neighbors "watch his every move" and Bangalore is a "dangerous place" due to robberies, crime, etc. Even the potholes in the road scared him, he said. This drew a chuckle from the doctor and myself, as Bangalore is known for its large and jarring potholes by the locals, which are due, it seems, to increasingly heavy traffic and inefficient municipal roadworks crews who were slow to fix them.

Sanjay said his troubles began when a "lady at work" reported him for harassment just because he "said hello" to her. She had turned the others against him and he had been fired. After the man had left the room with his parents, the doctor within the OPD explained that the patient's version of termination from the employer was much more complicated than he had asserted. During the session with the patient, however, the doctor probed further and found a "Truman Show"–like syndrome in this gentleman. This syndrome, re-named after a popular Hollywood film starring Jim Carrey, is one where one comes to believe that the whole world is watching oneself (Gold and Gold 2014). This is a grandiose delusion of reference that is found across the globe, but varies in cultural content. We will see this casually diagnosed in other cases (it is not an official diagnosis).[4] In this case he spoke of how the whole world was listening and watching him, but not with "good intention." Rather, his life was entertainment for a watching world. He singled out the West, and the US and the UK in particular. When pressed as to how he came to know of these things, he said that it simply became known to him. It was possible that he, as an English-speaking middle-class person, had watched the film and found it provided answers to his already existent delusions, according to his doctor.

Sanjay was on two antipsychotic medications for many years, but was put on a new drug the day of his visit, starting with a low dose. His parents, and evidently a sister in Delhi, had expressed exasperation at his "intolerable" condition. The parents pleaded with the doctor for help when the patient was out of the room. They "put [their] whole faith" in the doctor, proclaiming that no other doctor had helped their son previously. They were desperate. They also countered the son's claims that he was doing well and interacting with the family in a sociable way, as the doctor had queried this, as was part of his routine clinical interview with patients. The father spoke of "all the rubbish" that comes from his mouth. And the mother apologized for her son to the doctor for "having to hear" his delusions of paranoia. The doctor, of course, said that an apology was not necessary and that it was "simply the disease talking." But the doctor was also circumspect in evaluating the potential for cure. He suggested the new medication could help. But given the long-term delusions and previous non-responsiveness to medications, no assurances were given except that he would follow up every month for several months with the patient. The doctor also asked the parents to get the patient's blood tested monthly for the first six months of treatment.

This case could have been placed elsewhere in this study, with its themes of family tension and desired normalization. I choose to place Sanjay's short case here for its congruence with the themes of betrayal and a dyadic struggle that assumes near-cosmic proportions, dividing the world into a neat us vs. them, or in this case, an "I" against the "rest" that we see in the previous two cases. And while this could be taken as a presentation of "grandiosity" (I'm the center of the world's attention, à la the Truman Show syndrome, and famous actresses are enamored with me) conjoined to paranoid schizophrenia, its context speaks to the broader social pattern of achieving a singular identity over and against the one provided by the social milieu. This is not to romanticize the solution this man chose in dealing with a workplace that no longer wanted him. Indeed, staying indoors within his parents' home had only led to vitamin D deficiency and further familial stress, as he increasingly became a burden and embarrassment for his parents. Recall the parents' apology to the doctor for his delusions. In this apology, some acknowledgment of context and intimacy is revealed. The son is not wholly other, and his delusions do not make him unaccountable, despite the doctor's protestations to the contrary (it is "simply the disease talking"). No, the son's disavowal of both his parents' struggles and embarrassment, as well as that of his coworkers, which evidently extended to the general public, suggested a bifurcation of the social into a totalizing, indeed, cosmic or global narrative of betrayal. While not discounting the organic or biological dimensions of his illness, the social milieu in which it was expressed shared thematic resonance with the cases of attenuated cultural fluidity in favor of "reform." But in this case, the social pressure of narrowing one's identity into a fixed form was replaced by the patient's desire for a withdrawal from the social, or a narrowing that is self-induced in reaction to the pressures of normalizing medical and familial discourse. This thematic will receive greater attention in the subsequent chapter. But for now, I wish to point to permutations of India's serialized discourses, be they medical, familial, or religious.

In the next case we see a combination of the agentive or intentional withdrawal we just witnessed in the case above, coupled with the aggressive religious imaginary that brings judgement against the Other's desire. A woman in her late sixties or early seventies came with her husband to the OPD. The husband complained that his wife was suffering from "excessive dreaming." She kept to herself for long hours and would not want to interact with others in the family, he claimed, adding that "her behavior is not improved," and "she doesn't like people for no reason."

The couple came from a large extended family and were well dressed and English-speaking, suggesting they were from the middle class. According to the husband, she refused to interact with her grandchildren and did not want to meet people, with the exception of two or three individuals that she liked. He exclaimed with frustration in front of her that "she is not a normal human being—she hates everybody!" Moreover, she "doesn't want to talk to her mother-in-law . . . and spends her time playing games on her smart phone. She interacts with nobody and doesn't want any social commitments." The husband requested counseling from the doctor to be arranged. Then after the husband had said all this, the wife told her side of the story. "I stopped talking to the children for [my] health [*sic*]. I don't want the trouble they brought as I had suffered for fourteen years. The remedy was not talking to them. As a result, my health has improved." The husband then interjected, "She shouts at me . . . I just want a normal lady—a proper housewife." The wife quickly countered, "I withdraw to get peace of mind." This sought-after quietude, she explained, makes her "feel happy." She added, however, "I do play with my grandchildren, just not the two children." The mystery avoidance of these children became clear when she said, "I will not speak to his daughters." It then became apparent, which was confirmed later by the doctor, that she was the man's second wife.

I could sense that this was an unhappy marriage, given the couple's body language and, in particular, the husband's strong statements. But after the woman had left the room, and the couple had been told to go for counseling, the doctor explained that she had suffered from paranoid schizophrenia. She used to "hear voices," and had an "unfaithful husband," which worsened her mental state. Her delusional experiences were quite specific. She would often smell something "fishy." This occurred when an "electric current would enter her body around the pelvic region." To my admittedly psychodynamic-oriented ear this sounded quite sexual in nature and suggested an orgasmic response (see Obeyeskere 1981). But in India people often gave religious significance to these experiences. Indeed, she had seen a *Pir* (Sufi Muslim holy man) who offered her holy water to chase away the evil spirits that were causing this symptom (electrical charge in pelvis), suggesting further to me that this charge was, indeed, transgressive in nature. After taking this holy water and experiencing its "cooling" effects, she had felt some relief of her symptom. She would also burn holy papers with sacred mantras (incantations) printed on them. At one point, the doctor explained to me, she had experienced an elaborate hallucination of the baby Krishna living within her mouth. This seemed like a vivid recreation of the Krishna myth whereby he opened his mouth to his mother, Yashoda, revealing the universe, instead of the stolen butterballs she expected to find in her mischievous child. But we might also speculate further that this internalized Krishna had deeper, indeed, cosmic significance.

Krishna's *lila*, or play, as described in epics such as the *Mahabharata* and *Bhagavata Purana*, is resonant in theological and philosophical significance, and its analysis goes beyond my more modest suggestion in this context. But what we can observe, in a very basic manner, is the duality that exists between appearance and reality. While Krishna appears to be Yashoda's biological child, he is really the avatar of Vishnu, God-incarnate, and thus his actions are incomprehensible to human understanding. His play is thus partly didactic, to throw our human certainty and rationality into doubt. The conventions of human propriety do not hold with Krishna, as his ways are mysterious. This is more famously illustrated within the *Bhagavad Gita*, when Arjuna,[5] forgetting Krishna's divine nature, is given the vision of his infinite, terrifying, and sublime formlessness. The repetition or permutation of this drama, whereby Krishna is now internal to the mouth of the patient, now bearing the trace of the divine within her, is inexplicable to her husband. And by extension, the conventions of patriarchal law, which demand of her subservience to the mother-in-law, the husband's kin, and children, even in the knowledge of his being unfaithful, are called into doubt through her vision. Krishna's play is also hers. Her *lila* is, to human eyes, unfathomable and deep.

While I can only speculate as to the significance of her hallucination or "vision," it does align with the theme of cosmic struggle we have already witnessed, whereby the duality between good and evil is, in this case, cast more as a reflection upon what is real and imaginary. And, on the other hand, also to what is permissible and appropriate. Her refusal to submit to the normalizing demands of her husband, and perhaps the clinical intervention, to some extent—though this is hard for me to say, only witnessing her encounter at this stage and not during her initial treatment for paranoid schizophrenia—is, perhaps, a kind of "positive withdrawal" (Corin 2007) from a scene of great pain that had evidently lasted for over "fourteen years." Her refusal of the step-children's company is not hard to understand, in this sense. Like in the case of Sanjay above, a withdrawal from the social field can be protective, to some extent. Hauntings and hallucinations can, paradoxically, be consoling at one level (Luhrmann and Marrow 2016; Padmavati and Corin 2007) whilst attracting the clinical gaze by family members and physicians at another. She felt happy and at peace in her withdrawal, and perhaps her effacement of the everyday with her spectral interlocutors, akin to the case of the "personal symbol" in Obeyesekere's work, allowed for an objectification of an internal affect through which her subjective experience became lucid, or at least bearable (Obeyesekere 1981; Corin 2007; Luhrmann and Padmavati 2016; Sood 2016).

The treatment of hallucinations within the clinic was taken seriously. Part of the training for residents and fellows, in fact, centered upon the recognition of hallucinations and/or delusions as symptomatic of organic illnesses, or as part of a symptom cluster in the case of psychiatric diagnoses. For instance, in another case, a female patient, aged thirty-six, presented hearing persistent malevolent voices. Within the house, she often heard noises that she interpreted as "robbers." She interpreted these noises as threats to her personal safety. But her hallucinations also took on a delusional and paranoid quality in that she also claimed hearing her neighbors talking ill about her from several houses away.

For eleven years she suffered from irregular menstruation and conceived only after the intervention of a gynecologist. She also had hypothyroidism, which could account for some of her general ill health including of her state of mind. But this, as the doctor examining her explained to a resident he was training, would not account for the particular form her hallucinations and delusions were taking. The question put to the resident was whether hallucinations belong to a syndrome or cluster of syndromes? The resident was told that hallucinations usually have an organic cause that can be pinpointed, rather than being their own cause and symptom as part of a psychological illness. In this case, while it was highly likely that hallucinations were occurring, these were being organized into a pattern of thinking, or as delusions. But in her case, the delusions were increasingly paranoid and were gradually getting more "organized" thematically. That is, from random auditory hallucinations she now believed she was a target of intruders, malevolent neighbors, etc. As such, she went to a faith healer first, as many patients at NIMHANS continue to do, particularly among the working class. Some symptomatic relief was obtained once the "devils" were chased away by ritual means. But the delusions eventually returned with greater force and urgency. The patient was put on risperidone, a widely used drug for psychosis and schizophrenia, and CT scans of her head and neck, as well as other thyroid tests, were ordered to rule out any organic abnormalities.

In general, NIMHANS doctors were not overly eager to psychologize. Rather, they were methodical in testing first for organic causation when psychiatric symptoms presented. This was even true when patients came on referrals from other psychiatrists or neurologists with a given diagnosis of psychotic, manic, somatoform, or affective disorder symptoms. As pointed out earlier, the medical training at NIMHANS had always emphasized the Kraepelinian model favoring bio-organic causation, over and against the Freudian psychodynamic etiological approach to mental illness. That said, as we have seen in the cases thus far, it was the functional disability of patients to harmonize comfortably within their social milieu that brought them to NIMHANS. And moreover, we have seen in this chapter how the idioms of symptom expression, or the basic symptom repertoire, were derived from a common set of cultural and religious symbols that organized the world into benign and threatening forces (Nichter 1982). And while demonology and possession have a long and, indeed, central place in South Asian thought (Smith 2006), the forces of modernity (urbanization, inequality, serialized forms of identification, etc.) seemed to be changing the frequency and intensity of illness presentations according to the patterns I observed in the clinic, as well as the lamentations of certain culturally sensitive doctors who worried about the pressures of "reformists" within the religious sphere, along with the structural problems and iniquities facing both urban and rural populations. Risperidone, as one doctor explained, is a "Band-Aid upon a gaping social wound," a phrase repeated several times to me during the year.

In another case where reformism and modernism collided with the presentation of symptoms, a middle-aged working-class Muslim woman returned to the clinic to see the doctor who treated her for years. This doctor, one of the many eminent psychiatrists at NIMHANS, pointed directly to the psychosocial context that exacerbated, if not caused, the patient's symptoms. This, he explained to me, was a case of "domestic violence" that had gone on for "several years." As a result of the abuse, the woman suffered from migraines, "hysteria," and seizures. Her symptoms, debilitating and refractory though they were, had emerged out of physical and psychic abuse suffered domestically. But this presented a kind of double jeopardy within the trajectory of her treatment. She had been stigmatized as "psychotic" and as a "mental patient" within her family and community. But, the doctor emphatically told me, she showed no signs, in reality, of psychosis, and suffered no delusions or hallucinations. Through NIMHANS, marital therapy had been attempted but the husband always failed to show up.

The doctor felt that this was a problem of a more liberal "South Asian" Muslim culture colliding with a more reformed, modernist, and "puritanical" side of Islam that was spreading in India. The woman had worked as a beautician before, as in the case mentioned earlier, and had also visited *dargahs* and temples in her youth. She, in other words, practiced the "tolerant" strain of Islam that had mixed more easily with a fabric of shared cosmology and social intimacy that permeated beyond the now serialized and bounded forms of identification that were taking root in the country (Flueckiger 2006). The husband, like in the cases of Susila's charismatic Christianity and Salma's reformed Islam, having been influenced by reformist Wahhabi ideology, accused her of being a "bad" Muslim and took out his anger and frustrations upon her, which only worsened her symptoms, making her mental health spiral downwards. Tragically, as her doctor acutely felt, NIMHANS was in a position to only help her with her "symptoms," not help to mitigate their cause.

This pattern was not unique to Islamic modernists, but also appeared among Christians and Hindus. Although it was not always the case that women were the targets of normalizing reformist discourses within a patriarchal society, I witnessed a disproportionate percentage of working-class Muslim women suffering similar symptoms and social pressures within the OPD, perhaps owing to the social precarity and class marginality that Muslims faced, as compared to other communities, indicating the nexus between economic stress and psychosocial causation of illness (Patel and Kleinman 2003). The rising tide of communalism, as marked by the political rise of the Bharatiya Janata Party (BJP) and its affiliates, had also exacerbated stress and insecurities within the Muslim community, particularly after the installation of Narendra Modi, an ardent Hindu nationalist, as prime minister. Most of the doctors at NIMHANS I met were also intellectuals and social analysts, coming from elite and liberal-secular backgrounds, and were increasingly wary of the rise of right-wing populism and the trends towards policing social and religious boundaries in a nation that, in their words, prided itself on inclusivity and religious pluralism. Reforms led to feelings of betrayal and absolutism, which, in turn, exacerbated paranoid symptoms whilst also delimiting the range of therapies, particularly within the traditional spheres of faith healing, that were more freely available in the past. The absolutism arising from reforms, we might also note, worsens stigma by turning formerly permissible expressions of psychosocial stress into "bad" or "evil" practices that are increasingly proscribed forms of religious and somatic symptom expression. One might even say that the gods and demons were now more judgmental, as the following case illustrates. Modernity, as Deleuze might say, had "deterritorialized" and "reterritorialized" the more protean deities into more moralistic and rigid entities, disseminating their uncanny malevolence in so doing. That is, a modern rupture with the past that produced a potentially violent suppression of cultural practices ensured that the past would press itself into a haunting present.

A forty-six-year-old male Hindu priest named Hari had suffered from mental illness for the past ten years. He appeared to be normally functioning and very devout when he visited the OPD. Hari's case illustrated the tenuous and fine line between mental illness and cultural belief. In describing his entry into religious life, he said that the "goddess came on him" at some point in his life. He used to do *pujas* with his neighbor in his youth, before becoming a priest. One day, and in a dream, Lakshmi (the goddess) took him "by the hand" and guided him to become a priest. He worked as a priest in his village, which was, by his account, fairly orthodox. But beliefs in the various gods and goddesses, as well as visions of the same, were not considered strange or out of the ordinary for priests and other ecstatic religious practitioners.

In this case, Hari had been spiritually inclined since childhood. At one point, however, he felt that someone had done "some black magic" on him. Exorcism rituals were performed on him within a local temple as a remedy. But for ten months he felt numbness in his body as the "dark force" was being purged away by the counter-sorcery rituals. This treatment apparently helped him after many months.

The effects of the healing rituals were not permanent. Hari began having disturbing dreams where a "dark force" was targeting his mother. In his dream he would hold his father and mother tightly, but would awaken with anxiety. As a result of the recurrent nightmare, he had significantly decreased sleep, was socially withdrawn, expressed fear, and felt that "something bad will happen." But he also had dreams whereby the gods came to him and told him to chant and do *pujas* while standing on his bed.

Hari's family lived in a small town in western Karnataka, his native place, and were concerned about his state of mind and staged an intervention in the decade before 2014, when I met him in the OPD. At the time of the intervention, he was taken for psychiatric care, given injections and electroconvulsive therapy (ECT), and put on antipsychotic medications. After fifteen days of treatment, his sleep and social interactions returned to "normal." Since then he had occasional episodes, though while on his medications he functioned fairly well. When he stopped his medications, he would experience "mild irritability." Hari's wife, however, blamed her husband for his delusions and wanted him treated. The wife, in turn, was not spiritually inclined in the intense manner that the husband was, which caused recriminations, accusations, and counter-accusations within the household. Hari believed his wife's attitude was part of his "tension" and fear, as she did not dress "properly" given her "husband is doing prayers" and is some sort of "Brahmin priest." This schism within the family had ramifications upon Hari's parents and in-laws. The couple had an eighteen-year-old daughter who was mainly taken care of by her grandmother (Hari's mother). Because of the wife's "non-religious character," the "wife is an outsider" within the husband's household, according to the doctor who was treating Hari. In this case, the reformist pressures, in a sense, came from the wife, who could not accept the intensity of Hari's beliefs. However, even his own family had forced him into psychiatric treatment, worried about his state of mind a decade earlier. But in this case, Hari's family, ironically perhaps, seemed to supplement their own discomfiture with Hari's religiosity through the accusation that his wife had worsened his symptoms due to her transgressions of that same conservative religious milieu.

Hari's father had passed away a year before his visit to the OPD. For six months he said he experienced "sadness." Then around the six-month mark, he heard his father's voice calling him as if alive. This helped him recover from his sadness, though was a cause for concern that his psychosis might be returning. Hari continued to receive "visits" from the gods in his sleep. This alone was not a major concern, nor all that unusual for a priest. More concerning to Hari and his family was his worry about the forces of "black magic" that affected him and continued to threaten family members in his thoughts.

Hari was, at the time, perhaps, between forty-five and fifty years of age. He seemed to be high functioning and did not appear to suffer from a severe mental illness, based upon his presentation and ability to express himself clearly. His thoughts were, perhaps, delusional, and there was indication, as well, that he had auditory hallucinations of his father's or the gods' voices. But his main symptom seemed to be extreme agitation and anxiety about the malevolent forces that black magic had wrought upon him. Given his religious convictions and worldview, and the shared milieu of beliefs that surrounded him, it was hard to draw a line between pathological delusion and the far ends of faith associated with visionary experiences. But given that even Hari's family had concerns over religious obsessions, there was clearly some normative line that he crossed from time to time, which had led to the interventions and treatments.

For the past three years he had worked as a priest in an Anjaneya temple (to the god Hanuman, as he is widely known from the *Ramayana* epic) in Bangalore. He continued to hear his father's voice and was becoming somewhat withdrawn and depressed on account of his marital discord and familial worries. Indeed, his family, out of concern, had to coax him to come to NIMHANS for treatment. Prior to his visit, he had been taking lorazepam for his anxiety. Hari was not diagnosed with paranoid schizophrenia despite his fears of "black magic." His lucidity and high functioning seemed to indicate non-schizophrenic illness to the doctor who treated him. Perhaps, it was suggested to Hari and his family, mania or an "affective disorder" was affecting him, but this was hard to confirm, it was explained to the family. As he was free of ostensible symptoms at the time of his visit to the OPD, he was not given any other treatment by the doctor that day, but he was asked, along with his family, to consider family therapy, given the tensions in the household between the wife, husband, and mother-in-law.

My impression at the time was that there was nothing particularly pathological about Hari's ability to hear the voices of the dead relatives, or the gods for that matter, particularly as this often happened during dreams, but not exclusively so. Perhaps the telling sign of something being amiss was his family's concern, coupled with his own withdrawn and depressed state. While the thematic of spiritual malevolence is hardly unusual in this milieu, there were characteristic modern dimensions that figured into or exacerbated this malevolence. That is, the representational economy of malevolence was driven by a sense of haunting related to social changes or the epistemological vertigo that resulted when explanatory frames collide. On the one hand, Hari and his wife came from different worlds, to some extent. Her modern dress and behavior was, to Hari and his family, immodest and improper, especially for the wife of a priest in a conservative provincial South Indian town. This seemed to trigger both his anxiety and his family's making of her an "outsider." This, in turn, led to their daughter being raised by his family, sidelining the wife, almost certainly exacerbating the tension between husband and wife. On the other hand, Hari's own family was concerned with his mental state, having, it would seem, a sense of normalcy even within this traditional context that was breached by his intense religiosity. The kin, in other words, have, by their very actions of convincing Hari of his psychiatric illness, shown themselves to be shaped by modern biomedical understandings of mental health.

Hari was obsessive, anxious, and apparently haunted by malevolent forces beyond what was expected of a priest in his community. The unseen and untold story here might have been that at the time of his marriage, his delusions were, in truth, concealed from the bride. In any event, now that his symptoms had worsened after marriage, and especially after the death of his father, whom he held "tight" in his dreams, and his delusions of "black magic," the modern ways of this same bride, who might have been deceived, were now blamed for his symptoms. The implication seemed to be that Hari believed her irreligious ways had redoubled the "black magic" being directed towards him. A generalized malevolence now enveloped him at the same time that his wife withdrew from him, leaving him threatened on all sides: the gods, his kin, and his wife's alien and modern ways. Therefore, whatever psychiatric diagnosis he had received, an affective and/or anxiety disorder, or perhaps mania and depression, the cosmic struggle between the modern and the gods, and by extension, the demons that shaped his inner torments, was made real through his symptoms. An archive of cosmic struggles made sense, at least to Hari, of his inner compulsions. Again, we might also observe that sensations of betrayal may also animate his demonology.

But where does the betrayal lie? Is it in the concealed illness at marriage, in a sense, a reaction formation? The transgression against the gods by the secular and modern? Or is it in his family's ultimate betrayal in making him into a patient, whilst also damaging his marriage? I could not help thinking about the father's comforting voice in overcoming Hari's depression and sense of loss. Yet, precisely, this very consoling ghost was improper, melancholic, in Freud's sense (Langford 2002), and had to be abandoned, leaving him more haunted than ever. As he was deemed somewhat of a threat to his own daughter as a "mentally ill" person, so, too, was he threatened by his own father's voice, in the eyes of his family. This was not a permissible voice, but one that had to be properly mourned and made inaudible. Was there a betrayal of his father in Hari's own eyes for this exorcising of his ghostly presence? Was the pleasure associated with his father's voice impinging upon him a pleasurable form of self-punishment—a return of the Law, or secondary *jouissance*, in Lacan's (1977) sense? These unanswerable questions notwithstanding, we can witness a kind of duality or doubling of Hari's selfhood in this struggle of opposites. Renouncing or being urged to renounce an intimate object, or a shadow-self that is unacceptable as a result of this intimate object, is also witnessed in the following case.

Sati, a young middle-class Hindu woman from North India, presented with a diagnosis of schizophrenia. But her specific and fascinating delusion was that another woman was living inside of her. Here dualism was materialized in a corporeal sense. Sati could hear the woman's voice and saw that the woman was pregnant, given that she was "lactating" and her breast size and overall weight had increased. The doctor examining her mentioned that 5 percent of the women who took antipsychotics experienced symptoms of increased breast size. But Sati felt there was an actual corporeal presence: a lactating pregnant woman inside of her that explained her weight gain. The woman inside her was parasitic, "eating her blood," and thus blood is "not reaching her brain," causing her symptoms of irritation and a "lack of concentration."

The doctor queried about Sati's social life. She came with her mother each of the few times I was able to observe her interactions in the OPD. Sati had worked as an intern with a prominent computer company in Bangalore, and had been good at her work, despite her illness. But she complained that her "concentration level was weak." Her psychiatrist at NIMHANS asked her to concentrate her thoughts upon things that were interesting yet distant from her delusions. This was part of her recovery, he insisted. She complained that she could not understand the things in her mind, and this was distressing. The doctor suggested that she write two to three pages each day, and that writing, more generally, had a therapeutic effect by helping to "focus the mind." This required discipline and practice. Sati, however, complained that she lacked confidence in her writing. The voices in her head interfered with her studies and mental focus, more generally. "Practice," however, was a key part of her recovery, the doctor insisted.

In many other cases I witnessed in the OPD, some of which are still to be discussed, the physicians, and especially Sati's doctor, would not entertain the writings that patients brought in with them to the clinic, in hopes that the doctors would find them important and revelatory, in some respects. This attempted meaning-making was abruptly short-circuited by the doctors I witnessed, with the explanation given to me that these writings were often full of elaborate delusions that should "not be encouraged" or validated by their analysis. Doctors, on the other hand, intervened with patients who suffered delusions, especially when they led to "excessive rumination" on those very same delusions, which often took ominous and paranoid forms. Reading, writing, work routines in the house, and exercise were common remedies for excessive rumination. In this case, the doctor saw Sati as an educated and otherwise high-functioning individual who, because of her age, still had an opportunity to gain some control of her thoughts and mind.

The doctor suggested that because she was young, only in her late teens or early twenties, she needed to have a "good recovery" so that this delusion could be arrested quickly. He explained that she still had a "chance for a normal life" with a "good recovery" from her first major psychotic event. A good recovery, he emphasized, would involve medications, activities such as keeping a daily journal, and exercise.

While not explored in the OPD, it was mentioned by the doctor to me later that Sati had some "issues with her father" that were unresolved and might require psychotherapy. Sati mentioned "tensions with friends" concerning her purported flirtations with boys. But this was not queried further in my presence. She had insisted that her friends had betrayed her, not she them, despite their accusations that she had flirted with their boyfriends, which she denied.

The onset of her illness began when studying for exams in school. She experienced a high fever which was followed by "great fear." It was after experiencing both fever and its panicked response that the symptoms of hearing voices and ultimately, the person inside herself appeared. As a result of the recent and sudden onset of her symptoms, as related to an illness, the doctor suggested an MRI to check for temporal sclerosis. If there was a brain anomaly, then a "migration psychosis" was more likely, caused by neuronal migration or misfiring in the brain. Whether this be the case or not, her treatment would involve an active retraining of the brain and mind.

Sati was admitted to the hospital and was told she would spend a few weeks in the ward. A week after admission, she, upon returning to the OPD, still had a strange sensation that there was a lactating woman living inside of her. The doctor had urged her to stay busy and keep her mind occupied in order to quiet some of the voices in her head. But she complained that the voices were still there in her "mind." The doctor again emphasized that she needed to read, write, exercise, and make things (like knitting and other crafts). But she complained once again that her concentration level was "very low."

The possibility of a "migration psychosis" was discussed. These symptoms were, in turn, coupled with depression, according to the doctor. As was the case the previous week, the doctor urged Sati and her mother to stay another month or so at NIMHANS in order to have a "good recovery" from this illness. This disappointed both the mother and daughter, as they were eager to travel back to their home in the north. Though the etiology of Sati's illness was still in question, the treatment involved the conscious and volitional training of the mind through writing, reading, exercise, and other activities. She was encouraged to suppress thoughts about the lactating person inside of her, having been told this was a delusion. In a sense, her road to recovery, from the doctor's point of view, involved self-discipline, and, indeed, creating an "objective" archive of non-delusional thoughts and reflections that would override, in theory, her delusional self.

This active and intentional production of selfhood seemed similar to the kinds of spiritual training that "patients" received in traditional and religious healing contexts in South Asia, in that the authority or archon-like quality of the healer was as important as his or her didactic instructions to their patients. A "good recovery" seems to semantically suggest itself through the very iterative process of its so saying (Luhrmann and Marrow 2016). While in other cases we have seen, and will continue to see, the archive of the self that patients bring to the clinic, in their diaries and notebooks, or elaborate cosmological delusions, was believed by doctors to strengthen these very delusions, and must, thus, not be entertained seriously, which, we might add, would facilitate transference to the doctor of the entire psychic drama and its presumed psychosocial origins in familial life; in this case, the archive shatters one delusion and replaces it with a more acceptable one. This is not a flash-of-lightning insight or psychoanalytic breakthrough, but rather a pedagogy for the self that aligns more with cognitive behavioral therapy, as well as traditional healing. But unlike traditional healing, the "demonic" is not exorcised by a spiritual counter to a malevolent being. Rather, the demonic is simply pushed aside and denied a place within the self. That said, I often was left feeling that the "good" in recovery was also a function of the perceived goodness of the healer, in this case, the psychiatrists. Patients often thanked the more insightful doctors with phrases like, "God bless Dr. —," or "I thank God every day for Dr. —." This respect for the doctor as guru, healer, and teacher was more pronounced, however, with less wealthy or less educated patients, than was the case with the educated elites, who oftentimes came to the clinic with suspicions and/or cynicism about psychiatric interventions.

In Sati's case, too, we see a splitting of her into a good and bad side, though it is not ostensibly moralized in the cosmic terms we saw earlier. Still, the lactating and blood-eating being objectified, one could argue, the sexual maturity that had aroused suspicions of flirtation with her friends, but which she strongly denied. Her libidinal nature, in other words, became a separate person altogether, leaving her weak, tired, and without verve and confidence. One might even speculate that the modern crisis of feminine sexuality in India is acute for some precisely because of the resilience of patriarchal familial dynamics and attitudes in society, demanding on the one hand chaste modesty, yet on the other it was highly eroticized in films and songs in popular culture. And this, as many scholars have argued, has a longer history in the splitting of the feminine through versions of the Goddess as benign, wifely, and motherly, versus manifestations that are "hot," aroused, dangerous, and passionate (see Hiltebeitel 2000; Ramberg 2014; Doniger 2010; Ram 2013). While the doctor in this case did not investigate psychodynamic factors in her illness, his admission of the patient for a fairly long period suggested that family and other social dynamics would be explored, particularly given the emphasis Sati had given to school stress, peer suspicion, and the more unspoken but briefly mentioned tensions with her father.

Constriction and Betrayal

The next two cases point towards the nexus of traditional and psychiatric treatment, on the one hand, and the contemporary conditions that drive symptomatic presentations in cosmological and categorical terms. A working-class Muslim woman in her thirties, Farhana, presented with headaches and strong "suspicions of witchcraft" having been directed towards her. She also experienced financial stress and suffered somatic symptoms, primarily headaches, but also other aches and pains throughout her body.

Farhana was convinced that her sister-in-law and her husband had done some "black magic" on her. Six months earlier she had tried to stab her own mother, who accompanied her to the clinic on this day, with a knife. She felt that people were "always talking" about her, and in negative ways. This feeling of suspicion was present whether she was with her natal family, her in-laws, or outside of the home. Thus, she presented with a more generalized paranoia about persecution and ridicule, but she did not have the florid hallucinations or delusions that were normally associated with paranoid schizophrenia.

An exorcism had been performed within a *dargah*, as it was determined that Farhana had been possessed by a *jinn* or some other undetermined evil spirit, as a result of her violent outbursts and claims of witchcraft. When she fought with her husband, she experienced pounding migraine headaches. Her husband, in turn, an uneducated man, was accused by her of domestic violence. As the husband did not come to the clinic with her, we did not hear his side of the story, or that of her in-laws. Farhana had two children; one son worked in a shop, whereas the daughter was in college. They were apparently asymptomatic. Farhana's mother was sixty-five years of age. As it was in the previous case, there were some "unresolved issues" with the father who had already passed away.

She was accompanied in the OPD by her sister, who was working as a nurse in Bangalore. Farhana's mother-in-law, she said, was "very irritating." She imposed many restrictions that "kept [her] up in the house." Prior to her marriage, however, she liked to visit *dargahs* and had greater freedom to move about within the community. But now, she "cannot do anything." There was, as in the cases discussed earlier, a disjuncture between the husband's interpretation of Islam and her own. They restricted her movements in a way that shows a clash between the more liberal and fluid boundaries of "South Asian" Islam with that of a more orthodox, Wahhabi-influenced kind. The husband found her ways unorthodox, and believing her "evil," restricted her movement with the assistance of his mother. Farhana's mother was also "irritating," she claimed. Thus, she said that she felt no closeness to either her mother or mother-in-law, and preferred to stay with her aunt, cut off from the husband's family.

She was put on risperidone, though she had no hallucinations, just ever-present suspicions and explosions of rage coupled with the somatic symptoms of pain, particularly manifested as headaches. The doctor, a very reflective man in his mid-career, quite precisely and deliberatively told me that "we see many cases like this where *poverty and social context* [emphasis mine] is contributing to the illness, but we try to alter brain chemistry in response to it as a coping mechanism." This comment was also directed to a resident in the room, which was often the case within this teaching and research hospital.

In his saying this, moreover, he verbalized my growing impressions from several months of sitting in on OPD sessions. In each case there was an etiology of psychosocial stress coupled with local cultural understandings and cosmologies/demonologies that made sense and shaped the symptom presentation. Unless the patients were willing to receive psychotherapy, and most would not, due to the stigma attached to being seen as a mental health patient, the medicating of patients seemed largely palliative, but hardly transformative in terms of patient insights into their condition or in altering stressful social dynamics. Medication also did not offer much potential to alter society in a positive way through mental health education, and hence a reduction of stigma. Indeed, mollifying the rage of the oppressed, and in many cases, working-class females, could be called conservative and normalizing, a prevalent recurring theme in this study. This was the turning of a social problem into an individualized medical problem, making a social victim into a patient. Beyond constructivist readings of pathologization (Foucault 2006; Horwitz 2002), a psychiatric reading at NIMHANS could reveal the production of "local biologies" being forced upon subjects whose social and economic precarity was, at the very least, comorbid with commonly seen mental disorders (Patel and Kleinman 2003; Cohen 2012; Das 2006). In this sense, the palliative or symptomatic care received at NIMHANS is, as mentioned in the previous case, not unlike the exorcism in that it repeats the gesture of abnormality requiring a talisman-like "cure." But this case also repeats the theme of legalism and bounded religious identities and their discontents in the form of a general distrust, even paranoia, in which the label of "bad" becomes a self-fulfilling prophecy.

Farhana's life changed dramatically after marriage, leaving her controlled by a more conservative and serialized form of religious propriety. It is hardly surprising, then, that she had a general distrust and paranoia of others, particularly of her husband and his sister-in-law, whose constriction and control had been felt as a powerfully alien force, a force that possessed her body but also her soul, now discovering its contours through the supplementary evidence of malignant forces. It is worth pondering, perhaps, whether the *jinn* or demonic forces are friend or foe in this dualistic struggle (Pandolfo 2018; Taneja 2018). Exorcism is clearly incomplete, as her "evil" persists, along with her accusations of witchcraft and violent outbursts and irritation at those around her. On the other hand, the spirits allow her to articulate a negation of the Other's desire, in Lacan's terms. But Lacan also suggests that the hysteric's symptom is to locate the "lack" or fatal flaw in the Other's discourse, and simultaneously, to suture that lack further, locking a dysfunctional relationship into a kind of "schismogenic" spiral (Bateson 1977). We see a similar pattern of constricted aspiration and betrayal in the next case.

A middle-aged Muslim woman, Sheila, came with one of her sons. She suffered from a mood disorder. She was quick to cry and often became overly emotional. She complained that she carried out "her duties like a machine." But her automatism was not due to the Kafkaesque world of industrial bureaucracy. Rather, it was due to her relationship with her husband's family, with whom she lived. She often had disagreements with the family and had learned to cope in this "hostile environment." But now her capacity to cope was becoming precarious.

The family lived in Hyderabad. During her early life in Hyderabad she enjoyed meeting people, visited *dargahs*, and had a "satisfactory" social life. The family, however, severely controlled and curtailed her movements outside of the home. Sheila was left alone in the house often and felt very depressed as a result. The husband's grandmother was very blunt in her disapproval of the woman, saying things like, "You are not the bride we wanted." Due to this constant verbal abuse, she "lost confidence" and sank into herself.

As in the cases of Farhana, Salma, and others, Sheila, prior to her marriage, was very active in social organizations and clubs. When, after marriage, the family shifted to Kolkata, these rich social contacts and activities were lost. She felt alone and, indeed, lonely. And even worse, she had little to do outside of the house in Kolkata.

Sheila complained of many aches and pains in her body. These were assumed, to some extent, to be somatizations of her depression, as nothing in her medical tests suggested the presence of "organic disease." She also had quarreled with a younger sister and felt estranged within her natal family, to some extent. Her son, who came along with her to the OPD, and who was taking her in within his household temporarily as she visited NIMHANS, said he did not know what to make of her somatic complaints. Moreover, he said that she "does not forgive easily." One odd symptom of her distress was that she would walk around the house naked, which her son found shameful and embarrassing.

Sheila found some relief in visiting *fakirs*, or Muslim holy men, but this was also somewhat restricted by her family. She eventually found "faith" in an interactive self-help spiritual program headed by a Hindu guru. This religious organization used the telecommunications application Skype as a medium to "heal people," I was told. She paid lakhs of rupees for the "healing hands" therapy offered by this guru.[6] But the guru, she felt, had damaged her "nervous system." Her worsening condition, she insisted, was due to his malevolent touch. Sheila harbored great anger towards the guru and said that he had "ruined her life." And while it was true that the loss of money, and the loss of face by being defrauded of a lot of money, would have been yet another cruel blow in her life, her problems were deeper and longer standing than her being taken in by a fraudulent guru. The claim that the guru had ruined her life was likely a displacement or supplement (Derrida 1976) to her already fractured sense of self.

As was oftentimes the case, and as seen in previous cases in this chapter, marriage and the entry into a more circumscribed and religiously conservative, not to mention patriarchal, family had led to her depression and automatism. She emerged from this automatism when she was able to reanimate her world through *fakirs* and even a Hindu guru, who was initially healing but turned malevolent and predatory. Sheila was caught between a rock and a hard place, not being the wife and daughter demanded of her by her in-laws, yet yearning for a less constricting social and spiritual life, and not obsessed with conservative and serialized boundaries between Hindu and Muslim, and male or female. This duality, created as an after-effect of the proscribed or arbitrary law with its capriciousness, was resisted through her spiritual wanderings and, perhaps, shocking behavior to her family. But while walking naked or transgressing the "orthodox," as we have noted, in expressing both psychic and social resistance to the Other's desire (modernist religious reform, patriarchy), she was interpolated by these forces, all the same, as she was surely imagining the duality of proper and improper within her acts of rebellion. A fantasy space opened up as a kind of virtual capacity, in the breach of her imagined self and the reality of her predicament. Moreover, arguably, her dalliance with a Hindu guru would have aroused some transgressive guilt with her, which, perhaps, was also marked by an ambivalent disavowal of her own desire, now in the form of the supplement: the guru was evil and to blame for her "ruined life," rather than the broader social forces that had impinged upon her, causing her automatism and subsequent wandering outside of boundedness and constrictions of her post-married life.

In addition to these contextual etiologies that are, admittedly, speculations based on pattern recognition from the cumulative weight of many similar cases, another issue raised by her doctor concerned the side effects of antidepressants. Ironically, one of the side effects of these medications could be "mood disorders" that also manifested in somatic complaints. While Sheila clearly had suffered long and hard as a result of the social upheaval in her life after moving to Kolkata, and being subject to a more rigid religious and patriarchal code, there was the very real possibility that her psychiatric treatment altered her perceptions and moods, even exacerbating the somnambulant automatism and bodily aches that were her primary complaints.

Two of her sons were now trying to help their mother by bringing her to NIMHANS and letting her stay with them in Bangalore, but were troubled by their mother's condition, knowing that they had kept some distance from her owing to her personality disorder and odd behavior. "Out of sight and out of mind" had been a coping mechanism within the family, according to the doctor. They were somewhat transparent about this and felt a degree of guilt mixed with their embarrassment and anger over her increasingly transgressive behavior. That they mentioned her inability to forgive also hinted at their sense of culpability, and the recognition that some of her transgressive behavior was, indeed, aggressive and directed at them. But now, faced with the oddity of her behavior, she provoked, perhaps, a guilty response among her sons, who displaced this sense of guilt by medicalizing her condition in bringing her to NIMHANS.

It also seemed possible to me that her desire to reconnect with her sons provoked a range of symptoms that were passively enacted through somatization. That is, her anger at familial abandonment was too much of a betrayal to face directly, even to the extent that her crossing a bridge too far (e.g., nakedness and following a Hindu guru) was protective, a kind of narrative allowing her to construct and slay a dragon far less harmful to her sense of self than the Real, in Lacan's sense; that is, her family's care for and love of her was conditional upon her subjection to a certain level of propriety. Pushing up against the boundaries of these polarities, the proper and improper, circumscribed even her resistance and capacity for self-making, where, as Hegel famously argued, "any victory is a defeat," and the only refuge is to be found in an "unhappy" retreat into automatism, with its implicit repetitions of the same (Hegel 1977). The next case similarly illustrates the contagion of death, not the living death of automatism alone, but the ways in which corporeal and social death (repetitive compulsions of automatism) are related.

Contagion and Compulsion

Lata, a Hindu woman in her early sixties hailing from Bihar, presented with severe anxiety issues. Her husband's brother lived in Bangalore, which made it easier for her to visit NIMHANS. Her main symptom was a fear of "pollution" through contact with dead things, particularly dead bodies. This led her to obsessive-compulsive behavior regarding cleanliness, in which her family members, and especially her husband, were subject to demands for repeated bathing throughout the day.

Lata's symptoms began when she was in her twenties. At that time, she experienced some complications during a pregnancy. To deal with these complications she went to see a "Baba" (spiritual master, usually a Sufi Muslim) who gave her some blessed flowers that he exhorted her to keep "clean and fresh." The Baba had instructed that nobody should touch the flowers lest their healing power be diminished. Anytime someone came close to the flowers, she shouted, "Don't touch them!" Lata became excessively worried that somebody had damaged the flowers through human contact. As a result, she was haunted by the thought that her baby was born "damaged." To counter the damage, she washed the baby excessively if any human had or was suspected of having touched it.

Lata had perpetual thoughts and sensations of human pollution and experienced relief from these only when washing herself or asking others to wash themselves within her household. In particular, she feared "dead bodies." If a funeral procession passed by, or even if she heard the drums of a funeral procession, the whole family had to bathe. Sometimes the family was asked to bathe four times per day. Though they tried to accommodate her obsessions in order to placate her anxiety, this had eventually exasperated the family, and particularly the husband, who had tolerated the obsession for many years but was concerned that it was getting worse with age. If Lata, he said, should even "see an ambulance on the road," she would insist on everyone in the household bathing. The sight of a corpse, even in images, representations, or photos, or whether she was in close proximity or not, brought on the compulsion to bathe.

While there were familial stress factors, there was no history of psychosis, mania, or depression in the family. And Lata, while having obsessions with cleanliness, was not psychotic. Rather, it appeared that she suffered from an acute case of OCD (Obsessive Compulsive Disorder) for about thirty years. She had been married to her husband for close to forty-seven years. Observing and speaking with Lata, the doctor saw no indication of delusional behavior or severe family discord, other than the frustration expressed by the family over her illness. That even the "sounds of drumming" (which accompanies funeral processions) would spark her fear of death's pollution was becoming increasingly burdensome, they explained. Joining her in the OPD were the husband and daughter. They registered their hope that her obsessions could be controlled with medical intervention.

It was not clear that the patient had "insight" into the obsessiveness of her behavior, or whether she simply believed her obsessions were a practical solution to the many risks of spiritual pollution that occur on a daily basis. Indeed, an obsession with bodily and spiritual cleanliness is not uncommon in Hindu India, with its numerous caste, ritual, and food restrictions and beliefs of purity and pollution. Moreover, the odds of being "infected by death" was very high, particularly in a big city where death occurs in each and every neighborhood on a daily basis. Furthermore, when I asked about how she found visiting the hospital at NIMHANS with its many ambulances, sirens, and ill patients, she admitted that it was a very difficult experience and that just being there frightened her. As NIMHANS also had a general hospital with an emergency ward within its large campus, death was not an uncommon visitor.

In her clinical interview one life event jumped out as particularly significant. Lata had an abortion when she was younger, early in married life.

The timing of the abortion and the onset of her symptoms seemed to correlate, within a year or so. If the fear of death, in other words, was in part a ghostly apparition, a fear of contagion from death brought on by its intimacy, now repressed by the trauma and guilt of abortion, then perhaps the obsession, like that of Lady Macbeth, grew out of a troubled conscience. This might lead us to speculate about the resonance of *preta* beliefs in Indian culture (Kakar 1982). If *preta* are the souls of prematurely dead infants and children, could such a belief extend, even if by proximity, if not explicitly, to aborted fetuses?[7] While the contours of her case are somewhat different than Sheila's, there are some parallels owing to the ways in which automatism and repetition compulsions overlap and point to a kind of living death, and one that is inaugurated by traumas associated with malevolent aspects of modern life. In Sheila's case, the trauma of being thrust into a judgmental world of conservative and bounded religious and familial life had left her lifeless, desperate for reanimation of her spirit through intimacies no longer available to her, despite her best efforts to break from her cultural shackles. In Lata's case, the trauma of abortion had brought death's intimacy to the core of her being. Her possession by another kind of death, through the compulsion to repeat, as Freud argued, was punitive and hailed, perhaps, from an ego-ideal she had transgressed. The overwhelming sense of death not only resonated due to a past trauma, but was constantly reinforced by the phenomenology of modern urban life, where death is everywhere—in the sounds, images, and population density of both the living and the dead. Death, for Lata, was not a doorway to a new becoming, but was a haunting, a perpetual onslaught, in which any lapse in the inoculation of washing hands would result in irreversible contagion. Ironically, Lata is increasingly more dead than alive, already claimed by the grim reaper that activates the automaton-like quality of the repetition compulsion.

It is difficult, of course, to determine the causative force of repressed or psychodynamic factors finding partial, albeit repetitive and compulsive, resolution versus the beliefs of a society that create an already resonant obsession with cleanliness and the separation of life and death, the pure and the polluted.[8] Perhaps this case would exemplify the concept of the "personal symbol" as developed by Obeyesekere (1981). Obeyesekere argued, in my opinion persuasively, that a shared or public symbol, even a myth, can have resonance within a population due to its origins arising in a shared personality structure emerging out of socialization practices and enculturation, or a combination of a Freudian (unconscious) and Weberian (conscious) model of meaning. But when thinking about the genesis or excessive resonance of a symbol that might exist for a few individuals, the public symbol takes on greater personal significance. So while a god's or ascetic's matted locks may have theological significance and normative meaning within a more coherent set of symbols and meanings that are conscious, those who identify strongly with the symbolism at a deeply personal, emotive, and, arguably, excessive level, are motivated more than others to abreact traumatic life events through such symbolism.

If Obeyesekere is correct, then public meaning systems are not only intellectual "webs of meaning" but also, in part, projected fantasies out of unconscious traumas, forbidden wishes and desires, or punitive objectifications of subjective experiences of ambivalence. Akin perhaps to a Venn diagram, the resonance of any symbol, therefore, is one of degree, not a dichotomy between public or private. This then means, of course, that any individual's personal symbol, though drawn from a more collective set of meanings, is also invariably different, even its repetition of the same principles. Here the psychodynamic models of Freud meet the organic model of life as "difference" out of "repetition," as conceptualized by Deleuze and his reading of Nietzsche (Deleuze 1994; Colebrook 2007; Flaxman 2012). Indeed, if this be so, then rather than leading to a necessarily transcendental model of subjectivity, the "intensity" of life's events emerges from singular "intensities" or out of planes of "immanence" irreducible to singular models, but rather on the analytic or virtual plane, or as life lived as such. But while this might be a productive line of inquiry in order to find proximity, yet variation, between the traces of trauma and public meaning systems, such as those of a *preta* or other ghostly presences, this affirmation of life as repetition out of difference, and against the reductionism of universalizing models of the psyche, particularly its Oedipal Freudian version (Deleuze and Guattari 1972; 1987), does not do justice to the painful urgency of the symptom, whereby repetition is not marked so much by the production of life as by an intimacy with death. If death's door, so to speak, can only be closed by repeated slamming, but always remains ajar, where is there room for the subject or self to be open to a future undetermined by the past? We must continually ponder this, particularly when comparing the romantic ideas of resistance up against the suspension and endurance of pain that these resistances often produce.

One doctor, as mentioned earlier, in many ways mentored me at NIMHANS, though I absolve him of my speculations and interpretations. I had met with him a few times prior to my twelve-month residence in the hospital and Department of Psychiatry. He, being very open to comparative and ethnographic studies, had encouraged that I observe and note culturally significant features of clinical life and illness presentations. He was also of the opinion that, as mentioned in the introduction, psychiatrists today were not being trained enough in cultural psychology or psychological anthropology, and that narrow specialization coupled with an institutional insecurity made doctors less interested in the whole social and cultural context of human experience in favor of more easily measurable kinds of evidence, such as a neurologist or cardiologist could apply. He was not alone in this opinion, as many others at NIMHANS, from both the younger and older generations, lamented this trend towards a more specialized medical training, rather than taking a more holistic approach. As such, I was asked to teach a seminar to have the residents and fellows exposed to anthropological ideas and methods.

One afternoon, during his office hours, he told me about a female patient from a wealthy Muslim family who was admitted to the ward with a *jinn* having possessed her. She had, he said, a "traditional" marriage to a man she did not love. They had children and agreed, despite it being a loveless marriage, to stay together for the children's sake, though she wanted to live with the man she actually loved. This was agreed upon, strangely enough. Her "husband," not in a legal sense, wanted for himself to marry in a "proper legal" manner. Therefore, he was married in a "traditional community" wedding to another woman. This woman, this doctor's patient, then wrote a letter to the new wife and asked that she be considered the "first wife" and that they could "share" the husband and live as sisters.

This, understandably, outraged the newly married husband (and wife) who said that their "agreement" was not to "disturb" the wedding or home life of the other person. That she did so, in writing to the new wife, was sign of a *jinn* inside of her. What else would have possessed her to do such a shameful thing, her former lover had asked? The patient returned to live with her family after these events. There, after this trauma, she had been suffering from fainting spells, which were psychogenic not syncope (fainting due to insufficient blood flow to brain), which had been ruled out after medical testing. To her former lover or "husband," she was possessed by a *jinn*, and therefore no longer suitable as a partner, though by implication, had she remained discreet about their relationship, nothing would have occurred.

My mentor found this case to be unusual in that a middle-class Muslim from a fairly prominent family would come to believe in her own *jinn* possession, something he associated primarily with the working class and poor. Aside from the class dimension, also troubling was the implication that when one goes against the normative patriarchal order, particularly as a female, then one is "mad," possessed, or both, as we saw in the case of Catarina in João Biehl's important book, *Vita* (2005). When one's thoughts and words match those of the husband, one is fine. When one differs, one is mad. Thus the "cure" by sorcery is doubled-edged. It offers a cure through an objectified symbolic construct, but the very construct, while absolving accountability and reincorporating the social into the symptom and its cure, is also conservative and violent, in the sense that its radical alterity is domesticated and/or exorcised (Nabokov 2000). On the other hand, the haunting and unresolved nature of its presence also suggests that this "cure" is never complete. Some excess always escapes symbolic closure, leaving an uncanny presence.

Our conversations often turned to the problem of cultural attenuation, more broadly, under the guise of religious reform. We spoke sometimes about the problems of cultural serialization and homogenization and the psychic effects it sometimes brings. That a rich tapestry of cultural fluidity, for lack of a better word, was not separable and neatly legible (as bounded categories of difference) against this reality, the modernist and reformist discourses of moral and religious boundaries, absolutist difference, and totalizing notions of right and wrong, as grafted upon a serialized form, was an alarming trend that exacerbated underlying psychiatric vulnerabilities and conditions. Fundamentalism and populism often went hand in hand, and were based, often enough, on the invented or constructed categories of knowledge and community that were once used for colonial governance, what Anderson felicitously called their "serialized" form (Anderson 1998). Thus, while many of our conversations were about psychiatry's predicaments, our talk drifted to social and political traumas, such as the Partition and other regional conflicts. These conflicts and traumas, in turn, were concomitantly linked in our discussions to the impact of colonialism upon the postcolonial psyche (Nandy 1983; Sarin and Jain 2018; Pinto 2020a).

Significantly, and along these lines, he told me of numerous examples from his clinical experience in which the slightest insults were taken as cosmological, unforgiveable, and therefore increasingly polarizing between Muslim, Hindu, Jain, Sikh, Buddhist, and Christian. There was one story, in particular, that epitomized how the micro-violations of daily life turned into the grandest stages of cosmic struggle. The doctor described how a woman was spat upon along the roadside by a bus passenger who was passing by. The woman's husband was certain this was a religious insult, as she was a Muslim. This insult made its way to the OPD, showing the significant trace it left upon a psyche increasingly primed for religious othering. The doctor spoke of low-cost housing and flats in which the working class lived, oftentimes surrounded by complete strangers. In one such case, the Muslim family expressed a sadness that they could not "be themselves" as Muslims in the new housing complex. I asked if this troubled them because they could not be themselves surrounded by an Other, who, in turn would other them. He said, rather, it was because they had reached the "level of consciousness" in which they were so *aware* of themselves as being different, and thus, requiring *difference*, wholly separated from the Other. It was their self-perception that really concerned him, rather than a worry that the others in the flats would be likely to gaze at their otherness. While, of course, these are inseparable dynamics, bound in social exchanges that are increasingly fraught with a bounded or serialized distrust, the emphasis on the internalized "we-self" (Kakar 1996) boundary was more consequential.

We spoke then about the role of faith healers in the health system. Dr. R. L. Kapur, an important figure in twentieth-century Indian psychiatry and former director of NIMHANS, had co-authored a monumental ethnographic study of mental health in India, *The Great Universe of the Kota* (Carstairs and Kapur 1979), along with his wife, also a clinician. They were advocates in the 1970s of a more holistic system of mental health care that would recruit from the ranks of faith healers and practitioners of traditional medicines, such as Ayurveda, Siddha, Yoga, and Unani. Unfortunately, he said, this was not implemented by the central government, which feared liability for unstandardized forms of treatment.[9] His ideas, as well as those of his wife, were controversial, but there were evidently a few seminal papers from the 1970s on this issue (Kapur 2012). In the second volume of this two-part study, the relevance of partnerships with traditional healers will become more salient. In short, the lines between clinic and society, as a whole, were at one point more permeable, just like the ways in which religious and linguistic communities used to pass through more permeable boundaries.

The closing of more permeable boundaries as a "force of law" (Derrida 2002b) seemed to generate the psyche, and not vice versa. The torments of betrayal, legalism, and malevolence were, as we have often seen, generated out of the impossible demands of singularity and seriality. Excessive moralism, legalism, and othering, as psychological supplements effacing traces of alterity with archives of difference, went hand in hand with a perpetual suspicion of the Other's failure. The following case illustrates a totalizing impulse and an increasing incapacity to live within the grey and indeterminate zone where compromise, forgiveness, and openness is possible.

Obsessions of Totality

Dinesh, a twenty-three-year-old Hindu male hailing from Odisha (Orissa), came with his father. In 2012, he had begun to ruminate excessively over a friend's "betrayal" regarding the purchase of a book. As he stewed over this betrayal, he would sit alone and watch "godly channels" (regarding spiritual life) and little else. Religious obsessions seemed to coincide with his discovery and nonacceptance of his friend's "betrayal." Dinesh said he called his friend over "a hundred times," and continued still to call him seeking redress. The "friend" had since broken contact with and interest in Dinesh, possibly resulting from his revealed instability, as evidenced by his overzealous phone calls. The loss of this friendship, however, caused Dinesh to have crying spells, his father reported, at least two to three times per week.

Beginning in 2014, he began to report that people were "talking bad about him" when he left the house. Dinesh, however, accused other family members after his betrayal by his friend. In 2013, he had become increasingly irritable, and, specifically, directed his anger towards his mother.

Until he became obsessed about the "betrayal," he was an average student. Thereafter, there was a steep decline in his academic performance. Dinesh was now "below average" in his studies. His father reported further that he was not taking his "household responsibilities" seriously. Moreover, both Dinesh and his father reported that he had "bad thinking" when he saw women. But Dinesh seemed slightly foggy and unclear when he spoke, as if fatigued or medicated.

The father brought results of an EEG that had been ordered by a neuropsychiatrist "for no apparent reason," the attending physician commented. I wondered to myself if seizures were, perhaps, suspected, though these would only account for inattention, cloudy thinking, and/or fatigue, and not the sense of outrage and betrayal that seemingly precipitated his illness. The attending doctor mentioned that there was some history of "schizoid traits" in his medical profile. He had very few friends and was, generally speaking, not very sociable. Moreover, he was less active, both physically and mentally, than a man his age should be.

Furthermore, he had an "odd way of expressing wishes" (this was unclear to me from the OPD encounter) and showed some autistic symptoms, such as watching religious programming somewhat excessively, as well as overreacting to what would otherwise be life's little daily traumas. And his obsessive rumination (and phone calling) suggested a compulsion to repeat.

The attending doctor recommended a detailed psychiatric examination at NIMHANS. I was struck by the obsessive quality surrounding the theme of betrayal—he was a "victim" and this, in turn, had made him excessively religious against the evils of the world, but also very self-critical and punitive, as indexed by his "bad thinking" when he looked at women. This was a case of "hysteria," in some sense, in that he was betrayed, wronged, and altogether victimized by a friendship gone bad. This led to the obsessive delusion that people, more generally, were talking "bad" about him. While it was not clear yet what his psychiatric diagnosis would be, and hysteria was no longer a viable clinical diagnosis, though still deployed, as we have seen, in the clinical context, we can note the contours of his own dichotomizing world, as well as his retreat into an obsessive religiosity as a narrative frame, perhaps, from which to interpret his predicament. But, as in the case with hysteria as discussed by, for example, Freud, and later, Lacan, the victim's discourse is hysteric when it is also punitive and inward-directed at some sort of sexual-themed trauma, in this case, his "bad thoughts" when looking at women, which must collide violently and punitively with his hyper-religiosity. Filling and supplementing the Other's lack, in this situation, becoming overly righteous after his friend's betrayal, also involved displacing the forbidden intimacy of identification with the Other. Thus, displacement of his own faults, and the supplement of others (their evil and bad ways), was a means of sustaining and nurturing a hysteric subjectivity, prone to compulsive moralizing and self-punishment, in tandem. He no longer could retain the ambiguity and ambivalence of a "bad object," a buccal ethic, as we discussed earlier, and had to purge it outwards, clinging to a "good" object with increasing and repetitive desperation.

The next two cases offer more detail and also concern feelings of betrayal, as well as an overriding affect of generalized suspicion and "bad thoughts" being directed at the patients. These cases encompass many of the themes seen in the individual cases throughout this chapter, providing a larger canvas for seeing patterns that have emerged concerning betrayal, malevolence, and rigid boundaries being exacerbated by modern forces.

Thought Transmission and Cosmic Struggle

Vasanthi was a young woman in her early twenties from Tamil Nadu. This case piqued my interest as it dealt with the Tamil conception of sorcery (*seyvinai*), which was a pervasive concern within the Adivasi populations of the Nilgiris that I was simultaneously investigating. Vasanthi was accompanied by her father to the clinic. They were, judging by appearances, from the working class. The discussion was in Tamil, with a translator present for the attending doctor, whose Tamil proficiency was rudimentary. Her primary complaint was of "black magic" (*seyvinai*) being done to her. She heard voices that caused her to "break things around the house." Vasanthi also complained that her thoughts were "heard by others." Her father described, with Vasanthi interjecting added details, that the symptoms began after a dog had bitten her, causing her to fall and injure her head. After this head injury she suffered from "fits" (seizures).

The doctor, hearing of her injury, asked whether a CT scan had been done to check for brain injury. The father replied that none had been done. At this point, the doctor sighed, and began to ask her about her symptoms. Her father listed her main symptoms as fearfulness, loneliness, and headaches, coupled with an intense suspicion of others. Vasanthi sat passively, without disagreeing or nodding assent.

In terms of cognitive function, her reaction time to verbal conversation seemed reduced, according to the father. She also began to fail her school exams. Vasanthi called it a "demotivation" failure, which suggested some self-blame. The father nodded as she said the word "demotivation" in English, which stood apart from the Tamil being otherwise spoken.

Things had taken a turn for the worse in the last six months, according to the father, when she refused his "order that she work." There were loud quarrels in the house between the father and the mother, and more recently, between a frustrated father and Vasanthi. She said, however, that "black magic" was "being done by the downstairs neighbors" to her, causing her "disturbances and anger," compelling her to break objects, refuse work, and quarrel. The family conducted some Hindu rituals to combat the *seyvinai* (sorcery).

But Vasanthi had also been treated with olanzapine, an antipsychotic medication, at some point. This was not her first encounter with psychiatry. In many cases, patients combined faith healing with psychiatry, so there was nothing unusual in this.[10] Moreover, there was a family history of mental illness. Her mother, we were told, had been treated at NIMHANS for the "same symptoms" years earlier. The question that jumped into my mind at the time was whether Vasanthi's symptoms were, in fact, modeled on her mother's behavior, particularly in light of the troubling tension and quarrels that Vasanthi noted. Was she identifying with her mother? Indeed, the doctor next asked about work and family life, trying to elicit more information on these dynamics. A series of short questions and answers followed in rapid succession:

Doctor: Do you enjoy shopping?
Patient: I go with my mother.
Doctor: Does she help? What does she cook?
Patient: *Sambar* and *rasam* [lentil and vegetable stew and spicy broth]
Doctor: Do you like [your] mother's food?
Patient: (shrugs and smiles)
Doctor: What films do you like to watch?
Patient: Rajanikanth [popular film icon].

Doctor: What do you enjoy doing?
Patient: Cleaning house.
Doctor: Describe *seyvinai*?
Patient: This is black magic.
Doctor: How do you know they wish harm?
Patient: I was told in the temple that I'd been the victim of *seyvinai*. I'm a regular temple visitor.
Doctor: How do you know whom you can trust?
Patient: I have faith [*nambikai*].
Doctor: Do you hear voices? How do they sound? How do you hear them and what do they say? Are they male or female?
Patient: Both male and female voices come.
Doctor: Do you hear the same voices each time or are they different?
Patient: They are different each time.
Doctor: When you listen to the radio, do you hear them still?
Patient: No.
Doctor: So you hear them when alone?
Patient: Yes, while I'm alone.
Doctor: Do they interfere with you when you are speaking to another [*pesum pottu*]?
Patient: No.
Doctor: What are they saying [*enna pesange*]?
Patient: They are commenting on my thoughts.
Doctor: What do they say about your thoughts?
Patient: [No response, and a slight pause.] I confronted the downstairs neighbor but they deny any doing of *seyvinai.*
Doctor: Are they lying?
Patient: *Nambikai ille* [I don't believe/trust them]. But there is nothing to do [*enna seyvatu*] about them.
Doctor: What are they saying [*enna pesange*]?
Patient: Whatever *I think* they speak, but not in my own voice.

Aside from her delusion of thought transmission, what was so clearly enunciated was Vasanthi's sense of doubling. The voices were her, but not her. They amplified her thoughts, but in a voice uncanny and alien, coming from "neighbors" (close to home, but slightly removed). Vasanthi felt an overwhelming sense of something uninterpretable—a presence that is clearly both her and not her, but does not say anything definite, other than speaking her thoughts in a foreign tongue, in a manner of speaking. While not a lactating female, as in the case discussed earlier, an entity that is not quite oneself but is an overwhelming presence caused Vasanthi to "slow down," become "agitated," and, to some extent, become an "automaton" or the enactment of a kind of living death, reacting to, and perhaps, interpolated by, the Other's desire. Family dynamics were clearly an important part of the equation, though much remained implicit, and was not made explicit, in this clinical interview. This retreat from normalcy, however we might be tempted to frame it as resistance to patriarchy or the arbitrariness of the Law, we have seen, is never without pain, alienation, and increased social strain (Nabokov 2000). Headaches and other bodily pains have been ubiquitously seen in multiple cases, as has the persistent sense of betrayal by others, exacerbating the stress the patient and family experienced. Vasanthi's case, of course, like the others, had its idiosyncrasies and questions surrounding underlying organic conditions. Which is to say, illness presentations were shaped, but not wholly determined, by psychosocial stress factors or cultural belief systems. The doctor's final questions were addressed to these organic concerns:

> Doctor (addressing father): Physical growth was ok? Was she thin or short for [*seriyana vazhantu vayasam*] her age?
> Father: A bit less than other kids.
> Doctor: Did she get her period at the age of twelve?
> Father: Not sure, but I think so.
> Doctor: What has been her response the past few years? Any sadness or suicide wishes? Was she consistently sad for several days?
> Father: She wasn't so depressed but did sleep excessively.
> Doctor: But what about the breaking of things? Why does she do this?
> Father: I have no idea or understanding [*teriyale, puriyale*].
> Doctor: Are the voices telling her to do this?
> Father: No.
> Doctor: Do you have a BPL card [Below Poverty Line]?[11]
> Patient or mother: [No response.]
> Father: No.

The father explained that the family was facing financial hardship. The father was a factory worker but the factory where he had worked had been shut down. They were from Hosur, within Tamil Nadu, on the Karnataka–Tamil Nadu border, but only an hour or less by bus to NIMHANS, depending upon traffic. Coming there was not a "huge hardship" for the family, he explained. This notwithstanding, the financial stress within the family undoubtedly contributed to their tensions and worries.

And we can probably surmise that the daughter's refusal to work, and the quarrels it caused with her father, were intensified by their financial need in the wake of his unemployment. In this sense, even if it was something Vasanthi lacked insight into, the predicament of industrialized labor and her father's precarity within it had, in turn, influenced the malevolence and "*seyvinai*" she experienced. The "not her" that spoke through her might have been an indirect means of dealing with the everyday violence of the social (i.e., economic insecurity and her failures to contribute to the financial security of the family, due to her cognitive limitations). Modernity's discontents were framed in terms of dark forces and betrayed (or thwarted) aspirations. But these, too, reflected the strong correlation between social violence, social defeat, poverty, and mental illness (Patel and Kleinman 2003; Luhrmann and Marrow 2016).

The doctor was concerned that the father understand Vasanthi's likely cognitive limitations, noting that she possessed slight physical abnormalities. Her stature was quite petite and she might have possessed slight "mongoloid features," he wondered aloud, suspecting something along the spectrum of Down syndrome. He asked of the father that the family do some genetic screening to see if anything turned up.

Of course, finding genetic markers could be very useful for patient treatment in some cases, so testing was often done, in addition to the functional treatment of illnesses. In this case, I suspected that the doctor was also trying to communicate to the father that their aspirations could and should be tempered by an organic understanding of Vasanthi's limitations; and, moreover, this was also an indirect way to defetishize the resonance of *seyvinai* beliefs, with their sometimes pernicious effects on patient accountability. That is, sorcery or possession could be indirect idioms of speaking to distress, without directly accusing family or other intimates of moral transgressions and ambivalent emotions (e.g., Nichter 1982; Kakar 1982; Obeyesekere 1981). The body, so to speak, is able to speak through its symptoms, in ways the voice could not, given the Law that anchors subjectivity (Lacan 1977) and must be obeyed, or the truth that must remain unspoken. But failed exorcisms could redouble stigma, rather than lessening it, leaving the patient facing the double jeopardy of lingering, troublesome, and unacceptable symptoms, on the one hand, and the failed morality of the person who cannot, or does not deserve to, find relief of the malevolent forces that claim them.

This subtle but deliberate intervention on the doctor's part struck me as very skillful and practiced, given many years of experience and knowledge of how the comorbid and complex interplay of psychosocial, cosmological, and bio-organic variables impacted upon each patient. And given the time constrictions of the OPD, doctors had to be practical and offer poignant, though fairly terse, advice to the patients and their families. In this case, he was, obviously to me, cognizant of the deeply rooted culture and yet very "personal" (in Obeyesekere's sense) nature of Vasanthi's predicament and illness presentation. But in the end, the organic and practical were designed, I felt, to cut like a knife against the cloud of uncertainty that emerged in the dialogue. Recall that many of the answers he received to his direct questions were simply, "No," or expressed a complete lack of understanding in terms the psychiatrist would recognize as having insight. While extended family and psychotherapy, particularly of a psychodynamic kind, might have unpacked and deconstructed the affect of generalized suspicion and "dark" forces, particularly as familial dynamics were better understood, he focused on more modest, but most likely more feasible, interventions. This, in practical terms, was to reduce her dosage of olanzapine from 20 mg to a slightly lower dose, in hopes this would make her less lethargic, sleepy, and "slow" to respond to others. He also advised the family to increase Vasanthi's "physical activities" and encouraged her to "help her mother more around the house." Her social skills also had to be cultivated, he urged the father.

It will be recalled that she did not hear the voices when talking with others. These voices were her own thoughts, now verbalized from an elsewhere. But excessive rumination, which, clearly in this case, was harmful, could be circumvented through a more active and socially interactive life. Finally, it will be recalled too that her own thoughts could be heard by others, which, thus, is symptomatically symmetrical to the voices being her own thoughts. In either case, she didn't trust her own thoughts as they were infected by the Other's overhearing, hypostatization, and materialization through their vocalization back to herself. The interiority and exteriority of her thoughts, vis-à-vis a demonological supplement, revealed a doubling at the heart of her sense of self, somewhat akin to the "poison" and "remedy" intrinsic to the "pharmakon" that is exteriority in Derrida's analysis of written text (1981). That is, to experience being "infected" by an "outside" through writing, an exterior source of presence, belies its origins from an "inside" or interiority that always already necessitates an exteriority to sustain itself through difference. The exteriority marked by this threat is thus acting as a supplement, or archive, to reimagine an interiority uncorrupted by the external. This symptomatic obsession is more clearly seen in the last case of this chapter.

Ramesh, a young man perhaps in his late twenties or early thirties, came with his mother to the OPD. He was articulate, talkative, and inquisitive. Ramesh asked me where I was from, and when I said the US, he mentioned that he had lived there for five years. Boldly, I thought at the time, he immediately stated that Americans were "much better behaved outwardly" than Indians were. Indians, Ramesh said, "would cut the queue and not follow rules." But Indians would not "hurt the heart," though their outward behavior was "rude." That is, outward behavior and inward intentions were not always aligned or transparent, he suggested. The relevance of this statement only became clear a bit later.

Ramesh's doctor made some general inquiries as to how he was doing, as he was returning for a follow-up from earlier treatment. His mother complained about his "compulsions," which to her seemed unreasonable. Ramesh would counter with statements that were disparaging and sharply critical of her. He told his doctor that he was "studying Tamil and law online," and found these things "interesting." It seems he had felt cheated in the family business by his employees and was learning the law to deal with this. The doctor, in turn, inquired whether it was necessary to "go to these lengths" to deal with "minor cheaters" in the workplace. Moreover, Ramesh seemed to connect seemingly unrelated phenomena, such as the need to study law in depth with the small-scale cheating of some employees who were skimming bits of profit in the family business. His study of Tamil came, it was revealed by Ramesh, with an intense devotion to mastering some old religious texts and his desire to "go deeper" into Vaishnavism (worship of God as Vishnu) through its literature.[12] Though not a Tamil, he was a devout Hindu.

The doctor asked Ramesh and his mother whether his acts were "impulsive or well thought out." He asked further whether he made all his decisions alone or took account of what others thought or did. In so doing, he emphasized that some semblance of "family harmony" was essential. It was becoming clear to me that Ramesh had a history of being combative with his mother and father. The mother exclaimed that Ramesh had told his father that he "was just waiting for him to die." When the doctor asked how he could speak to anyone like this, much less his own father, Ramesh answered that as "everyone is going to die, it was not anything wrong." There was reasoning in this, as he invoked Indian philosophical notions of transience and non-attachment. In this context, however, this seemed less pious and, at least to the mother and his doctor, as hollow and cruel.

The doctor explained that it was important that he learn to have close friends and family bonds. Ramesh replied, "Guruji is close to me." This was in reference to having a close confidant to discuss problems with. But his doctor tried to explain that the "Guruji" was different, as he was a guide but not a close confidant, friend, or family member. Ramesh countered, saying that, in fact, his guru was very close to him and cared for him intensely. Therefore, he could discuss "anything with him."

The doctor was worried that his frames of reference seemed to come from a rigorous if not overly legalistic mindset. While the literal father had flaws, his spiritual father was perfect, all-knowing, wise, and loving. This perfect oracle could be trusted, while the more human father could not. People, more generally, were untrustworthy and could compromise his sense of self. There was, indeed, hypervigilance regarding his own ego. This manifested in being overly critical of others as well as taking offense very easily. It meant he would always search for the flaw in the other with legalistic zeal for vengeance.

While my impression was that Ramesh might be a "hysteric" or "borderline personality" who, while not psychotic, had trouble relating to people, he had, in fact, elaborate delusions and a psychosis that was fairly well controlled with medications. At one point, echoing the "Truman Show syndrome," discussed earlier in the chapter, he felt that the massive Howrah Station (train station) in Calcutta was an elaborate "set" that was made to watch and observe him. But to unpack his delusions, and perhaps understand his personal etiology to some extent, his unhappy life in the US as a student is critical.

Ramesh was quite brilliant and had gone to study at a major research university in the US as a mathematics and physics PhD student. Remarkably, he was admitted when he wrote a letter explaining to the United States–based university that he was "bored" at the highly competitive and ranked Indian Institute of Technology, where he was studying at the time. The faculty he wrote to at the university, intrigued, asked for his dossier/portfolio, and upon examining his work discovered that he was indeed quite brilliant. But while he was studying in the United States, an undercover FBI informant had entrapped him by offering to help him get a fake ID. Ramesh had hoped that with this counterfeit ID (it was not clear whether he knew it would be fake) he could stay on and work in the university library for a while upon graduation. When he was caught in this dragnet he was forced to leave the country, but not before he was arrested and put in jail. When the local district attorney and his appointed lawyer, however, saw how he had been set up, and also that he was not on any list of terror suspects, he was released and charges were dropped, provided he left the country. Therefore, he came back to India, but he understandably became more distrustful of others after this subterfuge. It was not known, however, whether he had already suffered extensive delusions or paranoia while living abroad, before the arrest.

Regarding his religiously "orthodox" and legalistic interpretations, it seems Ramesh followed astrological beliefs and calculations to the letter (and number) and believed that the stories about Lord Krishna—for instance, when he lifted a mountain to save a village (a popular myth)—were actual historical events. His obsessive literalness regarding religious ideas translated also into his handling of the family business, where he prosecuted all and anybody who would even slightly cheat on the factory floor. The slightest infractions incurred his wrath, we were told.

In a sense, Ramesh appeared to be neurotic, rather than psychotic, at least in Freud's and Lacan's understanding, having internalized and fully identified with the symbolic "figure of the Law" (Lacan 1981; 1977). That is, his absolutism was absolute. Truth was unambiguous and literal. His sense of the law or truth was not tempered with reflexivity, an appreciation of grey zones or indeterminacy, or conscience. Rather, it was a mechanistic reality that he grasped on to in order to structure his life. This was legalism wedded to grandiosity, fueled by the rage of betrayal, and overlaid with cosmic significance. His grandiosity was fueled, too, by his intimacy with an all-perfect father, his "Guruji" (Kakar 1982). His guru, his faith, and his fervent study of the law established his categorical understanding of human nature, incapable of nuance, appropriate context recognition, and living within the grey, where creativity and compromise go hand in hand. As in the "buccal ethics" (Guyer 2007; Ghassem-Fachandi 2012) described earlier, he could not swallow both the good and bad within the object of the Other, but had to spit out the poisons of the world. His "pharmakon" (Derrida 1981) was truly a "gift," in his inability, in this instance, to swallow its concomitant "poison." But this slowly working poison worked from within the gift to enact his delusions and paranoia. In this case, his "archive fever" (Derrida 1995), while acting as a supplement, could not defer self-judgement indefinitely, as his delusions claimed more feverish control over Ramesh over time.

The preeminent Indian psychoanalyst Sudhir Kakar theorized (1981; 1982) that a wounded sense of self results in a form of secondary narcissism, following Heinz Kohut, in the Indian context in which larger-than-life heroes, such as gurus, film stars, and politicians, are put on excessively high pedestals. Intense identification with a perfect leader in turn nurtures a weakly formed sense of self, he argued. But any threat to that perfected "father" or "mother" figure is perceived as the gravest of insults. Kakar locates this affective lure of the great hero in the common childhood experiences of Indians, in which a prolonged period of intimacy, particularly between mothers and sons, is rather suddenly interrupted, resulting in a particularly traumatic narcissistic wound. The adoration of heroes, and indeed, identification with them, he argued, is rooted in a longing for this lost intimacy and the feelings of boundlessness and grandiosity that, once experienced, were lost through individuation. Kakar uses this psychodynamic model of object relations to explain why the slightest of insults to the idealized leader causes intolerable outrage and despair among their followers, as the latter's identity has been fused with the former as compensation for the lack inaugurated by the narcissistic wound. Kakar later (1996) extended this argument to explain communal attachments, and the violent boundaries that have been forged in modern times between, in particular, Hindus and Muslims. To Kakar, the narcissistic wounds have become increasingly conjoined with the anomie (following Durkheim) fostered by modern life, as well as the rationalizations and singularities demanded by corporate identities, or what we have called, following Anderson, the "bound" and "serialized" identity structures facilitated by bureaucratic measurement and the subsequent rationalizations of identity these entail, with their alienating consequences (Hansen 2001; Willford 2018; Taneja 2018; Zizek 1993; Appadurai 2000).

In the case of Ramesh, we do not see him calling for preemptive violence or communal discord directed at any corporate identity. But a similar structural logic seemed to be in operation: threats and enemies must be prosecuted to protect the "truth" and righteousness, more generally. But this righteousness is legalistic and mechanistic, much like the boundaries wrought by reformist movements that sought to attenuate the more fluid and protean cultural boundaries between Hindus and Muslims, Sufis and Wahhabis within the Muslim lifeworld, or charismatic Christians versus a Catholic form of Christian adaptation to South Asian culture. In the political context of contemporary Bangalore, as was the case in many urban centers within the country, doctors sometimes emphasized that "fascistic tendencies" were on the rise, producing or exacerbating, as we have witnessed, fractured and wounded identities. In the case of Ramesh, his latent fractures were possibly exacerbated by the foreign trauma and the profound sense of betrayal and distrust that gushed forth from it.

More broadly, the doctors sometimes told me that a fear of difference, of minorities, and a generalized sense of menace from a mysterious Other, was increasingly seen conjoined to other clinical symptoms. Even NIMHANS itself, as an institution, was not spared the consequences of identity boundary-making, or serialization. Though it was a national or federal institution during the height of the pro-Kannada movement in the late 1980s and early 1990s (Willford 2018; Nair 2005), patients from outside of the state who did not know Kannada had trouble with the intake interviews and registration forms when coming for care. The forms were written exclusively in Kannada, which had been mandated by the state government at the time.[13] Doctors, however, lobbied successfully to remove this barrier to care, with its apparent discrimination against locals and non-locals alike. Bangalore, a polyglot city with almost equivalent numbers of Kannada, Telugu, and Tamil speakers, and situated close to the tri-state borders of Karnataka, Andhra Pradesh, and Tamil Nadu, had many patients visiting NIMHANS from all three states, as well as numerous other parts of the country. As a recognized national center, language restrictions would have greatly impacted the quality of care for non-Kannada speakers.

* * *

To conclude this chapter, it is important to remember that the serious and debilitating nature of the symptoms examined in these cases cannot be reduced to the psychosocial strains caused by modern life. In every case, though with slight differences, we have witnessed significant delusions, hallucinations, and cognitive impairments. As it turned out, bipolar disorder and schizophrenia ran in Ramesh's family, as we had also seen in other cases examined where genetics likely also played a role. While my focus has been to point to shared themes as they related to predicaments of modern life, particularly the social and cultural strains brought on by rationalization and reform, I am not arguing for a radical constructivism that mental illness is simply a sociocultural construct. To do so would romanticize the resistance and suffering that each patient seemed to be enduring, with, at times, catastrophic consequences to themselves and their families. I have tried to convey the various doctors' concerns with the psychosocial factors, which, perhaps, were amplified by my presence, knowing my disciplinary lens. Despite the emphasis on the psychosocial, the psychiatrists at NIMHANS, as discussed earlier, were fully committed to the organic, genetic, and neuropsychiatric dimensions of mental illness. However, their collective concern with the psychosocial was marked, and belied a concern with the increasingly narrow training of specialists in the country (Ruddock 2021), at the expense of more humanistic and social scientific approaches to understanding society's ills.

This chapter aimed to accomplish an understanding of a continuum of effects associated with the excessive hold of identity or a singular imaginary that creates or is created by legalistic demarcations of right and wrong, self and other, collective and individual. In some cases, we have seen the aspirations of the patient constricted by the reformist and legalistic mindset of modern ethnoreligious boundaries. In other cases, we have seen the possessive force of singular, serialized, and rigid boundary-making, leading to cosmological dualism between good and evil, right and wrong. In both instances, the capacity to live with nuance and a creative existence within grey zones of indeterminacy was constricted. The attenuation of more protean and fluid lifeworlds, conjoined to latent psychiatric vulnerabilities, proved disabling, indeed, malevolent. In the case of reform and religious purification, we have seen how aspirations, particularly of women, rendered them "mad" or "bad." But we have also observed the emergence of a totalizing mindset with a rigid love of the law take root in several of these clinical encounters. These rigidities in turn are buttressed by the dangers of "betrayal," which arguably form the archives and supplements of difference that are further damaging to the social fabric of the family and wider community. The key link, perhaps, between the psychiatric symptoms and the excessive boundaries generated by the themes of betrayal, the Law, and ethnoreligious constructs, is a social and, perhaps, legalistic demand towards some kind of impossible and categorical singularity (Hansen 2001; Kakar 1996; Aretxaga 2018; Willford 2014; 2018; Derrida 1995).

I would suggest going one step further: that the biological aspects of psychopathology induce the aporia or absence of agency characteristic of an overwhelming force overtaking the individual, exacerbating the need, symptomatic though it is, of supplementary meanings and identities. In this organic vulnerability, or fractious psychic wound, the suggestibility of a demand takes on added resonance (Malabou 2012). In that sense, the doctors seemed committed to a biocultural psychiatry (Kleinman 2012; Patel and Kleinman 2003; Cohen 2012; Gomez-Carrillo, Kirmayer, et al. 2023).

These categorical demands for singularity, of course, are buttressed by bureaucracy and material relations of power. However, against a power-centric reading,[14] in which "illness" is the mere thinking of power, we take note that the demand for singularity betrays insecure origins and is ultimately unstable. As Appadurai (2000) has cogently suggested, "dead certainty" paradoxically takes root in moments of greatest social and existential uncertainty. While this chapter has focused upon religious and quasi-religious themes of malevolence, the ghostly, and thwarted aspirations by various types of social betrayal, we can witness the salience of these themes where the emphasis and illness presentations are different, yet the singular pressures of conformity and normalization overlap with the more cosmological, leaving the stigmas of difference countered by the forces of rebellion and depression.

Chapter 4

Living with Urban Stress

Anxiety, IT, and Burnout in the New Economy

Previous chapters have focused on familial stress, stigma, and the cosmological emphasis upon the polarizing singularities that increasingly mark identities under stress. We have explored the fissures and predicaments of care and abandonment, as well as the symptoms that are anchored by sentiments of betrayal. Moreover, I have suggested that the occluding of grey zones, where ambiguity can be tolerated, in favor of an absolutism where identities are categorical, is both a reflection of the political serialization of identities as well as a symptom of its inner logic, or a kind of madness within the political that is heightened within the psychopathologies witnessed at the clinic. In this chapter, we extend this idea, and examine how the singularities and monotonies caused by the routines of urban life and work also make intolerable demands upon those caught up in the maelstrom of the informational economy and its increasing bureaucratization of experience.

As in the classic arguments of anomie (Durkheim), "one-dimensional life" (Marcuse 1964), and the "iron cage" (Weber), we see a flattening of experience and a loss of anchored social moorings, or a machinic routinization and its dehumanizing impact as manifested within the clinic. Stress, furthermore, had both physical and psychological comorbidities, being exacerbated within bio-social bodies (Cohen 2012). Moreover, we conclude by considering how doctors faced with the epidemic of stress are increasingly wary of the routinization of their craft, whereby the pharmaceutical palliative is offered for symptomatic relief but the underlying stress is left unaddressed by the medicalizing discourse of psychiatry, with its increasing neurological and psychopharmacological orientation. This, to many doctors, is a question not only of sound and ethical medical practice but also a question of advocacy and human rights.

One dimension of mental health care that remains critical for those who cannot or choose not to access psychiatric care remains traditional forms of healing. This chapter also considers, in brief, how yoga and faith-based healing fit into the overall medical pluralism and systems that provide care. Many individuals with mental health issues, particularly those of little material means, either choose to go to or are left by desperate families at healing shrines. Among the popular shrines are *dargahs*, which are tombs for Sufi saints that often attract those believed to be possessed by malignant beings that contribute to madness. We will visit two such shrines that draw, among devotees, people thought to be mentally ill and/or possessed.

When reviewing the multitude of cases I witnessed within NIMHANS, the majority of patients were working-class or poor. These patients utilize the subsidized health care system in India, finding generally high-quality care at a major center for research and treatment (Ruddock 2021). While structural violence was part of the social fabric that brought them to psychiatric care, or in some cases delayed it, the kinds of care that many received was palliative, and sometimes normalizing, as we have seen. Moreover, the doctors oftentimes expressed regret that their interventions, even when ostensibly efficacious at symptom reduction, did not alter the underlying structural dynamics within the family, community, and economic conditions. A smaller number of cases, however, were of professional, middle- and lower-middle-class individuals working within the fast-paced information technology sector, of which Bangalore was a leading center within India (Nair 2005; Willford 2018; Gupta and Mankekar 2017). The alienating effects of routinized data-driven careers were manifested in "burnout," fatigue, and depression, as well as in a number of somatic complaints. Workplace deadlines and the "bottom line" thinking of management were often noted with dread by those suffering from this burnout. Moreover, I was often told by doctors at NIMHANS that suicide rates in Bangalore were very high by national and global standards.

The explanations usually offered for this high suicide rate pointed towards the anomic side of urban life. That is, as many were drawn to the city from smaller towns and villages in search of professional opportunities, they lived in dormitories or flats, away from networks of social support. Loneliness and feelings of social disconnect thus combined with the monotony of a repetitive job. Call centers were, and continue to be, a large presence in the city's workforce. Many who were drawn to the city were, therefore, strong in English-language skills, and were lured by the promise of upward mobility through the information economy. Not only were these jobs oftentimes dead-end positions, either entering data or making calls to international clients, but they also had long hours, mostly during the night shift, so as to reach Europe and North America during work hours. Upward mobility within these call centers was oftentimes nonexistent, and the work conditions often grueling with poor pay. Rather than being valued as high-skilled employees, as they had been promised, they performed in automaton-like labor lines, with the product being assembled data services rather than machine parts (see Upadhya and Vasavi 2008; Nair 2005; Mankekar and Gupta 2017). At least two or three stories per week would emerge in the local print and electronic media about the "mental health crisis" that was emerging within this rootless and alienated community (Lang 2018). Addiction and depression were oftentimes the primary symptoms discussed in these media forums.

Let us consider a few cases related to "IT burnout" to highlight the wider range of issues that were at play, pointing also to the larger cultural shifts that were impacting upon peoples' lives in urban India. These cases also intersect with those already discussed but show more emphasis on the workplace demands upon identity than upon the familial and kinship-related stigmas and shame we have seen. Indeed, the more a part of the urban and educated classes one belonged to, the lesser the reluctance to speak about mental illness among patients and their family members.

Stress and Illness

Arun, a thirty-year-old male, came with his wife to the OPD complaining of memory problems. He quarreled often with his wife and was, as a result, receiving "cognitive training" (which included CBT) at NIMHANS as a form of psychotherapy. Arun was a software engineer and had a very stressful job at a leading information technology company. The stress of the job, coupled with a poor diet, had led to a heart attack in 2011, four years before I met him in the clinic. As a result of his heart attack, he had suffered damage to his memory and cognition. After six months of cognitive behavioral therapy Arun was feeling reasonably well, though he needed to "train" again in his line of work. He was now back at his company, but was doing some "basic training" to assume a much more modest position within the organization. To the credit of his employer, they supported his desire to return to work, even though it meant a demotion.

Arun's mental function appeared to be impacted still by the heart attack. He spoke slowly and responded slowly when spoken to. His body movements also appeared to be slow. Arun, however, was quick to criticize his wife when she requested information from the doctor about cognitive behavioral therapy and various medications that were prescribed. He had become "argumentative" since the heart attack, the wife explained, out of frustration with his memory problems. This was not a case of burnout or job dissatisfaction, but rather pointed to the consequences of a stressful job within a leading IT company. Arun's agitation and depression, however, were an indirect consequence of his job, as it had led to his cognitive injury. That he wanted, after all this, to return to work rather than leave this world behind, I found puzzling. It was as if, though his cognitive capacity would not allow for his prior high-status position, his sense of professional identity was still bound up with the brand he once worked hard for. This singularity of identity undoubtedly also added pressure and, apparently, agitation to his rehabilitation process.

Sampath was a young software engineer with severe depression. I had met him prior to his clinical interview in the ward, where he had been admitted due to "suicidal ideation." Sampath was still warded, but wanted to be discharged as soon as possible, he explained to the doctor in the OPD. His physical signs of severe depression included a flat expression and slow movements, though his cognitive abilities appeared to be fine. In addition to the severe depression, he devalued himself by comparing himself to others who were more successful, focusing particularly upon his siblings.

Sampath's depression and his reduced initiative were strongly related, the doctor felt. Moreover, Sampath said that the CBT that had been tried at NIMHANS "did not work." He felt as depressed as before, and perhaps even more so for having "failed" even in this. It seems that Sampath had been surrounded by "strong people" most of his life and felt a deep sense of inadequacy. His wife accompanied him to the session. In the clinic, she expressed anxious worry over her husband's "bad turn" and apparent hopelessness.

But Sampath said he simply wanted to be discharged after "two years of continuous treatment." While he had not been warded for two years, he had evidently been treated for his depression for this lengthy period, with the symptoms gradually increasing, despite treatment. Electroconvulsive therapy (ECT) had been conducted four times, and he had tried various medications. But Sampath said he had "no relief" after all this. On the one hand, he was very angry and frustrated that nothing was helping him; on the other hand, he felt even more upset that he was told he "needs to participate and initiate more in therapy work." Evidently, he was largely passive in psychotherapy. As a result, he felt he was being blamed for his failure to participate in his recovery.

At one point, Sampath cried in the meeting and said he would "just like to end it" (meaning his life). The doctor immediately interrupted this proclamation and emphatically said, "No, no!" But the doctor did not indicate that he would discharge Sampath. When Sampath said he was "more anxious and depressed after therapy," the doctor said that anxiety can be a "positive sign of progress" being made towards recovery. This made a lot of sense from a psychodynamic perspective. Freudian theory predicts that the closer to a breakthrough one came, presumably the stronger the resistance would be. The doctor, though not a psychoanalytic-oriented doctor, was invoking this idea, perhaps to encourage Sampath's participation, as well as to reduce his sense of failure for having made little noticeable progress. But in this case, Sampath did not show insight on his part that would suggest any movement, let alone improvement, in his condition. Rather, a vortex of hopelessness was palpable and impossible to escape, even for a moment of levity. There were no smiles, jokes, or hopes expressed by Sampath, or by his wife, who sat silently by his side. The only wish or desire expressed was, indeed, to terminate care and, perhaps, life. But Sampath was eventually compelled to continue with the psychotherapy and asked to return in a couple of weeks. A noticeable look of concern on the doctor's face betrayed his expressed confidence in the psychotherapeutic treatment he prescribed and asked the patient to trust. Sampath was nowhere close to being out of risk for self-harm at this point, despite the long-term care he received.

While young professionals are not the primary clientele at NIMHANS, I witnessed a high enough percentage of them in the OPD to warrant the observation that the stress of working in Bangalore's hypercompetitive IT industry was exacting a toll on many young people. Heightened expectations for professional success were tempered by the reality of social immobility in a city that is extremely expensive to live in; this was conjoined to a profound loneliness and alienation, as many of its young workers were living cut off from sources of emotional support. Sampath at least had the obvious care and attention of his wife, as well as the attention of the accomplished medical team at the hospital. Many in the lower echelons of the IT industry were less lucky.

Bala, a thirty-seven-year-old mid-level manager in a local IT company, came to the OPD one day with serious and recurrent depression. Like Sampath, the symptoms had started years earlier. Bala had previously suffered significant episodes in the past fifteen years prior to his visit on this day. On his own volition, he had reduced his antidepressant medication from 150 mg to 75 mg. But he had a lot of stress at work, he explained, which culminated in the development of an ulcer. He claimed, however, that he was "doing well" on the lesser dose of antidepressant. To manage his stress better, Bala practiced Ashtanga yoga,[1] and did better, he claimed, when he was "disciplined about the yoga." He claimed to do two hours of yoga each morning before work, which surprised the doctor, and pleasantly so. This practice involved some breathing and posture exercises. After three months of yoga, he felt his stress was abating.

Bala did not have personal financial worries, or at least claimed he did not have any. But he said he hates having to "lay off people at work." This caused him a lot of stress. At the time of this visit to the OPD, he had suffered a recent recurrence of the "severe depression" after dropping his antidepressant dosage to 50 mg. He had, apparently, even tried dropping it down to 25 mg, believing the yoga was more effective than the drugs.

The ulcer, which Bala said was a result of work stress that year, had caused him to seek out a lifestyle change, prompting him to redouble his efforts in yoga. He was also taking homeopathy to help with the ulcer. But Bala was reluctant to go back on the higher dose of the antidepressant for fears that he would not "have the energy to wake up early and do yoga." The doctor convinced him, or at least attempted to do so, that a "minimal therapeutic dosage" was necessary. The doctor said that Bala may be fine with 75 mg, rather than the original 150 mg that had been prescribed, but that 50 mg was "too low." Bala, for his part, expressed worry about the continued use of medication, and possible long-term side effects. The doctor, however, told him that, like in other "chronic conditions where medicine is required, the benefits outweigh the risks." Bala nodded in response to the doctor, but the question of compliance hung in the air, animating the doctor's advice, knowing that his patient had already proven willing to adjust medications on his own. Before Bala left the OPD, the doctor also mentioned that he wanted to check for "autoimmune thyroiditis," because this, too, could cause depression.

At the time, I recall thinking that the doctor's armory included, of course, knowledge about the therapeutic levels of various medications required to ward off recurrences of illness. At the same time, Bala exhibited resistance and skepticism that biomedical psychiatry offered a long-term solution to his stress-related illnesses. His turn to yoga and homeopathy were of his own self-healing agency, as was his experimentation with reducing his dosage. That he was committed to self-healing through lifestyle changes was undoubtedly a positive step, and met with some approval. But in being reminded to maintain a "therapeutic" dosage level, given Bala's recent setbacks with depression, coupled with the test for thyroid function, the doctor was reasserting biomedical authority over his skeptical patient, in effect asking Bala to trust his medical judgement.

In contrast to Sampath, Bala was taking the initiative, but perhaps in excess, from the doctor's perspective. Whereas Sampath was cynical or critical to the extent that he offered passive resistance to his psychotherapy, Bala's resistance was to the highly specific pharmaceutical treatment he received, though both men, from English-speaking and middle-class backgrounds, harbored skepticism about the expert knowledge of biomedicine. This concern over the side effects of medications is also seen in the following case.

David, a male patient in his thirties, English-educated and a software programmer and consultant, suffered a complex partial seizure following a high fever.[2] As a result of his seizure, he was taking anticonvulsants, but as a side effect of the medication, he said he had feelings of "numbness" in his fingers. His "primary issues" were hypertension and seizures, though there were signs that he had manic episodes and insomnia.

David had periods of "excitement" that would come and go. During these periods he worked excessively long hours. But he also was "stressed out" when manic, and could not sleep well for days. After a period of rest, he said he was "usually fine." But one manic period that lasted six months led to extreme exhaustion and stress. This, in turn, affected his blood pressure, and made him more vulnerable to cold and flu viruses. His fever was a result of this exhaustion.

Because of the deadlines he faced in his line of work, David often would work later than he had to, beyond the scope and expectations of his "official" work hours. He did so, he said, on account of "needing to finish projects." Moreover, with the traffic being as bad as it was in Bangalore, he also wanted to leave the office after the evening rush hours. David lived in another part of town that could take an hour or more to reach during rush hours, but only twenty minutes or so if there was no traffic.

David, like Bala, was trying to practice yoga to relax. The doctor reminded him that he needed to find a balance between "work and leisure." Doctors, in fact, oftentimes suggested yoga as a de-stressing method that could be an effective adjunct to whatever medications were prescribed. There was no conflict between yoga and biomedicine in that sense. But, as in the previous case of Bala, there was a skepticism about the deleterious effects of long-term use of pharmaceuticals, and a trend towards AYUSH as well as spiritual healers among the educated middle classes in urban India (Halliburton 2009; Langford 2002; Kakar 1982; Ecks 2013). These trends notwithstanding, David was told to continue the anticonvulsant and blood pressure medications. David worried, however, about the effect on his kidneys that these medicines could have. Moreover, it was not clear whether he had had only the one febrile seizure associated with the fever, in which case he did not have epilepsy. The psychiatrist deferred to the neurologist on this question and advised David to continue the medications until instructed otherwise.

As in the previous cases of Bala and Sampath, the relentless pace of urban life, its deadlines, stress, but also the monotony, perhaps, seemed to contribute to a kind of burnout. In David's case, one of the consequences of the information economy was the expectation that projects and deadlines superseded scheduled work. This was not in any way a unique situation, as global high-tech workers, and even academics, routinely think of their labor in terms of product outputs, not hourly labor. In the Bangalore context, the high stress of success, without, in many cases, an emotional support system, made these workers' lives precarious, though in a very different way, obviously, than those of the working class and poor. David, Bala, and Sampath, though different in many ways, were running on the fumes of stress within the new economy. The question of leading a "balanced" life was always in the forefront of their minds; and, at least, in the case of David and Bala, there were attempts to push back at technocracy through a perhaps healthy resistance to the biomedical psychiatric solution, as they perceived it. The doctors, far from being against traditional methods of stress management, were encouraged by this initiative, and equally concerned, in the case of Sampath, where it was absent. But they were also insistent that psychiatric treatment continue. Indeed, after David had left the room, the possibility was raised by the doctor that he might be bipolar (BPAD), though, in the doctors words, and in David's self-description of his symptoms, his episodes were "very brief." His six-month episode stood out as a warning sign of mania, as did his periods of insomnia, which left him exhausted and subject to the other illnesses that might have induced his febrile seizure. And this session in the OPD left unresolved the question of epilepsy. If epilepsy was diagnosed, then comorbid BPAD symptoms were not uncommon. But taking the patient's concerns first and foremost, it was also clear that his stress levels were a direct result of his occupation within the increasingly stressful urban environment (Srinivas 2018).

Anxiety over work and deadlines not only led to burnout but could also lead to panic attacks and dissociative states. One afternoon, Madhu, a man in his early forties, presented in the OPD with early onset bipolar symptoms. He suffered anxiety attacks that immobilized him. Madhu had recently moved back from California with his young wife and child to work in the IT sector in Bangalore. Prior to this, he had worked in Silicon Valley. Beginning a decade earlier, Madhu had suffered heart attack–like symptoms in California. He consulted with a neurologist there who suspected a seizure disorder. He was put on sodium valproate, a common anticonvulsant, which could also serve as a mood stabilizer. Madhu, though the suspected seizure disorder had led to his prescription, was never diagnosed with epilepsy. But while taking the sodium valproate, his heart attack–like symptoms had stopped. And when he stopped the medicine, the attacks came back. The psychiatrist at NIMHANS suspected anxiety or panic attacks were occurring, not epileptic seizures. His primary diagnosis at this time was BPAD.

Madhu was particularly concerned about the occurrence of a sudden anxiety attack while at work or elsewhere, outside the house. During these attacks, he felt he must "do something right away" to "drive" the anxiety away. Alternatively, he would shut himself into a room in his house until the attack subsided. These attacks could last minutes or hours. Madhu's wife accompanied him to the clinic and appeared to be very supportive.

Two days prior to the OPD visit, he had suffered a "massive attack." During this time, he felt he "would go mad." When asked what he feared the most by the doctor, he said "losing control." Therefore, he isolated himself during the attack so that he did not run amok, which is what he feared the most. Interestingly, he said that driving his car calmed him. Thus, on the weekends he liked to take a country drive, finding this relaxed him. But he avoided driving in the city with its relentless, chaotic, and heavy traffic. Indeed, he feared having one of his "attacks" while stuck in a traffic jam.

It was not clear what role, if any, being back in India played to contribute to, or mitigate against, Madhu's anxiety. But he had suffered a road accident before his illness had set in. I wondered, and imagined the doctor did as well, based on his careful query, about a PTSD effect from the accident. I had seen similar anxieties at NIMHANS in other patients who had suffered accidents. His "relaxing" self-therapy of driving country roads, I imagined, could have been an attempt to master the trauma through repetition. As in the case of other phobias, oftentimes the best treatment was not to avoid the phobic object but rather to work through it. Madhu's fear of driving in the city suggested the trauma was alive and at work in causing his panic attacks.

It was not clear, in Madhu's case, whether work was a primary causal factor behind his panic attacks and anxiety. Madhu lived in a wealthy area of town, appeared to be firmly placed within the middle class, and had worked overseas within the burgeoning Silicon Valley bubble economy. His return to Bangalore would have come with high expectations and, one could imagine, high stress levels. Transnational existence, as we have seen, poses its own stressful conditions. Sometimes, these concern family separations and the concomitant anxieties these produce. What has not been discussed much in the literature, or within the clinical context, is the stress associated with moving back to the homeland after adjusting to life abroad, particularly with the kinds of expectations that such a move might present, either at work or at home (Chua 2014). Being abroad, particularly within the prestigious information economy, might raise the specter of failure upon returning home precisely because it sets up an expectation of great success.

Concerning Madhu's BPAD diagnoses, there was little said about it. While anxiety attacks could be a part of this diagnosis, the primary symptoms of mania coupled with depression were less evident. Perhaps the mania and depression were relatively controlled by the sodium valproate, despite the panic attacks and his persistent anxiety that these could occur at any moment. The question of epilepsy remained unresolved as well, though from the description of Madhu's symptoms, these anxiety attacks appeared to be psychogenic and not epileptic. It is not uncommon, after all, for hysteria-like symptoms to be mistakenly identified as seizures. At this point, no EEG evidence was part of Madhu's psychiatric file to confirm epilepsy. Therefore, the doctor ordered an MRI to establish a baseline, and to see if there were any abnormalities related to his earlier accident. Madhu was told that a new MRI should be done every five years to see if there were any changes occurring.

Madhu's case left many questions unresolved. There were many other cases where the symptomatology and presentation of illness were ambiguous, though pointing to various modern stress factors associated with urban life, mobility, and the expectations and aspirations of young Indians. Transnational and national mobilities for work were often stress-inducing, as were the family separations they often caused (Chua 2014; Upadhya and Vasavi 2008). Moreover, it was not the case that the repetitive work of IT was always to blame for the stress and burnout that some experienced in the city. The following cases point to the anxieties of mobility associated with the economic transformations that are driving more migrants to the megacities of India.

Anxieties of Mobility

Amarjit, a pregnant woman in her early twenties from the Punjab, came one morning to the OPD with her mother and cousin, who said they were concerned about her anger and excessive fears. Her mother said she was increasingly fearful of Amarjit's aggression. The young woman's symptoms of fear and aggression began to crest four years earlier. At that point she had stopped psychiatric treatment, leading to the "tantrums" that were largely directed at the mother.

Despite Amarjit's problems, a marriage proposal was arranged for her three years earlier, though she herself was "not interested in it." Around this time she was treated again for her aggressive behavior. Prior to her OPD visit this day, she was asymptomatic and again stopped treatment. At this point, she was married but her side of the family did not tell the husband's family about her bouts with mental illness.

Amarjit seemed to adjust to married life without too much difficulty, according to her mother. But then her husband was sent to the United States for work. After this, she suffered crying spells and went to stay with her mother, leaving her in-laws' house. In fact, she had insisted that her mother move to Mumbai to live with her. But upon her mother's arrival, Amarjit reported feeling "suffocated" at home. And she apparently showed "no interest in anything," according to the mother. Nonetheless, Amarjit felt a bit better after her mother's arrival.

Amarjit wanted a child and eventually became pregnant. Once she was pregnant, she became disinterested in her "household work" and began to have more crying spells. Amarjit said at the time that she "missed her father." At this point, while pregnant, she left her in-laws' house and husband, who had since returned to India, and moved back in with her natal family.

The in-laws and husband were now worried and suspicious about Amarjit's "mental illness" and sought out her medical records. But the woman's family was "not keen to give" these to the husband's family, fearing they could be used as legal grounds for divorce, citing deception on her family's part. Amarjit was not happy living with her in-laws and husband, but also fought with her mother at her mother's house. She was not sleeping much, and bouts of aggression were directed at the mother. At one point, she called her husband back and asked him to care for her. The husband then took her to a psychiatrist in the month prior to the OPD visit on this day. But she refused the treatment of this psychiatrist and said she did not "trust the doctor," or her husband, for that matter.

Amarjit had slapped her mother's face many times, suffered from daily crying spells, and was afraid of the dark. She would also wake others in the household after they had fallen asleep. Amarjit was said by her mother to sleep only three or four hours a night.

Her cousin, a woman around her age, who had also come to the OPD this day, lived in Bangalore, and also suffered from mental illness (schizophrenia), but had done well with proactive treatment of her illness. The cousin, the mother said, was "overly concerned with her own family." Still, the cousin wanted Amarjit to come and stay with her in Bangalore, particularly now as she was in the third trimester of her pregnancy and needed to be looked after. Amarjit, who had now received four years of intermittent psychiatric treatment, said that she felt "suffocated" in her cousin's house, and complained that there was not enough "water" in it. Moreover, the house was "smelly," Amarjit complained. Amarjit said that she "was fine in Ludhiana," in the Punjab, where she grew up. The cousin countered by saying that she felt fine there because "nobody will tell her" of her "bad" or odd behavior. There was also an incident that had occurred back when she was living with her family in Ludhiana in which she quarreled with a tenant that was staying with the family. This was pointed out by the cousin to counter Amarjit's claim that she was "fine" prior to marriage and moving. Amarjit, however, explained that "the tenant had not replied properly" when spoken to. Moreover, the fact that she had been aggressive with her mother prior to marriage suggested that significant emotional problems were pre-existent to her marriage, though the move to Mumbai might have exacerbated her symptoms, particularly when the husband had gone overseas, leaving her with her in-laws and, eventually, back in her mother's care.

Amarjit, in fact, claimed that she had "no problems with the in-laws," but "facts suggested otherwise," the NIMHANS doctor suggested. She refused to go and stay with them, "without reason," the doctor pointed out, perhaps hoping she would reveal more about her relationships within the household. The doctor pressed further, noting that there, in the in-laws' house, she would "not interact normally." Amarjit, the doctor pointed out, was not "engaged" with either the others in the house or with the household as a working unit. She was, according to her own mother, extremely forgetful, and would not interact much with her in-laws. One could sense that the mother wanted to defuse tensions with the in-laws, fearing that they would be compelled to seek a divorce. That neither the mother, cousin, nor Amarjit herself would lay blame on her in-laws was significant. Indeed, she had said she had "no problem" with them, yet she had called her mother to Mumbai.

The doctor asked Amarjit if she would be willing to stay in Bangalore with her husband in her cousin's house, particularly as this was the last trimester of her pregnancy. The cousin reported that she had a "strong fixation to certain days," meaning, I surmised, that the significance of certain dates seemed odd and obsessive. But what this signified in terms of the semiotics of her illness was unclear to me. The doctor did not query further into the question of fixation or obsessiveness. The doctor, however, asked if the in-laws were now aware of the mental illness. He also warned that after the delivery of the child there was a 30 percent chance of relapse into her psychosis. Therefore, being close to NIMHANS would be beneficial, as her treatment and general condition could be closely monitored. Amarjit's cousin then said she was aware of her cousin's illness "from many years back," and said she had become very demanding and simultaneously insecure.

The doctor thought Amarjit might be "mildly psychotic," but that the generalized mistrust that she expressed towards various family members might also suggest that the "social context axis" was complicated. He was convinced that there was something "off" with her that exceeded discomfort with her in-laws. Amarjit's conflicts with her mother had manifested earlier, prior to marriage, and the cousin seemed to notice things from an earlier age as well. Her fears of the dark, inability to sleep, and quarrelsome personality seemed to indicate to the doctor that a mild psychosis was present. Her lack of trust seemed to suggest possible schizophrenic traits. On the other hand, no "florid delusions" or hallucinations were reported that would confirm psychosis or schizophrenia. It was also clear that her social predicament was not ideal, given whatever psychiatric vulnerabilities she might have possessed. Whatever of her illness, if any, existed before in Ludhiana, she now felt the evaluative and negative gaze from all sides. Her "suffocating" at home seemed to confirm this notion. The one mention of her father in the OPD was only of missing him. The quarrels with the mother and the non-presence of the father in her symptomatology were intriguing, but not queried. Perhaps, the father was no longer living, and this detail had already been noted in her file by the resident who had performed the intake interview. In any event, Amarjit's symptoms seemed to worsen with mobility, at least as she perceived it. She claimed to be fine back in Ludhiana, but had suffered in Mumbai, and now in Bangalore. Moreover, her husband's work-related travel seemed to have also precipitated some very strong emotional reactions in Amarjit. These symptoms were not mitigated with the arrival and care of her mother, with whom her relationship was fraught, and perhaps more so than before her marriage. That her mother seemed to blame Amarjit, to some extent, for her inability to "engage" in the house of her husband's family perhaps also bothered Amarjit more than was apparent. Therefore, while we might be tempted to interpret her hostility to her mother in Oedipal (Elektra) terms, that is, as pertaining to her father, who was conspicuously absent in the discussion, it was also the case that her mother was "suffocating" her. The cause of this suffocation, be it in blaming Amarjit for her poor relations with the husband's family, or for forcing the mother to leave home and care for her, resulting in passive aggressiveness on the mother's part, meant the doctor's suspicions that the social axis was complicated and required more analysis seemed appropriate. Moreover, and as it pertains to the topic of this chapter, this complicated familial context was exacerbated by the mobilities of work and the geographic dispersal it forced upon familial relationships. Feelings of frustration and betrayal, if not outright fear, seemed to lay under the surface of these geographically induced or exacerbated tensions.

The tensions precipitated by geography and political as well as cultural boundaries were witnessed in earlier chapters in, for example, the cases of Ramesh (chapter 3) and Shanti (chapter 1). We will recall that Ramesh suffered a major blow while living in the United States, while finishing his studies in physics. The betrayal that saw him arrested had precipitated feelings of generalized betrayal, as well as obsessive religiosity and legalism. In Shanti's case, her delusions became acute while living in Canada with her husband, leading her to be sent back to her parents in India, and away from her husband and children. In both cases, a kind of dualistic and legalist struggle seemed to define their polarized universe. This was more pronounced in Ramesh's case, with his devotion to spirituality and the law matching his highly technical and, perhaps, engineer's sense of the truth as singular. He, we recall, categorically defined Indians versus Americans, and divided his social world into allies and enemies, based upon where they aligned on the truth to non-truth spectrum. This is to suggest that legalism was not only associated with the repetitive routines of IT work and life in the impersonal city. What I have called legalism, or a categorical attachment to "truth" and its concomitant inability to live with ambiguity, was a generalizing trend seen throughout the cases within the OPD, which we have witnessed in the normalizing efforts of family members to "fix" the problematic symptoms that called attention to the structural paradoxes and inequities of daily life, particularly associated with an increasing sense of malevolence. This broader ecology of malevolence, though sociocultural, combined with clinical vulnerabilities to produce "local bodies" (Cohen 2012) more prone to excessive literalism.

One interesting feature of transnational life, in both Shanti's and Ramesh's case, and to some extent, too, in Amarjit's case, discussed above, was the notion that "home" was a site of potential stability and calm, after the traumas of displacement. But in these cases, there really was no going back. Home became ambiguous, unhomely, and perhaps uncanny, and comfort was never obtained. And while it was probably the case that forms of, and vulnerabilities to, psychosis predated overseas or migratory life, the experiences of displacement seemed to make visible the crack lines in a more pronounced way.

Home, as Freud would always insist, was the site of the original trauma of selfhood and separation, and hence alienation. Traversing time and space in geographic terms seemed to usher a series of transferences and displacements that made symptoms more visible (Sarin and Jain 2018). The famous short story by Manto on the Partition, "Toba Tek Singh," we might recall from the introduction, captured the displacement perfectly that for the mentally ill there is no place that is home. And when the contingencies of borders and states, with their exclusionary violences, come into view, the illusion of home becomes ever more elusive.[3] The romance of home was, like the resistance of the modern and serialized, a stabilizing fantasy of self-containment and control. Yoga, excessive religiosity, and legalism seemed conjoined as forces that attempted to surmount the contingency and velocity of everyday urban existence (Cohen 1998). Even the doctors, sometimes, would look for anchoring devices that ritualized daily life, and could serve as a bellwether as to dysfunctional distress within families and between family members.

Moreover, urban stress and its velocities of movement were strangely at a standstill in those cases of burnout described earlier in the chapter. Routine and repetition were a kind of antidote, albeit a stultifying one, to the stresses of life. Madhu would counter the panic attacks with country drives, perhaps creating a routine to keep himself preoccupied—to literally drive away his anxiety with a kind of routine act. Moreover, in his case, the act of driving was also an attempt to master an earlier trauma. In some cases, routine and repetition seemed to open a doorway to deep depression and immobility, as in the cases of Arun and Sampath, discussed at the outset. Bala and Sampath, we will recall, resisted the medicalization of their symptoms through resistance to psychiatric medication, seeking alternative pathways to destress through yoga. This resistance to the everyday was also witnessed in Nalini's story (chapter 2), whereby her journalistic career of meeting deadlines was countered not only by bouts of depression but also by resistance to the everyday demands of family and work that she experienced as a single mother. In short, the stress factors of urban life, geographic traversals, and the repetitions and drudgery of work seemed to interact in various combinations, but always producing symptoms of anxiety, depression, and a kind of literalism that was extremely constricting for some, and a point of resistance to others.

In some of the cases, the relevance of Simmel's (1971) classic essay, "The Metropolis and Mental Life," seemed apparent. Simmel had argued that the velocity and compression of social interaction within the city contributed to self-protective affective withdrawals into a "blasé" state, whereby the other could not demand social recognition without intense multiplicity, fracturing the self in the process. But "blasé," Simmel argued, could easily slide into othering, and ultimately, hatred of the Other from whom one protected the self. This argument prefigured a later argument by Appadurai (2000) that during times of social mobility, across nation states and within nation states, as driven by the global economy, social uncertainties produced anxieties of self-identification that were solidified only in the demonizing of the Other (Zizek 1993). When all that is solid melts into air, to paraphrase Marx, the solidity of self-identity is a desperate construct, in its most pathological form, that requires the production of Otherness as its necessary supplement. This can take legalist and archival forms (Derrida 1995), as the instability at the heart of such sentiments drives an economy of feverish evidentiary archiving of the

Other's intolerable presence. For Simmel, this intolerable presence was unavoidable in the metropolis, both literally, in terms of the frequency and intensity of social interactions that one experiences, and also phenomenologically, in the sense that the psychic impressions left by these interactions would be too much to bear without a psychic shield. Otherwise, the result might be psychosis through contagion. Ironically, the psychic shield that protected against contagion was its own refractory symptom. On this point, we may recall the patient who was afraid of death's contagion, which was exacerbated by life in the city, where death's presence was literally everywhere, and not only residing within Oedipal guilt of a parent's death.

Of course, urban stress was also economic, as was the case with rural stress in contemporary India (Vasavi 2012). We briefly touched upon the farmer suicide phenomenon in our introduction, and we have seen that working class and poor patients comprised a large, if not the largest, segment of the NIMHANS clientele. But life in the city was increasingly expensive and required, of course, the certainty of income. Moreover, the tools of modern navigation, particularly transportation and cell phones, were necessities. But as such, they also added not only financial stress, but another intensity to daily life. Addiction took many forms, with phone and internet addiction being one of the many that appeared in the OPD. The following case illustrates how the financial and technological had direct impacts upon familial dynamics.

One day a woman and her husband appeared in the OPD. They were both in their thirties. Mala, the wife, was said by her husband to have some paranoid symptoms as well as anger issues. The husband said Mala had broken an "iron box" recently in a fit of anger. He said that Mala had anger issues with her daughter, a teenager, as well as with him. The doctor asked Mala if she was angry with her daughter. Mala answered that her daughter "refused to study" at times and had not been working for the past two years. The daughter was "just in the house," implying that she was not productive. The husband then responded by saying that Mala's "cooking was no longer tasty," which drew a smile on the doctor's face.

There were significant financial stresses facing the family. In particular, managing "school fees" and the basic costs of buying daily food had become a challenge. The husband accused Mala of not managing the finances of the household wisely. She refused to spend money, he claimed, despite there being enough for them to eat well. Mala responded that she had no mental illness symptoms. Her husband, to the contrary, believed that there was "something wrong with her." Talk then turned, perhaps strategically, upon prodding by the doctor, as to whether normal "festival and household celebrations" were being "properly performed." This seemed to be a theme I would hear from time to time: that is, the doctor would ask about participation in relevant cultural events, perhaps to gauge social withdrawal and disinterest, if not dysfunction, in familial life. This question, I noted, was addressed to working-class or lower-middle-class families more than it was to educated and presumably more secularized elites. In this case, the husband and wife said festival and household celebrations had not been interrupted. This moment of consensus did not last, as the husband, pivoting back to his complaint, said that the "homemaker role" for Mala had been stressful.

The doctor did not find any evidence of psychosis in Mala. The treatment plan, however, was for family psychotherapy as well as screening for thyroid and hormonal issues. Hormone therapy might be useful, the doctor suggested, perhaps, wondering if menopause had exacerbated familial stress. Mala and her husband were urged to bring their daughter to the next visit to the OPD. Aside from the financial worries that they faced, which certainly was directed at the daughter's lack of productivity, there emerged, at this point, a troubling issue that the husband had voiced about Mala's "safety." This caught the doctor's attention. But it turned out that the husband was questioning Mala's mental health when referring to "safety." She was caught, evidently, checking her husband's phone incessantly and feared he was having an affair. The husband claimed that this was "paranoid behavior." Mala denied that she was paranoid, but did not deny checking his phone. It was possible, however, the doctor suggested, that this was a "very early stage of schizophrenia," and that she was capable of "covering it up" at this point. The husband's concern, however, focused more upon Mala's ability to manage the household, having noted her tasteless food and stingy "marketing" (grocery shopping).

As in many cases we have seen, a social problem was recast as a psychological one, and that normalization, in male patriarchal terms, was the gold standard for assessing "madness" (Pinto 2014; Addlakha 2008; Lang 2018). For the present discussion on urban anxiety and stress, however, we can observe how cell phones are not only a necessity but a potential vehicle through which anxiety is generated. The financial worries, of course, were paramount, though the phone became a site of psychopathology and obsessiveness, according to the husband. The phone became a link to modernity, with both its promises of prosperity and its subsequent haunting traces of temptation, mistrust, and betrayal. And as we often hear in the headlines, new modes of communication through social media become the vehicles through which gossip and rumor spread, leading to forms of ostracism that can have very harsh consequences, as in the case of the teacher who was forced to resign after clashing with her students. It was yet another medium of archivization.

We can find many avenues through which modern life in the city is not just alienating and impersonal, one-dimensional (Marcuse 1964), and routine, as per Weber's nightmarish vision of bureaucracy run amok, or Kafka's more visceral stories of the relentless yet meaningless application of the law. Modern life also has many new goalposts and measurements, be they educational or financial, as well as being signified by the acquisition of materials and certifications. Whether it be driving a car, getting a driver's license, or scoring well on a school exam, the objective measures of success are oppressive and omnipresent in the accounts witnessed in the OPD, and in India's broader competitive and hierarchical social fabric (Subramaniam 2020; Ruddock 2021).

The sense of trust that was challenged by modern measurements was therefore exacerbated by the failure of these measurements to provide satisfaction, leading to feelings of perpetual betrayal among those who came to the clinic for care. These, what we might think of little failures in well-functioning individuals caught on the hamster wheel, were catastrophic and represented betrayals that took on hysteric and cosmic proportions, and exacerbated tensions within families. Failure to obtain a driver's license in one case we witnessed was personally shattering, and led to a sense of betrayal. In the case of Ramesh, the legal problems he faced seemed to hasten his legalistic and spiritual obsessions. This is not to downplay personal traumas or individual vulnerabilities, be they genetic or epigenetic, influenced by poverty or unrelenting stress within biocultural bodies (Das 2006; Cohen 2012; Kleinman 2012).

Within the stress of urban life, and the inevitable failures and betrayals it generated, the popularity of "god men" and gurus was notable. Seeking perfect surrogates to the failed intimacies of daily relationships, sibling and spousal rivalries, and the insults to self-esteem that came from the assessment culture in the urban economy was highly seductive, and concerned the doctors at NIMHANS (Kakar 1981; 1982). I often heard doctors complain about the "fraudulent god men" who preyed upon the increasing insecurities and emotional needs of their patients, entangling their disciples' lives within the transference and countertransference of these relationships and leading them to emotional, and even financial, ruin. Patients' feelings of deception and betrayal by gurus and god men/women could be devastating, the doctors worried. Moreover, as in Ramesh's case, the notion that the guru was the center of the disciple's world contributed to indifference and even distrust of human relationships that were not supercharged with expectations of a transcendent perfection.

While it is not my intention to analyze the historical and spiritual foundations of guru worship in India, as this is far too theologically complex an issue to undertake here, the topic of false and fraudulent gurus was thought to be a significant problem. This could lead to coercive and predatory behavior, which would be particularly harmful to those already psychologically vulnerable. Moreover, financial ruin was also a risk, as devotees gave away belongings to their gurus. Another factor to consider, the doctors pointed out, were the dangerous methods of treatment that religious faith healers sometimes utilized to cure people of mental illness or, in some cases, "fits" (seizures) (Chandrasekhar 2008; Sebastia 2009b). We can recall, from the previous chapter, the disastrous "healing hands" therapy she received from her guru that had worsened Sheila's symptoms and left her with financial precarity. The dangers and seductions of gurus, while often noted, was not an indictment of the cultural institution of the guru per se. Rather, the implication being raised was of the "false." That is, by labeling the false and fake, or fraudulent, the general assumption was that there were sincere and even godlike gurus who were genuine and authentic. But finding the saint within the decadence of urban life was not easy. And, moreover, the worry about the false and fraudulent extended, we might recall, to psychotherapists who were practicing with dubious qualifications, and whose techniques and practices were potentially unsound, and even dangerous. Authentic psychiatry, like authentic spirituality, was rarefied and needed to be carefully assessed in order to avoid the pitfalls of charlatans. This said, faith healing was not discounted entirely for its efficaciousness. Many patients sought traditional medicine through yoga, Ayurveda, and spiritual healers at the same time that they sought psychiatric care. And among the poor and working class, traditional healing practices predominated. To complicate matters further, the charlatan and the doctor operationalized the power of suggestion, its illocutionary force, into a healing performance, akin to Lévi-Strauss's (1973) classic formulation for sorcery's efficacy (Stengers 2009).[4]

We will recall, on the other end of the spectrum, doctors at NIMHANS were oftentimes concerned with the narrow pharmacological and neuropsychiatric emphasis on treating the "symptom" over and above treating the person. The "Band-Aid" approach to psychiatry, against its more holistic multi-axis understanding of the role of the psychosocial in causing and shaping symptoms and the repertoire within which they presented, meant, to many doctors, that the healing of the patient would also come, to some extent, through the idioms of care that were part of the cultural worlds they inhabited. Or, put plainly, the stress and support systems within society were part of the same social context in which the self is constructed and maintained (Kleinman 1988). Therefore, the sociologically and psychologically sophisticated doctors would urge their students, the residents and fellows, to visit healing shrines to witness the varieties of madness that were manifested there, as well as the modalities of care that these sites offered for the predominantly poor, who found solace in these ambiguous zones of care coupled with abandonment. In the next section we follow the biomedical into the traditional, visiting two healing *dargahs* that were popular as care centers near Bangalore and Chennai, respectively.

Visit to *Dargah* in Chintamani

While the large numbers of patients in the OPD at NIMHANS suggested a shift was occurring in attitudes and awareness about mental health, a large percentage of people do not seek psychiatric care. Those afflicted seek spiritual healing, believing their symptoms to be the result of evil or malevolent forces (e.g., Sebastia 2009b; Kakar 1982). Sufi shrines marking the tombs of saints (*dargahs*) are believed to be particularly efficacious in this regard. *Dargahs* are sites not only of religious healing, but also religious and linguistic pluralism persisting within the increasingly bio-medicalized and polarized religious landscape (Flueckiger 2006; Taneja 2018; Gold 2014; Gottschalk 2000).

The day began with enormous traffic out of Bangalore. After getting out of town, the countryside opened before us and was pleasant for our drive, about ninety minutes or so to Chintamani, a small city in Karnataka famous for its *dargah* called the Murgh Malla. Along the way, we, led by a doctor at NIMHANS,[5] found a roadside restaurant and filled our stomachs with a mid-morning snack of tea/coffee and hot *dosas* (rice and lentil crepes) with spicy *sambar*.

The *dargah* was about a ten-minute drive out of the town in an area surrounded by dramatic and strikingly beautiful hills laden with large boulders and interesting geographic features. There were several old Hindu temples upon these hills, suggestive of the syncretism of the area. There was a famous Goddess temple nearby that also drew lots of pilgrims. One of the legends I heard, in fact, was that the saint entombed in this *dargah* had been blessed with a vision of the Goddess, and with this was able to heal people. There were palpable and strong Hindu-Muslim crossings here. Moreover, though in Karnataka, the area was also close to Andhra Pradesh and Tamil Nadu, and lots of devotees from both places came to the *dargah*. Therefore, it was not only religiously plural, but also linguistically so.

As we entered the vicinity of the *dargah* we could see pilgrims from all parts of the region. Small shops surrounding the shrine sold images of the *dargah*, of the saint for which it was named, and of other figures such as Mahatma Gandhi and Tipu Sultan for tourists and pilgrims. Incense and flowers were also sold to be given as offerings within the shrine. Small canteens lined one side of the shrine selling refreshment and meals. And while there was a large presence of Muslims, naturally, in this area near the shrine, the atmosphere was not mono-religious or exclusive, as imagery of Hindu gods was also prominently visible and ubiquitous.

After parking a short distance away in an official parking area for the *dargah*, the doctor informed the administrative office of the shrine of our presence and interest in visiting the sacred space. The doctor, a psychiatrist, had been there before a few times and had brought residents/fellows to the shrine to illustrate local healing traditions for them. As a result of this familiarity, the officials gave us a semi-"VIP" tour of the shrines, which gave us access to the two main mausoleums housing the saint and his wife, also believed to be holy, as well as access to certain residents of the shrine who suffered various maladies but had found some measure of relief living there.

Entering the shrine under a large, corrugated tin-roof area that provided shelter for hundreds of residents and pilgrims, it became obvious that we were attracting attention. It also became clear that many of the residents were mentally or neurologically disturbed or challenged. Moreover, it was apparent that the majority of those living under this roof were poor and without familial support. There was a high percentage of elderly women living in the shrine, perhaps abandoned widows who had no place else to go once their families could no longer care for them. This was suggested by the psychiatrist. Some women laughed hysterically, in the colloquial sense of the term, possessing matted hair and unkempt clothes. One woman surprised me when she spoke fluent English and seemed to be educated, though her disheveled appearance betrayed her social circumstance. She specifically tried to engage in conversation with my anthropological colleague and myself only to be told to be quiet by male officials working in the shrine. The sick and abandoned were lying on straw mats and blankets on the concrete floor of the shrine, leaving little room for walking.

As this was not a festival time, nor was it during evening prayers, the shrine was not overly crowded. But with the hundreds of residents living on the premises, I wondered what would be the impact of a large group of pilgrims or transient patients or, as the case was often to be, possessed individuals who came for exorcisms. Indeed, I expected to see exorcisms being performed, as this shrine was famous for driving out evil spirits (*pey*, *jinn*, *bhut*, etc.). But on this afternoon, only a more permanent population of people suffering from various mental and psychical illnesses could be seen.

Despite the Mental Health Care Act of 1987 (Sebastia 2009a), which supposedly prohibits the housing of the mentally ill within non-registered mental health care facilities, it was clear that hundreds of patients did, in fact, live permanently or semi-permanently within the shrine. Indeed, we were told by some patients that this was their last refuge and the place where they had found some peace (Sebastia 2009b). Some of these individuals had travelled to the shrine themselves, making a pilgrimage, as it were, to find a spiritual home. Others had been abandoned by their families who could not bear the costs of care, or the stigma attached to mental health within their families. Within the shrine, they received the protection and healing power of the saint, as well as a roof and hot meals. It was clearly much better than the alternative of being on the streets, homeless, with nothing. The psychiatrist leading our team pointed out that though the human suffering here was so palpable and acute, these people at least had some of their basic needs met. Moreover, from the stories we heard, some had found their symptoms alleviated by their faith in the healing power of the shrine.

At the same time, many of the residents of the shrine were interested in speaking with the doctor, or, in some cases, their relatives were. He had brought a few of his business cards with contact information, and as he spoke with a few individuals, he suggested they visit NIMHANS for treatment. He would explain that the treatment would be free for those of lesser means possessing a Below Poverty Line card.[6] But alas, many of them, though interested in biomedical treatment or counseling, could not afford the journey by bus and were unsure how they could physically endure the trip. In one case, a man suffered hemi-paralysis and needed to be properly diagnosed, but would find it impossible to make the two-hour journey by bus without extensive assistance. He expressed interest, however, to be seen by the doctor. In the cases of neurological conditions or other movement disorders, there was little by way of treatment that the psychiatrist could offer on site. Thus, it was necessary for a neurological evaluation through a visit to NIMHANS. Among the more psychiatric-looking cases, it was clear that some of the afflicted were depressed, dissociated in some ways, speaking to themselves, and manic. But no medicines would be administered on this day. The goal, if any, was to encourage people to also seek biomedical care, if this was at all possible.

My attention, however, was directed at the perceived efficacy of the shrine. One man explained how he could not walk well and had been to several doctors near Mysore, his native place, before coming to this *dargah*. Now his symptoms had abated, and he wanted to share this miraculous news. One older man could not even sit up, lying on his side with discomfort and pain. The doctor implored the family visiting him to get him treated at NIMHANS.

Among the audiences within the shrine there was a sizable group of people who were making a pilgrimage to the shrines of the saint and his wife, also deemed a saint. There were two separate shrines. Men and women were directed to go in separate shifts to view the tomb and elaborately decorated coffins. The heavy smell of incense greeted the devotee when entering either shrine. One had to bend low under a very short doorway to enter the tomb-shrine. These innermost shrines were simple, though some gold and silver had been added over time to the entrance. It was not unlike the sanctum of a Hindu shrine, in many respects. After touching the cloth that draped the coffin, which had sacred verses written in Urdu, and offering flowers, the devotee was also blessed with holy water by a local *Pir* (Sufi teacher), dressed in traditional clothing. The *Pir* would dip a bushy frond on a long stick in the bowl of holy water and then sprinkle a bit on the head of each devotee as they left the shrine. A sacred gold flag also pointed towards the main shrine, similar to the practice within a Hindu temple. While the majority of visitors were Muslims from the region, a fairly high percentage were Hindu. In fact, later I was told that this shrine was equally popular among the two main communities. This seemed to my eye aptly described, as we passed by long lines of devotees from both faiths, as evidenced by their facial markings and clothing (Flueckiger 2006).[7]

I could not but feel some sadness seeing so many abandoned, suffering, and mentally unstable people in one place. This tempered the mood of a place thought to be sacred. But with the faith invested in the shrine by the visitors, I also felt that the power of suggestion must have worked as a talisman and solace to those suffering from a range of illnesses or despair in their lives (Halliburton 2009; Flueckiger 2006; Taneja 2018). Indeed, it struck me that those who resided there might not actually suffer diagnosable disorders, but had found a spiritual home that accepted them without condition. There was an unmistakable smell of urine as well as bird droppings under the large tin roof. Monkeys were also seen everywhere. Though I was told the area was cleaned daily, the poor and "mad" who resided there had little investment, apparently, in personal hygiene. And without a constant water source, one wondered how people could bathe regularly. Bathrooms existed, but not on the scale needed for such a large and popular shrine. We were told that only long-term residents were supported by the generosity of various patrons of the shrine. A simple communal meal was offered to all residents twice each day.

I also wondered about the patronage and other forms of financing needed to keep such a large shrine functioning. A few large and strategically located collection boxes were placed to capture donations. But this was not a shrine that the wealthy normally visited. I suspected that the challenges of housing, feeding, and bathing this many people must have been overwhelming given the actual resources available. The Murgh Malla *dargah* was like hundreds of similar shrines within the country that were believed to have the spiritual power to drive away the devils or spirits that cause madness. These shrines, be they Hindu, Muslim, or Christian, as some scholars have argued (e.g., Sebastia 2009b; Kakar 1982; Raguram, Ramakrishna, and Weiss 2002; Gopikumar et al. 2016; Halliburton 2009), are hardly marginal or peripheral to the care of the mentally ill within India, but their survival is in question given legislative and economic pressures. The point being made here is that not only were pockets of religious and linguistic pluralism surviving in the Deccan (Willford 2018; Srinivas 2001), but various approaches towards healing those troubled by various mental disturbances also continue to exist and even thrive. The Murgh Malla and a few other powerful shrines across the religious divide, if anything, achieve greater popularity in the age of televisual media. News of miracles today spread much more quickly, as do the images of particularly powerful healing shrines through the print and televisual media (Srinivas 2018). These shrines, in turn, attract ever-larger numbers of devotees as their healing fame spreads and/or the sources of psychosocial stress in urban Bangalore and other places increase.[8]

Dargah in Kovalam

The *dargah* in Kovalam, a coastal village south of Chennai, is Tameem Ansari's grave. Tameem Ansari, we were told by an assistant to the *Pir* who was head of the shrine,[9] was a saint from nine hundred years earlier, purportedly a companion of the Prophet, who settled in Kovalam after traveling through India. When he died, the saint had told his disciples that he wanted to be put into a coffin and set out to sea. However, his disciples, years later, decided to reclaim his body, and miraculously were able to do so as it emerged from the sea, according to legend. The disciples, finding his coffin, built the *dargah* around it, and made it into a place of pilgrimage. When these disciples died, their twelve bodies were interred and are also considered to be the graves of saints. According to a Wikipedia page on the saint:

> Tamin ibn Zayd al-Ansari was a Muslim saint whose dargah is located in Kovalam, Tamil Nadu, 30 km from Chennai. Al-Ansari was born in Medina, Saudi Arabia and is a Sahabi (companion of Prophet Muhammad). He visited Asia continent during the caliphate of Umar ibn al-Khattab and stayed in Sindh for 18 years. The first Thursday after the full moon of each month is a day of devotion. Though the dargah is open from 5am to 10pm, some devotees spend the night there.

A short biography of the saint published online had the following background:

> The most famous Dargah Shareef of Sahabi-e-Rasool Sallalahu Alaihi wa Sallam which attracts the largest number of people in the entire India is of Syedina, Hazrath Tameem-ul-Ansari (Rizwan Allahi Tha'alahi Alaihim Ajmaeen), also called as Hazrath Tameem Ansari (Rizwan Allahi Tha'alahi Alaihim Ajmaeen). The Dargah is located in Kovalam shareef, near Mamallapuram, about 30 km from Chennai. Syedina, Hazrat Tameem-ul-Ansari (Rizwan Allahi Tha'alahi Alaihim Ajmaeen) was born in Al-Madina Al-Munawara and joined in Islam in Al Makkah Al Mukarrama before the Hijrath of Huzoor-e-Kareem Sallalahu Alaihi wa Sallam. Before his Pardha (Wisal), he had instructed his disciples to cast his Janazah Mubarak (remains) into the sea after his death. After the last instructions from Syedina, Hazrath Tameem-ul-Ansari (Rizwan Allahi Tha'alahi Alaihim Ajmaeen) as stated above, his companions or disciples did the same and it is said that the Janazah Mubarak was in the sea for about 5 years and it was guarded by the big fishes during this time. Eventually, one big fish brought the Janazah Mubarak nearer to [the] sea shore of Kovalam." (Mohammad 2017)

The man who told us the story was the assistant to the "Baba" or *Pir* (holy man) who counseled the people who came to the shrine with various troubles and ailments. The Baba sat in front of the main shrine to Ansari and said prayers together with the people who came to share their troubles. He would then sprinkle holy water and bless them, using a frond, as was the case in the Murgh Malla shrine discussed above. The *dargah* was thick with smoke and the smell of incense. Crowds had gathered by 5:00 p.m. within the courtyard and street leading up to the shrine. Inside the main sanctum, crowds of people were sitting anywhere they could find room. The devotees were both Muslims and Hindus, men and women, about equally divided by religion and gender. Some were clearly troubled, tears in their eyes, and faces downward. But nobody was agitated or spoke incoherently when we were there. There was an older-looking shrine off to one side where the graves of the twelve disciples of Tameem Ansari lay. Some of these disciples included women and children, we were told. Inside, each grave had been draped with a cloth and was covered with flowers. Incense burned before each coffin. Sitting on the ground, a group composed of mainly women sat with their heads facing the graves. Some wept and others rocked back and forth in intense prayer. The intensity of their prayers was a powerful and moving sight to behold. Inside the courtyard of the main shrine to Tameem Ansari, devotees circumambulated the shrine in a manner very similar to what one would see within a Hindu shrine or temple (left to right). Along the circumambulatory route were little alcoves with candles and *kuttu vilakkus* (oil lamps) burning, together with incense. There were also, along little Islamic architectural-style porticos surrounding the shrine, small locks stacked upon other little locks, taking up every inch of space. Locks were, in turn, locked upon other locks. Locks were also tied to the windows with little pieces of cloth. Locks could be purchased at the entrance of the shrine by devotees as a kind of prayer-offering to the shrine. Each lock represented a wish and a prayer.

We were told by a staff member from The Banyan, a non-governmental organization (NGO) focused upon mental health care that ran a care center for the homeless and mentally ill across the road, that both Hindus and Muslims would be equally present on any given day within the shrine. The Baba's assistant, who spoke with us for some time, said the percentage of Muslims to Hindus was about 60 to 40, with Muslims being a slight majority. It was pointed out to him that a lot of practices and instruments of worship were very much like that found in a Hindu shrine. He responded that "all are the same—and worship the same god." He further emphasized the "harmony within" the saint's shrine. Indeed, as we spoke, a Hindu woman was receiving blessings and healing from the Baba. I asked if many of the devotees were able to do the Hajj. He responded, saying that doing "ten visits to this dargah was equivalent of doing the Hajj," and that as the people were "too poor to travel to Mecca," this was "just as good." He also said that this was "the most important *dargah* in the area, and one of the greatest in India." His point about poverty among the devotees was convincing as we could see that among the crowd of those within the shrine, almost all appeared to be working-class and poor.

I asked the Baba's assistant what happened when the illness or affliction was not cured by the *dargah* or through the intercession of the Baba. His answer surprised me, as he said this was "not really ever seen," as 99 percent had "their prayers answered" and were "healed" within the shrine. He pointed out that one could begin to feel a difference in one's life even after a short period of ten minutes. As we had been there for well over half an hour at this point, and felt uplifted by the sanctified atmosphere of the site, it was not hard to believe him. Moreover, his faith was secure, and, as such, it would have been nonsensical to ask about doubts and failures among the clientele who beseeched the saint for divine assistance.

Rather than asking about doubt and uncertainty, I pivoted to question what sort of problems people brought to the *dargah* that sought divine remedy. The assistant said that *seyvinai* (sorcery) was rampant now. My associate, who was also from The Banyan, asked about *pey* (malignant spirit) possession. The Baba said that the *pey* were driven out by the power of a sacred tree, which the devotees would circumambulate. I asked then about *jinn*. The man, who wore a green skullcap, said that this was "correct" and added that he was "very happy [I] knew about the correct term for these spirits." He then elaborated on these spirits, noting that they lived in the stomachs of people, consuming them from within, and did not want to leave their bodies. But the power of the saint was too great for these nasty parasites to withstand. I asked about forms of Islamic treatment that used numerology, such as *taviz* and *falita* (Flueckiger 2006).[10] He seemed surprised and delighted that I knew of these concepts and terms, and said, "Sir knows everything"—of course, a polite exaggeration on his part.

I was struck by the informality and casualness of the shrine. Nobody corrected people in their dress or styles of prayer. Anyone could enter, and the unusual behavior of the mentally ill or possessed did not raise eyebrows. Outside the shrine, but still within the compound, was a tin roof offering shelter over a large cement floor. Mats were stacked up in one corner. We were told that every night, the shelter became completely full of residents who lived within the shrine, or were being healed for a period of time within the shrine. But the Baba's assistant also pointed out that a lot of people were abandoned at the shrine; and, moreover, they found it hard to know personal details in these cases. The mentally ill, as was the case in Chintamani, were the most abundant among residents abandoned. They received shelter, spiritual cures, and daily meals that never failed to materialize through the charitable offerings people made at the shrine.

As one approached the *dargah* along a narrow road, there was a *masjid* (mosque) adjacent to it, as well as an administrative office. Inside the office was a closed-circuit television that monitored different angles within the healing complex. I asked what this was for, and he said it was to protect against petty theft within the shrine.

The *dargah*, like other healing sites, Hindu or Christian (see Halliburton 2009; Kakar 1982; Obeyesekere 1981), is a traditional site where madness can be revealed and cured within a repertoire that is culturally fluid, meaningful, yet exculpates the guilt and shame that madness might otherwise bring to the family. Moreover, familial dramas and tensions can be indirectly enacted and realigned, perhaps, in the anti-sorcery and curative exorcisms that are performed within their sacred boundaries. Within this liminal space (Turner 1974), the afflicted are allowed to express their symptoms, unattached to their personal and social identity, which is, as many have pointed out, significant in South Asia with its sociocentric ideologies of the person (Daniel 1984; Kakar 1982; Roland 1988; Nabokov 2000). The *dargah* is also a vestige of ambiguity and cultural fluidity, against not only the individualized form of selfhood that the assessment or audit culture demands within the modern, but also works against the serialized and bounded forms of identification that are driving the cycles of distrust and othering within contemporary South Asia. The enduring "deterritorializing" quality of the *dargah* against the machinic and "arboreal" (Deleuze and Guattari 1987) schemas of identity that are solidifying in India makes it a refuge and site of creativity, to some extent, against the uniform and ossified forms of self and group identity that seem to be contributing to feelings of betrayal. Efficacy within these sites seems to serve as a refuge against the modern. But not all is joyous or creative. These sites are places of human suffering and abandonment as well. They are sites where the drama of the "good family," with its sociocentric ideologies of care and filial respect, is staged in opposition to the "bad family" (Cohen 1998) that abandons the elderly, infirm, and mad within safe houses, be they psychiatric or spiritual.

"Tension" was a term that was often used by patients to diagnose the symptoms of stress in their lives, particularly within the urban swirl of keeping up with deadlines and demands of work, family obligations, and economic worries. Addicts were ubiquitous visitors to the OPD, and oftentimes were symptomatic of "tension." In cases too numerous to count, and too generic to explore in detail, the relationship between addictions (to cannabis and alcohol) and stress was evident. While addictions to internet and smart phones appeared to be prevalent among the middle class, addictions to cannabis and alcohol were far more prevalent among the working class, and especially among males. One of the common cures for addiction, however, was a vow taken to visit a site of pilgrimage. Sabarimala[11] for instance, a famous Hindu shrine in Kerala, was very popular in South India, and known for its power to cure addiction. In a few cases I witnessed in the OPD, the male patient would make a vow to walk over two hundred kilometers from Bangalore to this shrine, where the vow, successfully undertaken, would break the addiction. One of the doctors I shadowed who specialized in addiction confirmed that these vow-pilgrimages were efficacious in, at least temporarily, ridding the patient of their addiction. One patient I encountered claimed that he needed to complete the vow each year because the urge to take cannabis and alcohol would increase as the effects of the pilgrimage wore off.

The "Good" and "Bad" Family

Urban stress and its spiritual and psychiatric remedies witnessed in this chapter bring us to the question of the family as a unit of stress and support (Kleinman 1989; Pinto 2014; Marrow 2016). As Cohen's (1998) masterful study of dementia in India demonstrated, the ideology of the sociocentric, filial, and traditional extended family continues to resonate strongly. Indeed, one might argue that the dilemmas of modernity center on the family and the conflicts made visible by mobility (transnational and domestic), economic opportunities/challenges, and the concomitant decisions that these modern pressures create. Normalization, though a prevalent force for compliance within conservative norms and ideals, particularly in their patriarchal form, is not always possible. Dementia, for instance, as Cohen argues, is not treatable in the same manner as are other forms of mental illness. Epilepsy, also being a neurologic condition, is similar in this regard. Therefore, the questions of guardianship and long-term care inevitably collide with the ideologies of care and filial commitment. Abandoning the elderly by placing them in a managed care environment weighs upon the "bad" or unfilial family. For the poor, the healing shrines offer another alternative, as discussed above. At least in the case of the *dargah*, piety intervenes on behalf of filial attachment, or its lack thereof. Though we have already touched on the theme of abandonment as continuum, and not an absolute, in most cases, considering long-term care as entangled between ideals of care (good family) and abandonment (bad family) points to emerging discourses of rights and advocacy for the mentally ill. A look at two cases of long-term care and the dilemmas it poses for family members helps us to see the complex issues at play, along with their legal and spiritual ramifications.

John, a man from Mumbai in his late seventies, came with his brother to the OPD. John was said to "present with minor expressions of aggression to his care givers," in this case, his brother. He was a long-term patient and had been diagnosed with schizophrenia in 1977. For forty years he had been treated by psychiatrists and had somehow managed to "survive" on medications for an "alarmingly long period," according to the doctor who was treating him this day in the OPD. But his symptoms, evidently, had never completely subsided, despite ongoing treatment.

John heard voices and felt that people were following him. He also complained of various somatic problems that "stopped his movement." Chlorpromazine, a sedative in the benzodiazepine family, was the preferred medication for John, his chart revealed. He lived in a "half-way house" (a term that John did not like when the doctor used it) in Bangalore that was headed by a charismatic German social worker who for decades had accepted the mentally ill in his institution. Now this social worker was in physical decline, and for this reason, John's brother and his wife were considering taking him home to live full-time with them. John already had spent many days with the brother at his home.

John was mostly lucid, though he had complained of voices in his head while in the doctor's office. But he also seemed to possess enough insight to realize that these voices were not objectively real. This insight was contradicted, however, by his statement that there was a "living man inside" him. He said the words "the man" while holding the sides of his head, so as to indicate that the man lived within his head. This was, while not a symbiotic relationship by any stretch of the imagination, something he had learned to cope with over the years. The brother, an articulate man who appeared to be from the middle class, said he just "wanted his brother to be happy" and somewhat self-reliant, though he had no illusions of a cure at this stage.

John said he enjoyed shopping (so he claimed, though his brother countered that he is very difficult to shop with) and reading magazines. He mentioned *Outlook* by name, a news magazine popular with English-reading audiences. Though not a devout Christian, from time to time he attended St. Patrick's Church on MG Road, in the heart of the city. In the past six months, however, he had gone only once. It appeared as though his brother's money was enough to sustain him. John was well groomed and wore nice clothes, but kept no budget or expense log. The brother hoped John would become financially self-reliant, in the sense that he would be able to mind his expenses, but did not expect him to work.

While we were talking to John, the resident was present. The attending doctor mentioned that all "five axes must be present" and treated in diagnoses and treatment.[12] This was to suggest that there were various comorbidities that required constant monitoring and care, regardless of the apparently elusive cure. John talked a bit about his earlier years. It seems that he had lived and worked in Los Angeles in the 1970s. Prior to his diagnosis he was a reasonably high-functioning individual who possessed a good education, as was suggested by his reading habits. He was still mostly coherent, though you could see he was not quite right, and exhibited slightly slowed thought and movements. After several years of treatment, his condition improved in the early 1990s, but in recent years he had declined. This decline was in terms of both "cognitive and emotional function." For instance, he had trouble choosing clothes or things like watches. Certain patterns or insignias bothered him. In one case, after a full day of searching for some new clothes, he finally found some shirts that were to his liking. As the cashier was packaging a few pairs, John noticed a crest or label on the shirt or sweater. This upset him greatly and he cancelled the purchase, to the frustration of his brother and sister-in-law, who had patiently shopped for the better part of a day with him. Furthermore, it seemed that he often wore the same clothes day in and day out, not liking any changes in appearance. John exhibited increasingly compulsive or repetitive behaviors. This was true of hygiene products, as well; and he wore a "special watch" that was not working anymore, feeling reluctant to take it off. But John still interacted with various nephews and nieces and could hold a light conversation with family members.

The doctor mentioned that such a long-term patient had a greatly elevated risk for dementia. Therefore, it was very important to monitor John's medications and perform MRIs occasionally. While there might have been signs of cognitive decline, there were also signs that the schizophrenia was acting up. In conversation he often said unintelligible things. I heard John mumble something a couple of times, but nothing was particularly dramatic or demonstrative. But at home, he often lost the thread of the conversation and spoke of strange things that nobody understood. Towards the end of the OPD visit he chimed in, "I'm actually from Bombay," which had already been long established in the meeting.

Though John was "irregular" and had an odd sense of timing, he was relatively well considering the long-term treatment he had been on, according to his doctor. And his decision-making processes, annoying as they may have been to others, were still intact. The brother mentioned wanting to take his "sick brother" home with him permanently after the half-way house was no longer an option. This was commendable, the doctor said, given that he was an added burden to the family. And moreover, it was clear that this family had the resources for further institutionalized stay, if needed. Still, this case raised tough questions of guardianship for patients and their families dealing with chronic long-term illness. If the family was wealthy, as this one appeared to be, what would John's stake be in an inheritance? What would his decisions be with regard to his own money? Would a relative less kind than this brother appeared to be assume guardianship, with ulterior financial motives? These were questions that the doctors at NIMHANS always worried about but had little power to intervene in, despite some legislation that existed to protect the disabled from abuse. This legislation, the doctors complained, was in actuality "weak" and hard to enforce.

A middle-aged man with schizophrenia, Jyoti, had been treated for thirty years at NIMHANS. Jyoti, coming alone, was excessively deferential and friendly to the attending doctor, whom he had known for years, and even to myself, whom he had just met. He greeted us warmly, lowering his head slightly as he did so. Jyoti appeared to have some cognitive impairment when he spoke, but was able to communicate clearly. He claimed he walked fifteen kilometers per day on his parents' farm. The family, it seems, were influential organic and sustainable farming pioneers in the region. When asked if he was reading much, he said he had very low levels of concentration, which impeded his ability to read. On the other hand, he claimed he watched devotional channels on the television but avoided "romantic" shows or films. He proclaimed that he "only had faith in God." The doctor asked if he was "taking care of himself well." For instance, was he "cleaning" his own room and "washing his own clothes"? Jyoti said he wanted to work "on the land" and wanted to clean his own room, but was told by his sisters "not to worry" about these small things. There were domestic helpers at home who aided him with practical life-skills matters. The doctor, however, felt it important that as part of his therapy, he learn to clean his room and wash his own clothes.

When asked how he was feeling in recent days, Jyoti complained that he was "not feeling well." He experienced "tensions and headaches." Moreover, Jyoti said he was sleeping ten to fifteen hours a day, which the doctor said was "excessive." Jyoti was asked to sleep no more than ten hours per night. He carried a notebook of his own thoughts, a kind of diary. He offered to show this to the doctor, but was told to "put it away." The doctor, as in many other cases we have seen, did not want to call further attention to his "obsessive ruminations" over his own delusions. Rather, he wanted the patient to keep himself busy, physically and mentally, with tasks, so as to interrupt endless ruminations and, presumably, going down the rabbit hole these thoughts might precipitate.

Jyoti was highly motivated towards spiritual life and spoke of his desires to "serve God and other people." He would, we were told by him, give away his money to help laborers on the farm. And he specifically mentioned that the laborers were "innocent and good people who were being taken advantage of"—perhaps an indictment of his own family, the landlords.

The doctor said Jyoti had elaborate psychosis and schizophrenia. He had seen Jyoti having very intensive and paranoid delusions over the years. He made much of his own thoughts, excessively ruminating on them, which explained the doctor's reluctance to read his diary. Moreover, Jyoti was overly religious, speaking always of God and the need to remain on the path, so to speak. He at one point during the interview said he "prayed to God and to his doctor," and thanked both in prayer. He then said, "Thank God for Dr. —," saying the doctor's full name. He seemed to split the world into the righteous and the criminal, suggesting that there was an almost Manichean struggle between them in which his vigilance and discipline were required. This was another case of cosmic struggle, like those we had learned about in the previous chapter, in which the significance of the individual made a critical difference. The doctor advised Jyoti to "sleep less" and to "walk less." But on the whole, he told Jyoti he was happy he was doing relatively well, given the long-term nature of his illness.

The OPD offered, between patients and during coffee and lunch breaks, an opportunity for doctors to discuss their varied concerns about institutionalized medicine, politics, or trends in illness narratives that they encountered. After Jyoti had left the room, his case had reminded his doctor about various exclusions and dichotomies that were being drawn in society, or the hardening of social categories and cultural imaginaries, or what I have called their serialized and boundary-hardening forms, following Anderson's (1998) terms. As Jyoti had spoken of good and evil forces, the doctor told me that social exclusions could even infect the space of NIMHANS, a national center for health care. He said that a decade or so earlier, when the Speak Kannada movement had intensified in Bangalore (Willford 2018; Nair 2005), he would often encounter patients, whether Muslims or Christians, or Urdu or Tamil speakers, respectively, who had trouble with the intake interview and forms. These were deliberately all in printed in Kannada, which made it hard to get accurate patient information about patients who were not Kannadigas. This came up in the context of a conversation about the accessibility of care for all communities, across various linguistic and economic divides. The doctor spoke of the political "madness" that could only exacerbate and reflect the madness he witnessed in the clinical context, whereby people, as we have witnessed, became more attached to their identities in opposition to the increasingly bounded and inscrutable other.

At this point, after the patient had left, a conversation with the doctor and residents veered towards another case whereby, evidently, a patient refused to leave her father for any amount of time. But in this case, the father suffered from delusions of persecution and was schizophrenic. The daughter now shared his delusions as well as his diagnosis. The doctor made an elliptical comment about family intimacies being entangling, with regard to mental health. He again cited a work by Sartre called "Intimacy,"[13] mentioned also in another case, which dealt with the impact that mental illness had on a family. The woman in this case felt that if she left her father alone, he would, in turn, be harmed by her mother. But in such a case as this, one first step towards recovery for both the father and daughter would be, in fact, to have them separate for a while, the doctor pointed out. In her fear and psychotic panic, or we might say, "intimacy" with madness, she refused this separation.

This lesson as delivered between doctor and residents stuck with me, as did the intimacy of madness prove adhesive to those family members impacted by the illness of one or more of its members. It helped explain the conundrums that made care and abandonment, as two ends of a continuum, affectively powerful and conflicted (Pinto 2014). As the intimacies of family blurred the boundaries between parents and children, siblings, and partners, the doorway of contagion was palpable. As Mitchell (2000) argues persuasively, the somatic symptoms of hysteria are always mimetic and contagious, whereby identification with the afflicted is at the core of symptom presentation, and not merely in an Oedipal sense, but between siblings and spouses, and even within a wider community symptom repertoire. So, too, the transferential space of intimacy, perhaps, drove some to ward off contagion through an impulse to separation and abandonment, whereas for others, the pull was to offering the care for a sibling that might have been absent or challenged between parent and child. That is, the family member identified with the sick member of the family, understanding their predicament through transference and intimacy. But the implication, which complicated straightforward understandings of distance and abandonment, was that separation was not necessarily abandonment, but might be a useful interruption of the contagion and its transferential identifications that underpinned it. Moreover, the clinical encounter—which, after all, was my primary venue for observation—involved a short-circuiting of transference and countertransference. This happened through the doctor's refusal to enter into the narrative archive on his/her patients vis-à-vis their diaries and extensive, and perhaps, performative delusions. These diaries were designed, in part, to hysterically enact the doctor's expectation and wish, as understood by their patients, to become "patients" with recognizable and diagnosable symptoms (Mitchell 2000; Marrow 2022).

* * *

This chapter has examined the anxieties of modernity through occupational burnout, "tension," and the turn to "traditional" methods, both as resistant alternatives to biomedicine among the educated middle class and as the social recourse for the poor and destitute. Yoga and the healing power of the *dargah* may seem entirely different, but both point to the limits of medicalized care and the challenge of psychiatry in meeting the growing mental health needs of the nation (Sebastia 2009a). At the heart of traditional medicines and faith healing is the authority and, indeed, the illocutionary force of faithful practice, and a proclamation of efficacy that is affirmative and to some extent self-fulfilling. But this exclusion involves also negating the negative, be it a malignant being, repetitive symptom (occupational or possessive spirit), or toxic medicine that causes confusion and somnambulance. In short, the prospective treatment has a magical quality that supersedes contingency and the murky social provenance of the symptom. The cure, like mathematical reasoning, is abstract and removed from the stickiness of intimacy and the transferential interpersonal violence of the social. As Mauss argued (1902), magic supplements reason by enacting a causal relation when reason fails. This involves an abstraction, following Kant, in the form of grammatical or synthetic reasoning. But magical thinking is also palliative only through faith and its iterative archive. Thus the symptoms often return, requiring, in turn, more magic, be it in the form of pilgrimages, tablets, or ritualized cures such as exorcisms.

This is not meant to conflate middle-class burnout, particularly with its modern IT-related flattening of experience, with the florid delusions of psychosis and paranoia associated with schizophrenia. Again, we must underscore that there may be strong organic and genetic vulnerabilities that make any constructivist understanding of normalcy as the dictates of power seem vulgar and myopic. Rather, I point to a common thread in the Indian context: that introspection and analysis seem secondary to purposeful and agentive transformations, against the contagion or intimacies of madness. This short-circuiting of the self-archive as a creative and intentional act is shared across the faith-based, traditional, and biomedical psychiatric spectrum. This does not mean that "insight" and self-examination are absent, but rather that excessive rumination is thought to be sometimes harmful, opening up Pandora's box, with thoughts ushering in and out of the "doorways to (mis) perception" of the patient, to misquote Aldous Huxley.

It must also be recalled that in the Indian context there is a long philosophical history of deconstructing self-identity. Be it in Vedantic monism, in Buddhist notions of impermanence or non-self (*anatta*), or within the *Yoga Sutras* of Patanjali, among many other schools and practices, the self as ego or identity is ultimately illusory. Within these traditions, the practice of "*neti neti*," or "not this, not that," is a recurrent theme. That is to say, rather than examining one's unique history and how it constitutes a reality that one must come to understand, the Indian view has, much like Lacan might say, emphasized the illusory nature of self-identity in search of a higher self. Hindu thought, as well as the various other currents of Sufi Islam, Buddhism, Jainism, etc., have all contributed philosophical and pedagogical legacies that permeate the South Asian worldview. In short, the axiom to "know thyself" takes on a different ontology in Western and Indian thought (Kakar 1982; Fabrega 2009; Roland 1988). As Kakar (1982) has argued, there is a fundamental difference in the Indian view, in which the self is fluid and must adapt or harmonize with that which is constant (monism) in order to find the real Self (Atman), which ultimately requires dissolving the ego, versus the Western idea that the self is a constant, whereby external reality can be changed and addressed to meet the ego's inner needs (Cartesian dualism). In the clinical light, we might understand a doctor's unwillingness to engage in the examination of patient writings, such as diaries, or follow their delusions in search of hidden clues or etiologies. Rather, and surprisingly congruent with Lacanian thought, the self, as imagined, needs to be short-circuited when symptoms are disabling in everyday life. Cognitive behavioral therapy, which is favored at NIMHANS more than psychoanalysis, like yoga, is about utilizing the plasticity of the brain and mind to disrupt negative feedback loops that are psychologically and physically crippling. And as we have observed, the emphasis on routine exercise, work, and daily activities such as dressing, self-care in terms of hygiene, eating well, and sleeping the right amounts were of paramount importance.

In this sense, psychiatry and traditional healing in India share a common concern with establishing a habitus that will have transformative effects, as opposed to focusing upon the semiology of the text in each case presented. Rather, context trumps text, as does the emphasis on social harmony over individual surmounting of difficult social circumstances (Kakar 1982). This, we might recall from our historical context for NIMHANS, was part of its founder's philosophical orientation. That is, the monism of Hindu thought translated into a monistic non-separation of mind and body, or taking selfhood and embodiment in a different direction from the psychiatry that evolved in the West out of a strong psychodynamic and specifically Freudian legacy (Murthy and Jain 2009).

The complications, however, to this culturalist, indeed, ideological, account of Indian thought, cultural psychology, and its extension into psychiatry, is that not only does it gloss over differences that are substantial, it also erases, to some extent, the severity of conflicts, social violence, and intractable self-division that is witnessed in the cases presented. The doctors, all to varying degrees, acknowledge that when they give advice that might seem conservative, "harmonizing" or "normalizing," they do so not because they do not recognize these intractable and structural tensions in society, but precisely, due to the limitations of time and resources, as well as the societal stigmas attached to mental illness. My own representation of the rhythms and modalities of the clinic has tried to replicate these moments of pause, poignancy, and frustration, despite my inability to open up these life histories with the kind of nuanced detail that a psychodynamic approach would offer. This method of representation was my own limit, owing to the conditions of research, but also to some extent mirrored, and self-consciously so, the conundrum of interpretation the doctors faced several times each day they worked the OPD and wards. That is, while the doctors would assert psychiatric authority through the lexicon of diagnoses that the ICD established, and the efficacy afforded by the drugs that they prescribed, as well as the medical tests they ordered that looked for metabolic or neurological determinants, there was a trace of uncertainty that often remained. What were thought to be organic diagnoses, such as schizophrenia, acute psychosis, or cognitive deficits through brain lesions, were haunted to some extent by the fact that biomarkers were often absent or elusive, leading to diagnoses like "borderline personality," "schizoid traits," "dissociative" and "fugue states," and the persistence of the term "hysteria" in casual conversation, but more normally labeled "histrionic personality" following DSM and ICD terminology.

The residual presence of hysteria haunted the clinic, arguably productively, precisely because it conjured the uncertainties of psychosocial dynamics, the intimacies of contagion, and the uncanny ability of illness to travel from one person to the next. As in Derrida's (1981) famous discussion of the "pharmakon" that is writing, self-interiority can easily be supplanted by the archive of writing that is its supplement, or an exteriority that permeates this illusory interiority. Like Derrida, in that sense, the illusion of an interiority being invaded by an exteriority was the illusion of presence, or the sovereign self. Deconstruction, like Indian philosophy and psychiatric practice, grapples with illusion and its pragmatic effects. In the context of contemporary South Asia, where the illusions are becoming entrenched within serialized archives of difference, marking increasingly ossified boundaries as aided by technological mass communication, the pathologies and hysterias that were emergent and, indeed, prevalent, were hardening dualisms, over and against the tacit resistance to these forms of illusory, permeable, constructed selves, as established in the modalities of South Asian life. In that sense, the psychiatric clinic was, though not ostensibly, an arena where the politics of identity were playing out.

This is not to deny the reality of mental illness, but to underscore what was obvious to those working at NIMHANS: *the political and the pathological were conjoined*, particularly at this historical juncture. Indeed, I often heard, as we will recall, that the "grey" zones were increasingly intolerable to the moralizing and cosmological thinking that was emerging within the clinic. And while serialization was occurring on all sides: occupationally, in terms of objectifications of labor, religiously, and even in terms of the hardening of illness categories within the diagnostic lexicons through the neurologizing trends of psychiatry, the resistance to serialization, and with it, the Other's demand, was witnessed in the myriad of symptom presentations that could be labeled "hysteric." We must reclaim that term from its gendered assumptions and prejudices and, rather, see hysteria as a social symptom par excellence that enacts protest that is often self-defeating, refractory, and, indeed, painfully suffered within normative ideologies. Therefore, while it is important to recognize that ontic specificity of Indian modalities of selfhood, following Heidegger, their normative and pedagogical implications in social and cultural practice, the ontological difference that some might presume separates the Indian and the Western psyche, is perhaps overstated, based upon what I have observed as well as what the doctors at NIMHANS themselves say about the illnesses they treat. The human condition, in so far as we can imagine it, exists as one of division, negation, and alienation, as our Hegelian, Freudian, and Heideggerian legacies might have it within Western philosophy, though the valence of the struggle for insight and self-knowledge varies in its progression from pan-human predicaments, such as those that mark the emergence of individuation from parents and siblings, to the specific boundaries of the self, as constituted by specific social demands. Historicism and culture still matter, not as beginning and end, but as temporal progression, semiotic sensibility, and the constitution of content that comprises consciousness, fantasy, and phantasm.

These philosophical musings notwithstanding, we might then ask: what is the emergent flavor of psychiatric care in this context? Indeed, throughout these OPD cases we have witnessed the limits of psychiatric care not so much from a posturing of authoritative knowledge (though this can also have a suggestive function, we have seen), but rather, doctors are acutely aware and frustrated by the limitations imposed upon them by the institutional setting of the OPD and the patient wards. Though the primary intervention at NIMHANS was pharmaceutical, and secondarily psychotherapeutic, the conversations and case histories that occurred within the OPD, between patients, among doctors and their protégés, concerned the psychosocial contexts out of which their patients' symptoms emerged or were exacerbated. As one doctor put it, to repeat again, "We put Band-Aids on gaping wounds." Moreover, while research in genetics and psychopharmacology had evolved to an extent that vulnerabilities to serious and refractory forms of mental illness could not be understood as sociocultural constructs in their entirety, the status of biomarkers in the tracing of mental illness was greatly lacking in precision. Though the lexicon of diagnosis in the ICD-10 and DSM-5 indexed particular pharmacopoeias with an increasing degree of quantitative certainty, the neural and genetic underpinning of mental illness was still poorly understood vis-à-vis the psychosocial stress factors that triggered illness, and the cultural models that shaped symptoms and their recovery (Harrington 2018). Perhaps because of this troubling uncertainty, doctors were often committed to social causes, and in particular to the rights of their patients and to the potential abuses they suffered in society and within their respective families. The drama of the "good" versus "bad" family was, to an extent, staged in the arena of psychiatric care, or in its absence.

Of the recurrent themes that doctors—at least those I accompanied in my year at NIMHANS—were vocal about addressing, including the issue of "good" and "bad" families, abandonment versus care, and advocacy for patient rights, those concerning the need to educate and reform "obscurantist" traditions in society were prominent. As we might recall, the idea that marriage was a "cure" for mental illness was one such belief that doctors were passionately opposed to, as this would contribute to concealment of illness prior to marriage in hopes that the problems would go away after marriage.

Given the intimacies discussed above, and the overall impact mental illness had on the families' lives, the practice of concealing mental illness came up time and time again as an enemy of care. Concealment, of course, also related to stigma, and the contagious effect of stigma upon others in the household, which, in turn, would alter their social position and marital options. Moreover, doctors at NIMHANS, while not directly opposed to traditional treatments, including Ayurveda, faith healings, and yoga, were opposed to painful rites of exorcism that might cause psychological, if not physical, scars (Chandrasekhar 2008). And of course, stigma and the hardship it created would also contribute to abandonment within places of worship, such as in the *dargahs* discussed above. Some doctors were involved in educational outreach within rural areas surrounding Bangalore. Street pedagogy included hosting clinics in underserved areas, as well as staging plays using local actors to dramatize manifestations of mental illness and the kinds of abuse that patients and families endured when it was ascribed to moral faults, demonic possession, and most of all, social exclusion. The last point emerged in almost every OPD session witnessed. Social exclusion was an unnecessary cruelty linked to superstitions and ignorance, the doctors warned. Moreover, the prognosis of a mental illness was certainly worsened when social and familial life was diminished for the patients (Luhrmann and Marrow 2016). Therefore, it followed, and we have witnessed, that patients and their families were encouraged to engage in robust social life, including religious festivals and daily worship, as this was the arena where obscurantism occurred, and therefore was the front line of reform. Indeed, one of the debates that occurs in psychiatric treatment in India concerns the polarities of institutionalization versus a movement towards de-institutionalizing mental health care. As many advocates have argued, community-based care conjoined to psychiatric treatment produces much better results than does long-term institutionalizing of patients in hospital wards (Patel et al. 2018; Desjarlais, Eisenberg, Good, and Kleinman 1995; Narasimhan et al. 2019). On the other hand, leaving patients without the support of accredited and institutionalized care could leave them vulnerable to forms of traditional practice that were exclusionary, violent, and bordered upon neglect and abandonment. Or, conversely, patients could be left dependent upon pharmaceutical self-care as an outpatient (Lang 2018). The NIMHANS philosophy may not have been uniform, but it generally tended towards favoring medical pluralism, to the extent that expert psychiatric care could be empowering to patients and their families, whereas traditional treatments could be useful adjuncts, particularly if stress relief and social support were obtained through the latter. But when the individual rights of the patient for medical care were infringed by "backward" beliefs, they were less hospitable to prevailing social norms, and saw themselves as reformers and educators, as much as physicians. As such, the doctors were educated in the laws of the nation, particularly concerning issues surrounding marriage, dowry, and divorce, but also elder abuse and discrimination against those suffering from disabilities. Doctors were sometimes called in as expert witnesses in legal cases, and were at the front lines of media and scholarly accounts of improving care within psychiatric institutions throughout the country (Murthy 2018).

Dealing with "tradition" was nuanced at NIMHANS, and the most thoughtful doctors often spoke indirectly about two sorts of traditionalism that had to be addressed. On the one hand, there was a vast undereducated rural sea of populations that still held to beliefs in demonology and were unable to distinguish mental illness from spiritual contagions. Though vague notions of mental illness were certainly not unknown, the first, and in many cases final, recourse to treatment came in the form of faith healing and exorcisms. But there were also the varieties of neo-traditionalism that we have witnessed in the form of alternative therapies, on the more benign side, to the excessive fixations upon religious identity as a modern symptom.

Heidegger's (1977) diagnosis of modernity as the "Age of the World Picture," whereby representation and abstraction reduced the world into subroutines of quantum measurement to the peril of humankind's relationship with the Earth, comes into view; but in extending his argument, we could say, to the detriment of meaningful yet indeterminate and non-categorical forms of social intimacy in favor of transactional bureaucratic exchanges, it leads to the symptom of "flight." In Heidegger's analysis, the flight into "tradition" was the great technocratic peril of the age. He knew from his own personal folly the risk of a regenerative and redemptive politics rooted in blood and soil,[14] as did Weber, with the latter's warning of oscillation to charisma and meaning-based politics out of the "iron cage" of constricted mental life. Fighting the emergence of totalitarian tendencies as a form of psychopathology, in turn, required a political consciousness that the specialized terminologies of psychiatry, with its neuro, chemical-based, and genetic emphases, could not provide. This concerned the doctors greatly, who saw the "Band-Aid" being applied through the technical grid of diagnosis and palliative care, but were wary of the historical moment and the hysteric contagion of cosmological ordering as a byproduct of alienation and anomie, not to mention the loss of meaning and social intimacy within the new information-based economy. Moreover, and this may not have been in the doctors' minds, the very serialized form of symptomatology that their craft had become was yet another singularization and serialization out of complexity and etiology.

The craft and art of psychiatry also mirrored the redactions and categorical lexicons that were part of the ethno-religious and occupational winnowing of meaning, in which "grey" zones were increasingly intolerable. But in saying this, I am not arguing that psychiatrists were pathologically attached to these lexicons and technical operations. Indeed, they themselves were made uneasy by reductionism induced by the increasing specialization and technical measurements of diagnosis that were operative in their practice, as evidenced, too, by their oft-repeated concerns that the younger generation of medical students were being trained to narrowly to treat symptoms, not persons within a psychosocial milieu.[15] Therefore, as I have tried to show, the OPD witnessed a frequent tension between the practical, precise, and efficient operations that allowed the greatest number of patients to be treated, and the meaningful expressions and speculations that doctors offered about the historical moment and the not-so-distant pasts that informed and sometimes resisted it.

Chapter 5

Seizures, "Fits," and Neurology

NIMHANS has more psychiatrists than neurologists. India as a whole has more psychiatrists than clinical neurologists. Given this paucity of specialists throughout the country, NIMHANS is an important site for research and neurological care. As is the case with psychiatry, patients travel from all over the country to be treated for various ailments, with epilepsy being perhaps the most common. Within neurology, specializations such as epileptology are even more rare. Therefore, patients from all over the country make the long journey to NIMHANS when seizures are intractable. NIMHANS not only has some of the top epileptologists in the country, it also has some of the best neurosurgeons who perform delicate brain surgery. As a result, NIMHANS has advanced technologies such as MRIs and EEG monitoring facilities, which allow for extensive pre-surgical testing. As a government hospital, it offers high-quality care for very reasonable costs, and is free for those below the poverty level. Even surgery and post-surgery rehabilitation costs are borne by the institution when a patient cannot afford to pay.

My interest in clinical neurology concerned the areas where comorbid psychiatric and neurological diagnoses overlapped. The back and forth between being seen by either a neurologist or psychiatrist often hinged upon the presence of an organic disease such as epilepsy, as compared to a "hysteric" conversion disorder that might mimic the symptoms of a neurological disease. In previous pilot research in a North American epileptology clinic I was surprised to learn that upwards of 30 percent of the intractable seizure cases that were seen there were, in fact, psychogenic, not epileptic. That is, the seizures, while resembling epilepsy, and perhaps modeled after it, albeit unconsciously, did not show the characteristic epileptiform brain waves associated with epilepsy. These seizures, to a highly trained epileptologist, could be induced within a hospital setting by the power of suggestion. For instance, strobe lights and tilt table tests could be performed and the patient told that these tests are likely to produce seizures. Sometimes the seizures, even without EEG confirmation, could be diagnosed as psychogenic, or "pseudo seizures," simply through their semiology. For instance, if a person having a seizure closed his or her eyes in a hard grimace, this was a telltale sign. Seizures almost always occur with eyes open. There were other tricks of the trade that the doctors could use to diagnose these seizures. But the "gold standard" was the EEG coupled with simultaneous video monitoring. The synchronized video recording of the seizure and the corresponding EEG could confirm either epilepsy or the psychogenic attack.

Oftentimes those patients with psychogenic seizures I had observed in the North American setting had been taking anticonvulsants for years, being earlier diagnosed with epilepsy by primary care physicians or general neurologists less expert in epilepsy. To my surprise, however, when the patients were brought the "good news" that they did not have this dangerous disease, and could therefore go off the harsh anticonvulsant medications, they often resisted their diagnosis. Indeed, they would oftentimes demand more tests, not believing that their seizures were not "real." The doctors, for their part, would try to reassure the patients that their seizures were real and serious, in terms of the disruptive effects that they had on peoples' lives, but that stress management, counseling, and perhaps psychiatry were the best chances for a complete recovery. This resistance suggested the patients did not want to be seen as "crazy" or "mentally ill." This surprised me given that the psychogenic diagnosis was objectively good news, in terms of prognosis. Intractable epileptic seizures, on the other hand, were almost impossible to cure, and when it was possible to cure, it involved risky brain surgery, which in turn involved a long process of recovery after a major resection of the brain occurred. But I suspected that attitudes and stigma towards mental illness, as well as support groups, were less developed than was the case for epilepsy. In the case of the latter, education within society and support groups had grown substantially, and thus the stigma of epilepsy was far less than it had been in the past. Mental illness, on the other hand, was still stigmatized far more. Moreover, insurance coverage for neurological care was more generous, but considerably more limited for mental health treatment.

Doctors implied there were unconscious push and pull factors towards the psychogenic seizure. While stigma was a large factor, as suggested above, insurability and protecting a sense of self, by externalizing the illness, objectifying it as "not me" but rather a brain disorder that should be seen within the brain scan or EEG, and therefore, like a demon in demonology, a foreign entity that can be exorcised by neuroscience, offered the patient a shift in culpability. No, they were not mentally ill, they had a neurological condition. Thus, it was not surprising, seen in this light, that they resisted the diagnosis of a conversion disorder. Interestingly, I was told that a high proportion of cases came from those who cared for a person with epilepsy, or worked in the clinical context where they witnessed epileptic seizures. This supported the idea that a repertoire was emergent within the culture to embody stress and convert it into a physiological symptom. Whether this was an emergent culture-bound syndrome remained to be seen. But given the purported disappearance of "hysteria" in the West, as a set of symptoms and as a psychiatric diagnosis, it was striking that the trajectory in the West, with regard to hysteria, had gone from witchcraft accusations or demonology, through a period when hysteria was a common diagnosis during the height of the psychoanalytic domination of psychiatry in the first half of the twentieth century, to a period of its disappearance into other modern maladies and diagnoses, such as "histrionic personality," "schizoid," "borderline personality," and, of course, "conversion," "somatoform" disorder, and "psychosomatic" illness.

This digression into the North American context is relevant insofar as my initial interest in the Indian clinical context was driven by the questions that arose from the North American ethnographic material. Indeed, when discussing my ethnographic observations with a psychiatrist at NIMHANS, we will recall from the introduction, he remarked that this was "remarkable." He added, "You have found the re-emergence of hysteria in the West, where we assumed it had died out." He added further that in India, he believed the cultural lexicons and demonologies were more intact, and that the presentation of physical symptoms that converted psychic stress into somatic symptoms was culturally patterned by beliefs of spirit possession. Moreover, in the general public, "fits" and "seizures" were indistinguishable; therefore, the provenance of both was assumed to be a malevolent agent. Of course, he added, among the educated classes, particularly in urban areas, the attitudes towards epilepsy were changing. Therefore, it would be interesting, he added, for me to shadow neurologists at NIMHANS to see if the presentation and frequency of psychogenic seizures did, in fact, conform to cultural models and shaping.

Prior to the fieldwork at NIMHANS, I was advised to visit the "healing temple" of Chottanikkara, in Cochin, Kerala. This famous temple to the Goddess was said to heal "madness" and "fits" (Halliburton 2009). There, hundreds of patients visited the temple daily, most on pilgrimage to a sacred spot, but some with severe mental disturbances and "fits" that were thought to be caused by demonic possession. Within the temple is a sacred tree where one can see little dolls nailed to it with iron nails. The possessed individual is told to hammer the doll to the tree with the iron nail, using the forehead, which causes bleeding. This coupled with exorcism rituals would trap the malevolent spirit within the dolls, curing the afflicted. When I visited, I was not able to witness the exorcism rituals. I was there during the day, and these rituals occurred in the evenings (see Halliburton 2009). But I did see a large number of individuals who appeared to be afflicted, sitting within the temple with family members. Some rocked their heads back and forth, and others made gestures with their hands. These individuals, primarily females, I noted, seemed disheveled in appearance, with unbraided hair. The look of possession was not different from what I had witnessed in the *dargahs* described earlier. Within the sacred space of the temple, these individuals and their symptoms were calmed.

Having witnessed possession in many contexts (Willford 2006; 2014), I was not particularly surprised by what I saw in the healing temple. But I was thinking, all the while, about those patients who might have epilepsy or other neurological conditions but were thought to be possessed when they visited Chottanikkara, or other healing shrines. Where the power of suggestion might enact the placebo and nocebo effects of either curing or calling forth symptom presentations, in the case of the epileptic, the electrical discharge within the brain was not psychically controllable or amenable to suggestion. Therefore, a double jeopardy might be faced by those with "fits" who actually suffered from epilepsy. Would they be blamed for their failed cures within the healing site? Was their fate to suffer seizures and the moral blame for lacking faith? Or was their fate linked to previous karma and thus the fault of the afflicted? Indeed, this was a concern among neurologists and psychiatrists (Chandrasekhar 2008) who, while noting the psychological benefits of curing rituals in some cases (Raguram, Venkateswaran, Ramakrishna, Weiss, et al. 2002; Kakar 1982; Halliburton 2009), were wary of the cultural and social violence inflicted by the "ignorant" upon those suffering organic illnesses.

With these questions in mind, I devoted some of my time at NIMHANS to shadowing a renowned epileptologist. I was also quite interested in the porous borders of psychiatric versus neurological care. As psychiatry became more neurological, grounded in brain science as opposed to theories of mind such as psychoanalytic theory, psychiatrists did see and treat patients with neurological conditions. And vice versa, neurologists at NIMHANS treated comorbid psychiatric conditions. Both increasingly understood each other's craft and were certified to treat in each other's domains. Indeed, comorbid psychiatric symptoms were treated in the psychiatry OPD. But there were handoffs, where a referral would be made in either direction when it was thought important, particularly if the diagnosis was not obvious. Moreover, the technology, for instance, to test for psychogenic or "pseudo" seizures was under the jurisdiction of neurology. Thus, when a person might be suspected of having either epilepsy or psychogenic seizures, they would receive a referral to neurology to answer this question with certainty. And conversely, if a patient had seizures and depression and/or mania, as was often the case, they would receive a referral to psychiatry for treatment.

The following observations came from shadowing the clinical neurologist in the OPD. Though I sat through many days of neurology OPD, where the cases were not epilepsy, or the cases were routine follow-ups for epilepsy, I will, for present purposes, only focus more upon the "grey" zone of the psychogenic seizure, given the significant overlapping themes discussed in earlier chapters.

There are very few epilepsy specialists at NIMHANS. Among permanent faculty, the clinical neurologist I shadowed was perhaps the most active, seeing up to fifty patients a day, between the hours of 7:30 a.m. and 7:30 p.m. The doctor, a mild-mannered man of short stature, was perhaps in his early fifties or late forties. Unlike some of the neurologists, he did not wear a white coat, preferring to dress casually. He often wore short sleeves, which was also a bit unusual for clinicians at NIMHANS. I had come to him upon recommendation of one of the senior psychiatrists I often shadowed. He was, for his part, quite receptive to being shadowed, and would explain, in terse, clear, albeit brief words, each case that appeared in his clinic.

Upon meeting him first in his office I had mentioned my interest in the cultural dimensions of psychogenic seizures. He told me that in India, anyways, the term, "pseudo seizures" was still used. I explained to him that some doctors in the US had told me that "pseudo seizures" was not used to describe these seizures nowadays because it implied that they were not real, or faked, which was certainly not the case. The doctor said, however, that in India people did not make assumptions about false versus true seizures, as malingering was not common. Moreover, most people from rural areas did not know the distinction between seizures and "hysterical possession," using the term "fits" to describe both. He did mention, however, that psychogenic seizures accounted for about 10 to upwards of 20 percent of the seizure patients he saw in the OPD and LTM (long-term monitoring).[1]

The doctor had a brisk and to-the-point bedside manner within the OPD, but was laser focused on each patient, whether it was morning or, after a long day, in the evening. The actual OPD was almost identical to the Psychiatry OPD, which was just across the hall within the same building.

Sharing the building meant that referrals and cross-checking of information were easy. As with psychiatry, dozens of patients and their families would fill the waiting room in the mornings, taking a number. There were no fixed appointments. Therefore, as in the case of psychiatry, the wait could last an entire day. The social aspects of each case were covered by one resident in an intake interview, whereas another resident would screen patients for their symptoms, and prior treatments as well, before presenting before the doctor. While there were a number of residents screening patients, I did not see a more senior fellow take on a larger role as I had, on some occasions, in psychiatry. The doctor was urbane and polite, and very self-assured. In general, he was too busy to spend much time with each and every patient, given the daily patient load he faced. He said the neurology OPD, as a whole, sees well over two hundred patients per day.

"Pseudo Seizures"

A young woman named Gita, in the ninth standard, came all the way from Assam, and was diagnosed with epilepsy. During times of academic stress, and following poor results in school exams, she began to suffer from left-hand pain and stiffness. The whole arm stiffened and twisted during these "fits." Nobody was able to turn Gita's arm back to normal position when this happened. These events had occurred four times during the past year, and again, always while under stress. Gita's EEG was normal, according to the doctor. But at the local level, she had been diagnosed with epilepsy by a provincial doctor. For the past year she had been taking Dilantin, a common and older generation anticonvulsant. These attacks were always precipitated by stress and never occurred during sleep.

As I observed her in the clinic, Gita seemed a bit confused and sad. Her brother did all the talking for her with the doctor. After some time, her mother also joined in the conversation. During a pause, while they waited for further instructions from a social worker who spoke Bengali, I asked, with the aid of this Bengali-speaking social worker, whether she had been to a faith healer. The family said that they had gone to one and it had helped somewhat. The faith healer, or "Baba," was a Sufi healer. Gita's family was Hindu. The Baba was "more helpful" than the medications, the family explained. But there had been four attacks in the past year, and this was reason for concern. I inquired whether they believed a spirit (*jinn*) had possessed her. The mother and brother said, indeed, that they were very worried about this possibility. I then asked if they had any specific medicines from the healer. They answered that "holy water" (*pani*) had been given.

During these "attacks" there was no incontinence or loss of consciousness, both of which might indicate epilepsy. The family, however, was worried. I then asked if there were any inappropriate or "bad words" said during the attack. They answered in the affirmative that she would sometimes speak Urdu, a language they did not speak, and utter "foreign things" for a few days at a time. They thought this might be an Islamic spirit possessing her (*jinn* or *shaitan*). Given the onset of the symptom with her maturation age, one might, from a psychodynamic perspective, suspect suppression and repression giving cathartic corporeal shape to a hidden desire. This may have been relevant, but another factor was also mentioned. Not only was the bad language used, but there was also aggressive behavior seen during these attacks. The mother said that "aggressive behavior was there." It became clear that that possession was occurring when Gita indicated that she saw the entity that possessed her in physical form. This revelation led the doctor to believe that schizophrenia might also be possible, or some other transient psychosis was occurring. For this reason, she was referred to the psychiatric OPD for a same-day evaluation.

This, indeed, turned out to be a likely case of "pseudo seizures," on the one hand, but when I asked why epilepsy was ever suspected, the doctor had no answer other than to say that local provincial doctors were often "guessing." None of her attacks happened during sleep, which also suggested a non-epileptic attack. The revelation of hallucinations, however, only came about when I had queried about spirits and faith healers. Still, the doctor discerned that this was a case of pseudo seizures from the other clinical data points, as well as the descriptions that Gita and her family had provided. What struck me, however, was the family's assertion that the Baba had been effective, indeed, more effective than the medications that had been prescribed by the provincial doctor. This, too, was a clue. The symptom of hemi-paralysis in one arm also suggested that aggression and its control through the symptom might have been a factor. As Kakar (1982) had noted in a similar case, the paralysis of the arm made it impossible for his patient to strike his parents, protecting him from a more catastrophic unfilial event.

Stiffness and hemi-paralysis seemed to be a recurrent motif in the Indian clinical context (Marrow 2012), which I often heard about in rural contexts, such as the Nilgiris Adivasi communities, to be discussed in the second volume. Indeed, the very next case in the OPD was of a Muslim woman who presented with stiffness in her upper arm. She also suffered from "weakness" after sleeping. During these bouts with stiffness or weakness she never lost consciousness. The EEG in her case also appeared to be negative for epilepsy. Therefore, she was referred to psychiatry with a suspected conversion disorder noted in her charts. At this point, the neurologist said that he sees up to ten pseudo seizure patients each day! This, out of the approximately forty to fifty patients he might see in a day, was not unlike what I witnessed in the epilepsy clinic in the US. This in turn suggests that while the term "hysteria" no longer has diagnostic currency, the symptoms that were used to describe the range of behaviors thought to be hysteric, or a "conversion disorder," had not gone away with their relabeling (Mitchell 2000).

I shadowed the neurologist six times, each time for several hours. The doctor had impressive stamina, I found, throughout the day, treating each patient and their families with the same pleasant affect and alertness to the details of each case. Most of the cases he saw in the OPD were for epilepsy. Out of these, the majority were follow-ups from previous treatment, and therefore were brief, sometimes less than five minutes. Only the relevant details, such as lab results for medication blood levels and seizure frequency, were discussed. On some occasions, the doctor would advise further testing to ascertain whether the patient might be a candidate for surgery to resect the seizure-triggering part of the brain. He had a lot of success, he said, treating intractable epilepsies with surgery. Indeed, he believed in aggressive surgical treatment for epilepsy, particularly when uncontrolled by medications, and especially in a child's early and critical developmental years. If the seizures could be stopped early, the chance of normal development was greater.[2]

The doctor saw more patients with seizures than any other kind of disorder, though he was a general neurologist, and did treat other neurological conditions. As one would expect at NIMHANS, he possessed a detailed amount of knowledge about a wide range of diseases and never consulted any secondary source materials while in the OPD. The OPD clinics, indeed, were unlike the faculty offices of the doctors at NIMHANS, in that there were no reference books or charts available. The doctors only had the patient charts and whatever scans or test results were at their disposal. To view a computerized scan, the doctor had to step across the hall to another room where a computer was set up to view MRIs and other scans.[3] As mentioned, I was impressed by the doctor's stamina as I watched him for about four or five hours of his OPD without a break, whereas he was actually in the OPD for more than ten hours a day. While I felt exhausted trying to note details of each case, he seemed attentive to the smallest of details and asked incisive but reassuringly calm questions throughout the day, without any visible fluctuation of energy.

The doctor did break for lunch and coffee during his long shifts. He lived in faculty housing on campus and would go home for lunch. I tended to always eat in the faculty and resident "canteen" (cafeteria), which was the same food that the patients and families ate, though divided by a partition wall, giving the doctors some respite from their patients. The food was all vegetarian and offered a choice between North and South Indian cuisine, as well as some popular "Chinese" dishes, that were, in fact, Indian inventions, such as "Gobi Manchurian" (spicy cauliflower deep fried into little batter-covered balls).

As neurological exams in the OPD seemed to be even briefer than they were in its psychiatric counterpart across the hall, my notes seemed to be even more terse. The psychiatric OPD, in contrast, did explore some of the experiential issues within the patients' symptom presentation, as well as some family history. As there were fewer clinical neurologists, and even fewer epileptologists, the patient load for this particular doctor was heavier than it was for the psychiatrists. This was also reflected in the fact that he saw patients at a much quicker interval than did the psychiatrists. I counted in one session that he saw twelve patients in four hours, which might translate to thirty plus patients over a twelve-hour working day. As many of the relevant facts of the case were already discussed with a resident or fellow, the clinical interview with the doctor was expedited. Some patients who had waited up to seven hours or more would only receive five minutes with the doctor, and perhaps a bit more time with the residents, fellows, and social workers who did intake interviews.

I asked the doctor about the appointment system and how it worked. It seemed that patients would sign in first thing in the morning. Some would be seen immediately, but others simply had to wait it out the whole day. Part of this was based on the urgency of the condition. But there was also a numbering system. Visiting the OPD was, however, a commitment of a full day's time for the patients and their families. The impression I had, that NIMHANS looked like a small village with whole families camped out in various spots within the waiting room, or outside on the few green patches or benches they could find, was buttressed by the rhythms of care in the OPD. The canteen did a good business, too, with so many captive patients together with their families for long hours. The canteen, I guessed from observation, must have served several hundred people per day, just counting patients and caregivers alone, not to mention the staff and doctors of the hospital. That prices were nominal (thirty rupees for a full meal, or approximately forty cents in US currency) was also a plus.

When I mentioned that in the US, patients would never wait all day and would expect an hour, perhaps two at the maximum, for an appointment window, the doctor explained that an appointment system had been tried at NIMHANS in the past. But the poor patients, he said, would not "follow the instructions" and would "invariably misunderstand" and miss their appointments. Therefore, it was decided that to insist on an appointment schedule for OPD would inhibit access for the poor and illiterate, a core constituency for the hospital, with its free and subsidized services. But this did mean, he added, that those who had the means might prefer to go to a private hospital for

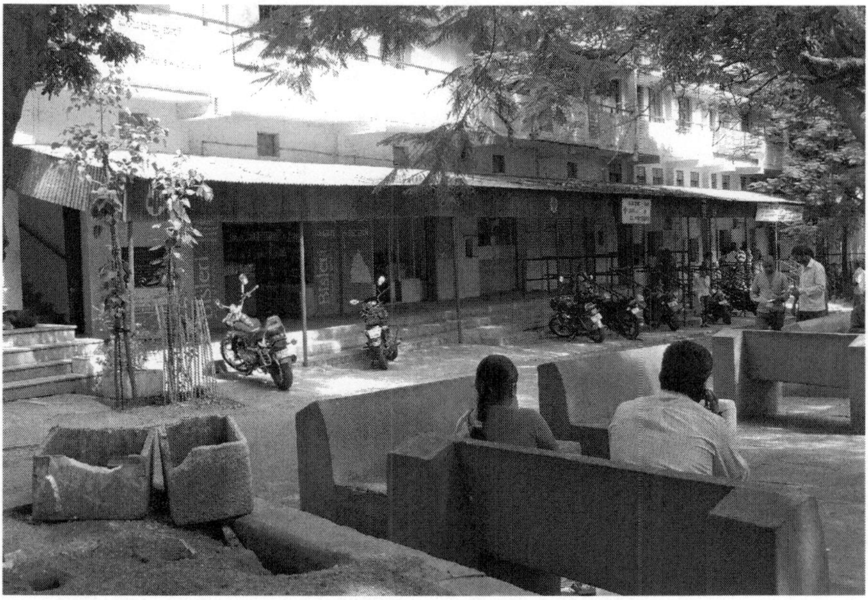

Pharmacy and sundry shops at NIMHANS. (Photograph by author.)

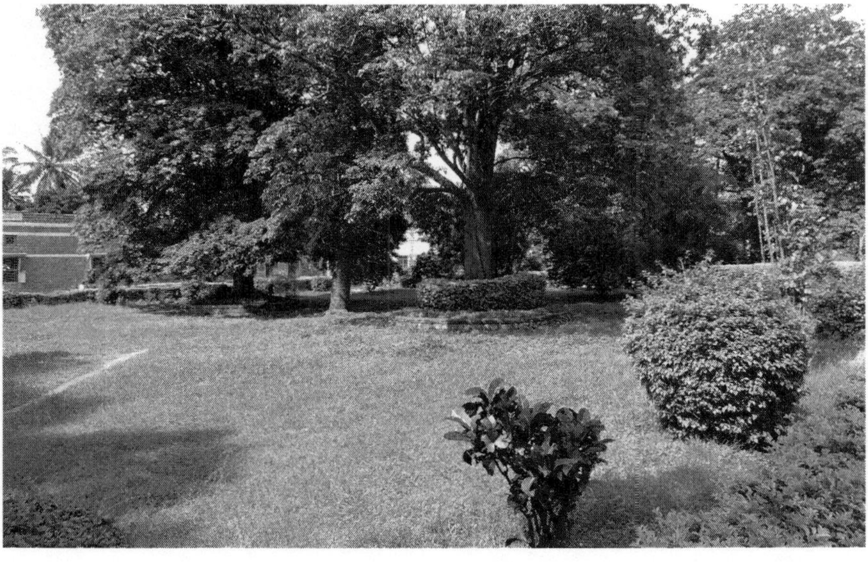

Green space adjacent to patient ward, seen in background. (Photograph by author.)

services, as they were reluctant to join the crowds for long hours in the OPD at NIMHANS (Ruddock 2021). This explained, in turn, the preponderance of poor patients relative to middle-class ones. While I witnessed many middle-class patients each week, they were a minority—despite the fact that some of the best doctors were based at NIMHANS. The neurologist said (as did the psychiatrists) that some of the doctors in private hospitals were excellent, but this was not always the case. Indeed, as we have seen, the doctors at NIMHANS were often very critical of the care that patients had received in other institutions prior to their arrival at NIMHANS, noting the false diagnoses, contraindicated medications, and over-medicating of patients that often occurred at the provincial level, or within private clinics where there was less government oversight and a greater likelihood of fraudulent practice.

I mentioned to the neurologist that multiple brain surgeries for seizures in the same patient were rare in the US, as far as I knew. But we talked about the different schools of thought regarding how aggressive one should be with early onset epilepsy, when the seizures were intractable. He said that aside from it being about seizure control, when it involves a young child, it was also about the urgency of achieving developmental milestones. Therefore, he favored a more aggressive approach, suggesting that it might be warranted so as to give a child a chance of normal development. In the US, with the more litigious concerns around malpractice, the doctors and hospitals were very cautious, only advocating surgery when a focal lesion was clearly marked through scans, and/or the seizures were clearly emanating from a focal part of the brain, as confirmed by advanced EEG testing. NIMHANS also followed similar brain-mapping procedures, which was why it might take one year of testing before surgery was performed. But, according to the neurologist, the philosophy was to advocate for surgery if there was hope it might allow the patient to develop normally.

We talked on occasion about the financial support that the poor received. The doctor mentioned that even the surgery, scanning/testing, and associated medications were largely free at NIMHANS for the poor. This often meant that the family could, in fact, have the surgery without financial hardship, though they might lose some income during the extended period leading up to and following the surgery.

Among the free antiepileptic drugs that NIMHANS could provide to those with a BPL card were: valproate, Dilantin (phenytoin), phenobarbital, and carbamazepine (Tegretol). Among the common drugs that were not free, topiramate, lamotrigine, and levetiracetam were commonly prescribed. For the very poor it was more of challenge to pay for these drugs. These could cost anywhere between INR 300 and INR 2,000 (USD 5 to 40) per month to purchase. As this amount could be prohibitive to the very poor, there was a special fund at NIMHANS to provide help purchasing these medications for families that were below the poverty line.

On one occasion, I had a brief conversation with the neurologist about medical tourism and the state of India's high-tech medical facilities versus the challenges of reaching the poor. The doctor said that all this "boasting of international clientele" coming to India for health care is "a load of nonsense." He went on to say that one must "take care of your backyard first . . . there is no point talking about foreigners coming here." He went on to explain how corporate interests were taking advantage of the move towards privatized hospital care. While he claimed that India had not reached the level of privatization and capitalization that exists in the US within the health care industry, this was also the growing trend in India, fueled by the purchasing power of the expanding middle class. The "poor will feel the pinch," he claimed. I asked whether foreigners coming to NIMHANS for treatment were expected to pay a different rate at public institutions, like NIMHANS. The doctor said that they would pay the same rate as Indian patients.[4] There was a sliding scale based upon income, but this would not amount to a separate category of "foreign" patient. He went on to add that most patients received free treatment at NIMHANS, given their low incomes.

We discussed the costs of studying medicine in India and abroad. I had asked the doctor about the heavy patient load and whether the replacement of doctors by newly minted neurologists was sufficient in India. He replied in the negative. There were limited "lines" or positions at NIMHANS, despite the fact that the patient load was expanding with each passing year. More investment in faculty lines was needed, he said. Moreover, getting into a government medical institution like NIMHANS was extremely competitive. Therefore, a lot of medical students would study abroad in order to "save on cost." I was somewhat surprised to hear that private medical schools in India were more expensive than studying abroad in some countries. Therefore, I asked him about the quality of these doctors who study abroad and whether they need additional qualifications to practice upon returning to India. He mentioned that the quality "varied a lot" in the overseas institutions. But the cost of attending a private medical college in India could be as high as USD 50,000–80,000, he said. This, in Indian currency, was an astronomical amount.

Our conversation often turned back to surgery interventions for epilepsy and the relationship between epilepsy and "pseudo seizures." He pointed out something fascinating and somewhat akin to "phantom limbs." It seems that there were documented cases, and in his own personal experience, where patients began to have pseudo seizures even after successfully curing their epilepsy through surgery. He attributed this to the expectation that they were now to "care for themselves" and had lost the "support network" that had become part of their daily life, as well as losing emotional sustenance, if not their sense of identity. I had previously discussed how my research had discovered that support for epilepsy was greater than that for mental health, and thus my hypothesis was that psychogenic seizures reflected that gravitational pull towards a category and identity that provided literal care, through insurability, emotional support, and an objectification of one's symptom as "organic" and located in the brain, and not in the self or mind. This was similar in logic to Obeyesekere's (1981) model of the "personal symbol," which serves to objectify an inner ambivalence by identifying it as a corporeal entity, such as a spirit or god manifested as a physical symptom. With the greater support and acceptance that epilepsy enjoyed in the US, as compared to mental illness, I thought of the psychogenic seizure as a new and more politically neutral name for what used to be called a hysteric conversion disorder in US society (Mitchell 2000). This mimetic form of illness was also contagious, as health workers and caregivers were more likely to suffer this symptom. We might recall the case of the dancer that was discussed in an earlier chapter who, while not having a neurological condition, according to test results, still had a hard time regaining her ability to walk. In that case, whatever the provenance of the illness, the patient had taken on the identity of disability advocate. Like the healer who turned their illness or personal crisis into a craft of healing (Obeyesekere 1981; Kakar 1982; Nabokov 2000, Ewing 1997; Trawick 2017), the epileptic or the disabled sometimes found it hard to overcome their symptom when a psychosocial investment had been made.

As our conversation continued, he also pointed out that many patients with epilepsy also have pseudo seizures. This might be a way to "gain control," he suggested, of the seizure disorder, as I had speculated was the case in the US as well.[5] I then mentioned that the category of psychogenic seizure might be a "catchall" diagnosis that lumps a lot of nonepileptic symptoms together, like the earlier category, hysteria, conversion disorders of various types, and other somatic complaints. If, as Mitchell argues (2000), the patient mimics the diagnostic category, performing it, in a sense, for the therapist, albeit unconsciously, then, like culture-bound syndromes, the idea of a newly recognized "seizure"-type could be productive of the very symptoms it purported to diagnose through mimesis. I noted that the presentation could vary substantially, in my experience, and that there was some risk in lumping things together under a broad category, be it hysteria or pseudo seizures. The doctor seemed to agree and said that there were actually many "disorders that were being lumped together under this category" in order to "pass off" patients to psychiatry. Once it was determined that the patient was nonepileptic, the diagnosis was used to simply pass the patient along.

I had, indeed, heard similar sentiments in the US when clinical neurologists, I was told, were sometimes impatient with psychogenic seizures, believing their treatment was within the psychiatric domain, and thus wasted their valuable time from dealing with intractable "real" seizure disorders. To be fair, most doctors did not share this view, at least not consciously. They took the seizures seriously, often noting how intractable and refractory they were. But the disabling aspects, aside from the physical risks they posed for bodily injury, were best treated by mental health professionals, not neurologists. A "pass-off" was indeed required as a necessary part of the treatment, as it was the moment of reckoning for the patient, whether they resisted this or not. Their resistance to the hand-off was evidence of psychogenic resistance, a key indicator of psychological resonance. From the patient's point of view, however, they felt the diagnosis as accusatory, telling them, in fact, that they needed to "deal" with "their" problem, as it was not an organic disease, but was an indicator that they needed help dealing with life's stresses. In other words, they could not objectify and externalize the cause as existing outside of their "self," where sovereignty over one's thoughts and actions were part of the American ideology of selfhood.

In India, according to the neurologist, there was less concern among patients with the psychogenic diagnosis, given that the line had always been blurred between fits and seizures, and their demonological causes, within the cultural milieu. But, he added, there could be resistance within the urban educated patients, who were more aware of epilepsy and its distance from mental illness. At this point, however, the stigma associated with both illnesses in society made an unconscious desire of the patient for one diagnosis over the other less important. Moreover, he said the authority of the doctor, for better or worse, was not questioned in India as much as it was in the West. Therefore, resistance would rarely be openly stated to the doctor making such a diagnosis. Again, however, we will recall in the previous chapter how the educated middle-class patients did, in fact, resist biomedical psychiatry in favor of self-healing practices such as yoga.

A key question that remains then is: To what extent does this diagnosis have explanatory power and produce clinical efficacy within either neurology or psychiatry? Do psychiatrists, after the "pass-off," explore and complicate the diagnosis? And where does the cultural shaping of the symptom, as a nocebo effect, come in? Or is there perhaps a power in the authority of the doctor to suggest a cure, much like that authority witnessed in the exorcism (Stengers 2003; Lévi-Strauss 1973)?

Viewing psychogenic seizures in the clinical setting is not an everyday phenomenon. While a number of patients described symptoms that turned out to be psychogenic, capturing the actual seizure usually involved video monitoring, or LTM (long-term monitoring). Patients were admitted to a special ward where they had constant video and EEG monitoring. When a seizure is about to happen, in the aura phase, the patient or observing family member is asked to push a button that marks the video and EEG, allowing for the synchronized reading. Watching the physical movements synced to the EEG, in turn, allows the doctor to determine the status of the seizure. Inductions are also a part of the process, as these are seizures by suggestion, more easily produced if the seizure is psychogenic. Deception is involved. Usually, this takes the form of vague statements by the physician that the "test" might produce a seizure. In the US, strobe lights and tilt table tests were the forms of induction I witnessed. The doctor told me that at NIMHANS, the forms of induction involved "suggestive words," lights, the use of placebos, and using a tuning fork. The tilt table test was not mentioned.

While I had witnessed many occasions of trance and possession that involved "fits" or seizure-like behavior during religious rituals, I did not view psychogenic seizures in real time within the clinic at NIMHANS, like I had in the US clinic, where I witnessed inductions through deception. But I was given an opportunity to watch videos of psychogenic seizures at NIMHANS that had been collected in the LTM. In one case, the patient clenched his fist and coughed repeatedly, while seemingly in a dissociative psychological state. In another case, a patient appeared to be catatonic for about ten minutes, which the doctor described as being "out of phase." In another case, a man had a glassy stare on his face and began kicking his leg in a kind of rhythmic jerk that went on for several minutes. After some time, a family member spoke to the man in Tamil gently, suggesting he stop. After a minute or so of consoling words from the family member, he regained normal consciousness and his kicking stopped. The power of suggestion worked both ways, in this instance, as he was talked out of his seizure. In yet another case, a male appeared panicked and coughed repeatedly with fear visibly present on his face. In yet another case, a young woman banged her head repeatedly during her seizure. I was told in her case that "parental strife" was a contributing factor. I asked about "teeth clenching" as a symptom, as I had read about this particular psychogenic symptom (Marrow 2012; Kakar 1982). The doctor said this was also seen fairly frequently at NIMHANS, though it was more common in North India.

I was struck by the differences between what I witnessed in these "pseudo seizures" and the semiology of the seizures I had witnessed in the US clinic. In the US, the seizures resembled tonic-clonic (convulsions) seizures, or in some cases, just tonic (stiffening). That is, they strongly resembled and "modeled" epileptic symptoms. In the NIMHANS videos, on the other hand, the behavior seemed much more focused upon specific limb movements, or in the case of the young woman, intentional acts of self-harm. The sample, however, was too small to draw any firm conclusions about the cultural modeling of symptoms, though it was suggestive, perhaps, that the presentation of epilepsy was more familiar in the US context owing to medical dramas on television. After viewing the "fits," the doctor commented that he suspected that in some cases, the "burden of well-being" caused those who had been cured of epilepsy through treatment to have these relapses of "pseudo seizures." He was suggesting that in those cases where epilepsy had morphed into pseudo seizures, it was a regression to a state where concern and care were provided, and the pressures of being self-sufficient, post-illness, were difficult to manage. We can recall, too, the child dancer from the second chapter, who continued to suffer paralysis, despite negative neurological tests.

The neurologist was not conservative when it came to recommending admission for patients who did not show signs of improvement. I asked if there was any shortage of beds for these admissions. He had already told me that cost was not a factor, but that there were, indeed, shortages of space. For instance, specifically in the case of the LTM, there were only four beds. Patients resigned themselves to whatever the doctor recommended with regard to admission, though, to my eye, they did not look terribly pleased to be admitted into the ward. But the doctor said that, generally speaking, the patients rarely questioned him and would turn "all decisions" over to him. I asked him specifically about whether patients resisted the recommendation for surgery. Unlike the US, he said, patients have "faith in the doctor" and submit to their medical authority. This was a "good thing," he said, with a smile. In the context of NIMHANS, with its very large percentage of poor and working-class patients, and their presumed medical illiteracy, the faith in the doctor was a potent talisman on the path to wellness. As I had seen often in psychiatry, the confidence and illocutionary force of the doctor's words to predict a remission of symptoms, or even a cure, was a notable cultural feature of the clinical environment at NIMHANS.

As a general observation, surgery seemed a more readily available option here than was the case in the US, where more caution seemed to exist, in my experience.[6] A senior psychiatrist that I worked with at NIMHANS, on the other hand, thought that NIMHANS was being too aggressive, perhaps, with surgery. He mentioned that lobotomies were performed in the hundreds in the 1960s and '70s, and that no statistical records had been kept to look at the long-term outcomes of these surgeries. I asked the psychiatrist whether he felt this would also be true for epileptic surgeries. He replied that "it could be better" in the case of epileptic surgery, but that recordkeeping is "not a strong practice in India." Thus, the rates of success suggested might be misleading, and based on short-term gains, whereas the long-term risks might be downplayed. In comparison, the US doctors, he said, worry about lawsuits and malpractice, which might inhibit useful surgeries out of an abundance of caution. But also, he added, there is more care in the presentation of data in the US and Europe. With so much at stake in the litigious West, presenting a "high success rate" was sought before advocating a surgical option, and this, in turn, meant that a more general conservatism around the question of brain surgery pervades in the West, as compared to India, the psychiatrist suggested. This seemed entirely the opposite of what I had assumed prior to my time at NIMHANS. That is, I assumed that in the West, where resources and expertise in brain surgery, as well as in the pre-testing that was necessary for pinpointing the seizure-producing lesions, was more plentiful, there would be a higher frequency of seizure interventions than was the case in India. Perhaps on a national level, this was true. But NIMHANS, we must recall, was a major center for neuroscience and neurosurgery in India, and thus would have higher numbers as compared to other major hospitals.

I also suspect that structural factors as well as cultural factors favor a more aggressive surgical approach. Patients less familiar with brain topography, such as working-class Indian patients, might not get that much in the way of explanation for going down the path recommended by the doctor. Moreover, as the neurologist himself told me, he would make a recommendation in the form of, "If it was my child, or if it was me, I would have the surgery." Given the faith that patients bestowed upon doctors, the recommendation carried great weight. I wondered, too, if the patients approached the disease as something akin to a cancer that should be removed with great urgency. I noticed that the neurologist never mentioned, in my presence, at any rate, the pros and cons of surgery to patients but only the possibility of "curing the seizures." Therefore, surgery emphasized the removal of a harmful disease, not the resection of a part of one's brain. This leads me to question whether the brain is seen as the "seat of the soul" in India. Or conversely, if cultural models of the self, or of malevolent agents that invade the person, favor surgery as a kind of analogous treatment to exorcism, then there is less a sense of dread in exorcising the malignant agents that have invaded the body, as these are deemed foreign to the self. In the bounded view of selfhood that permeates Western psychology and philosophy, perhaps the internal provenance of mental symptoms might in turn inhibit dramatic exorcism and surgery both, in modern times, though this is a project for another researcher.

As mentioned above, by the time the patient had reached the doctor in the OPD, there had been a pretty detailed workup by the resident and/or fellow, complete with lab, EEG, and MRI results, in most cases. The doctor usually heard a brief summary, not lasting more than 3–5 minutes. He then would check the MRI online, and in some instances also the EEG. Then a quick interview with the patient and a plan of action was drawn up and quickly discussed with the fellow/resident, who would either stay in the office with the doctor or would be called back in. The fellow/resident would then take the patient back to their office for a debriefing in greater detail. The doctor did not explain details to the patients. No physical examination, in most cases, was performed. Basic vital signs (heartrate, blood pressure, and temperature) would have been recorded by an assistant. A kind of verbal shorthand, in a hushed voice between the doctor and the resident/fellow, sped interactions along. I could not always follow these verbal interactions, but the doctor would offer a short overview to me between patients, or sometimes right before them, particularly if they did not speak English.

While surgery was not discouraged, the neurologist spoke of the problems associated with placing a "grid" on the brain. Prior to any surgical resection of the brain, the electrode grid is placed on the surface of the brain to more accurately measure seizure foci. The external EEG indicates focal activity, as does the MRI, if there is an abnormality, such as polymicrogyria, a malformation of the lobes. Positron emission tomography (PET) scans also can indicate seizure locations, but are rare and expensive in India, though NIMHANS was about to have the equipment installed in its imaging lab. The doctor explained that, on the one hand, there is a "telescoping effect" whereby the focus upon one area with the grid "deafens" one's awareness of any other "hot spots" in the brain, thereby suggesting more focality than might be the case. On the other hand, you had the "expedition" effect, where one goes "fishing" to find all seizure spots by placing multiple grids. Here the risk was from the medical complications of placing multiple grids on the open brain. In the former, the risk was missing additional affected areas, whereas, in the latter, it was magnifying anomalous EEG activity and assuming multifocal seizure activity in the case where one "hot spot" was the predominant cause of seizure activity. Moreover, laying multiple grids increased the chances of infection and complicated the skull's integrity more, requiring longer recuperation for the patient prior to their actual brain surgery.

Resources for pre-surgical testing were also limited. The LTM at NIMHANS had only four beds, as mentioned earlier. Patients on the waiting list might have to wait for up to one year. The medical residents generally ran the LTM, though all issues and problems were reported to the doctor. But the doctor did not spend a large amount of time in the unit, though he tried to pass through every day from 7:00 to 8:00 a.m. to check on patients and study the seizures that had been captured.

I once again asked the doctor what percentage of the patients in LTM ended up having psychogenic seizures. He said about 10 to 20 percent did, which mirrored what he said about all seizure cases seen at NIMHANS. And given the dearth in beds, and acute need for pre-surgery testing, this seemed a high percentage. At the same time, however, when I asked how long most people would stay in the LTM, he said it was usually just twenty-four hours, but sometimes as long as three days.[7]

We have already discussed the emergence of psychogenic seizures after epilepsy has been controlled, and have suggested reasons why this may occur. But the doctor told me a fascinating story about a case of psychogenic seizures that ultimately evolved into, or triggered, epileptic seizures. I had already heard from him (as well as doctors in the US) that epileptic patients often suffered from psychogenic seizures, and that this was a means to "control" or have some agency over the possession-like quality of seizures. But this was the first I had heard of a psychogenic seizure patient evolving into epileptic seizures out of a psychogenic event. This had been captured and recorded with the video EEG, according to the doctor. Though unusual, it pointed to the difficult line between psychiatry and neurology. Indeed, the doctor said there might be a more precise diagnosis in the future that demonstrates an organic base for what are now known as psychogenic conversion events. In that sense, the hope is that advances in neuropsychiatry would emerge to complicate the division between neurology and psychiatry, and biologize further our understanding of the mind as brain, which, in turn, would allow for better diagnosis and treatment as the vexing dualism of psyche and soma was overcome.

But the desire for a monistic neuropsychiatric understanding of the brain, mind, and body was still out of reach, and a grey zone persisted between the psychological and the neurological. Moreover, there is ample evidence that whatever neurological factors can be discovered to make people more vulnerable to psychogenic seizures, their range and variation, not to mention cultural shaping, mimetic, and suggestive qualities, make diagnostic certainty a challenge. As a result, while not an official clinical category, hysteria still has currency in clinical discussions. Hysteria, as we have discussed earlier, captures a range of illness presentations, and the notion of a hysteric conversion disorder covers a range of somatic complaints that seem to also be captured by the "pseudo" or psychogenic seizure diagnosis. The neurologist at NIMHANS was probably correct in noting that the term probably needed more nuance, given the range of cases already touched on in both psychiatry and neurology OPDs.

In the Indian context, it was not altogether clear how much these seizures mimicked epilepsy, versus being shaped by beliefs of possession or other cultural beliefs. For instance, there are specific beliefs among Irulas and Kurumbas, two Adivasi communities living in the Nilgiris mountain range, in spirit beings of the forest that can cause paralysis or hemi-paralysis. The symptoms could be described, therefore, as conversion disorders or culture-bound syndromes, rather than pseudo seizures. This topic will be explored in the second volume. In the North American context, seizures were no longer thought to be linked to demonologies; therefore the cultural powers of suggestion would favor the "cultural" model provided by epilepsy, as evidenced by the fact that those susceptible to psychogenic seizures were individuals who worked as caregivers and had been exposed to epileptic patients and/or family members.

As the Indian psychiatrist had pointed out, the question was whether "hysteria" was being rediscovered in a new presentation and diagnosis, where it was thought to have died out. Mitchell (2000), for instance, argues that hysteria reappears in various times and places but is called by many names. For her, following Klein, hysteria is marked by regressive behavior to a state of infantile desire for the intimacy and care of the mother after intolerable annihilating sensations of displacement have occurred through sibling rivalry. The initial traumas of childhood, however, become recurrent, symptomatically, over stressful life events to cause a reliving of these traumas. These can include gendered and political marginalization. Hysteria, in these terms, is a demand for recognition, but one that takes a regressive nonverbal form such as possession, in cultures where these beliefs exist. Lacan has argued similarly that hysteria is a symptom that illustrates the Other's overbearing demand manifested as a symptom of neurotically identifying with the Other's desire, whilst simultaneously recoiling from the Other's lack which commands this identification. In this sense, hysterics are speaking truth to power, as I. M. Lewis (1989) argues, and as has been argued to some extent by Obeyesekere (1981), but in a manner that is self-defeating, to a large extent, unless it can be parlayed into a position of respect and care from the Other. In short, there is a politics potentially hidden (or not so hidden) within the hysteric that cannot be captured by the neuropsychiatric desire for diagnostic certainty. It is, as Derrida (1998) concludes, a "resistance to resistance," through its refractory nature. The fungibility of the conversion disorder, and the elision of certainty, perhaps, like the spirit who refuses to be named in exorcism rituals, is a mark of defiance against the Law, or the Other. No archive of biomedical certainty can fully erase the political significance of the desire that is expressed through the symptom (Pinto 2022; Thiranagama 2022; Seale-Feldman 2022; Marrow 2022; Cohen 2022; Willford 2022; Funahashi 2023).

Returning to the neurologist and his domain, it was evident that similar concerns about rights and abuses within society, as was the case with psychiatry at NIMHANS, concerned him and other neurologists. Moreover, though surgery seemed more prevalent there, many protocols were established so that there was no rush to judgement and action. In addition to the LTM and multiple tests that were ordered, which could take a year or more as we have noted, case conferences occurred twice a month. In these conferences, four or five cases would be discussed in detail. Before any surgery was recommended, the entire team of neurologists would discuss these cases and reach a consensus about whether surgery was the best option or not.

On the question of abuse, the doctor told me a strange story of a "famous Ayurvedic doctor" practicing in Rishikesh and Haridwar, North India. He had hundreds of patients and had become a big celebrity. This doctor claimed he could treat epilepsy through Ayurvedic medicine better than neurologists could. Many patients had evidently vouched for him, and subsequently, his practice grew large. He also became well known as an advocate for Ayurveda and had famous political allies. His patients were told to throw away all their old biomedicines and just to take two pills that his own Ayurvedic lab produced. One was a black pill, the other a pink tablet.

At some point this neurologist had suspicions about the Ayurvedic doctor when a patient was admitted to NIMHANS having suffered *status epilepticus* (a long-lasting and dangerous seizure). At this point, the doctor had him admitted and ordered blood work. When the patient explained that he was a patient of the famous Ayurvedic doctor, and did not take anticonvulsants, the doctor expected to find no traces of medicine in his system. But the lab work came back and showed that the patient, in fact, had a high concentration of valproic acid (sodium valproate), carbamazepine, and phenobarbital, all mainstream anticonvulsant medications, in his system. This raised the doctor's suspicion about the so-called Ayurvedic "lab" that produced the pink and black pills. After further testing of the pink and black tablets, it was discovered that the "Ayurvedic" medicines were actually compounds containing these drugs. The black pills contained valproate and carbamazepine, whereas the pink pill contained phenobarbital! After this was confirmed, the Ayurvedic doctor was eventually arrested for fraud and was currently in jail. My neurologist guide at NIMHANS quietly chuckled and said he had helped to put the "famous doctor behind bars." While this was the most dramatic case of fraud, as was the case with the psychiatrists, the neurologist noted that quality neurological care in many parts of the country was scarce. Therefore, patients were often falsely diagnosed and given the wrong medications, or medications that might be contraindicated.

For instance, a boy presented with seizures and suffered some encephalopathy. There were recorded seizures on his EEG, which had been taken in the LTM. More recently, he had begun to show behavioral problems at home and school. It turned out there was often a link between behavioral problems and the taking of the drug levetiracetam, which had been prescribed to him by another doctor outside of NIMHANS. Therefore, this medicine was immediately removed on this visit to the OPD. Though he had fairly good seizure control with the medication, as he had a lesion on his brain associated with the encephalopathy, he might be a candidate for surgery, the doctor said. The family was told to proceed with a surgical evaluation at NIMHANS, noting that many more tests would have to be done.

This case gave me an opportunity to ask the doctor about the relative success rate for surgery at NIMHANS. He said it was along the "same lines internationally," or about a 75 percent rate of success. The success for MTS (medial temporal sclerosis) surgery was even higher, he said. But I then asked about memory being a post-surgical issue,[8] and he said, in response, that it was "a problem, particularly if the left side was involved." The success rate, he explained further, probably dropped to 60 percent, if patients were tracked for five years or longer. This, in my mind at the time, was a significant drop in efficacy. Efficacy was measured in terms of seizure control, and therefore, the drop over time meant the chance of seizure recurrence increased over time.

Some cases bordered with psychiatry, as already discussed, and whereas the first stop might be neurology, the neurologist was not reluctant to ask for psychiatric evaluations to complement his analysis. In one case, for instance, a fifty-two-year-old female suffered from pain in her left upper limbs and chest. There was stiffness in her back and neck, too. Some demyelination could be seen in the MRI, suggesting a neurological component was at play. But it was also possible, the doctor felt after examining her, that some of her symptoms were psychological. Therefore, he ordered a psychiatric evaluation, transferring her across the hall. Similarly, in another case, a boy, aged nine, had developed seizures. They came nocturnally. During these events he had "altered behavior" and would walk away with "unusual talk," according to his parents. At the time of being seen in the OPD, his scholastic performance was declining. And an epileptic spike could be seen in the EEG, suggesting he did, in fact, have epilepsy. But the nighttime events could have been "night terrors," he thought, and asked that the boy also have a psychiatric evaluation while there.

In another similar case, a young boy presented with delayed milestones and very rudimentary language skills. I noticed that he wore a charm, a *taviz*,[9] on his neck, which would be there to chase away bad spirits. It seems that fifteen times or so each month he would wake up at night and beat his head for five to ten minutes. When he was distracted by a family member, he might stop this odd behavior. He was also restless and exhibited some hyperactivity. There was no history of seizures, and his MRI and EEG were normal. Though he was on two anticonvulsants, prescribed by an outside doctor, the neurologist said with confidence that the boy suffered from "night terrors" and not epilepsy. The medications were removed and the family counseled on how to deal with night terrors. We see, then, that while a majority of cases in the OPD were for difficult cases of epilepsy, the doctor also would routinely catch cases where wrong diagnoses had led to the wrong medications.

Issues of abuse and rights, and not just incorrect diagnoses, were also noted by the neurologist. In one case, a twenty-eight-year-old woman presented with seizures twice per month. Her husband had abandoned her due to the epilepsy (it was not clear whether she was divorced or simply abandoned). This upset the doctor, who said that this was illegal and could be fought in the courts. In any event, she had suffered the seizures for the past several years. With Dilantin, her seizures had been well controlled. When she stopped the medicine, the seizures returned. The doctor studied her MRI and almost immediately discovered a lesion in the form of a brain tumor. A neuropsychiatric evaluation was ordered to check cognitive and neural function. A video EEG within the LTM was also ordered, and the patient was started immediately on carbamazepine. I asked about the tumor and whether it looked benign. The doctor said it did, in fact, look benign, but was causing her seizures. He added that it was "unbelievable" that it had not been caught earlier, as she could have easily controlled her epilepsy with surgery, saving her from a "life of much grief." This patient was probably heading down the road to surgery and recovery, as the tumor was in the frontal area, accessible to surgeons. In this case, while the seizures were a problem, the real "grief" she suffered was social abandonment.

Reflecting upon the future of medicine, increased specialization, and whether technological changes were impacting upon the way we think and write, the neurologist thought that the era of electronic devices might be producing changes in the way we process information and express ourselves, and that this would eventually be seen in MRI scans. I mentioned the book *Musicophilia*, by Oliver Sacks, which, among other things, illustrated how brain injuries affected musical abilities in surprising ways, as well as the ways that music could rewire neural pathways during rehabilitation from brain injury. He said he had read and appreciated it. I then asked whether repetitive and truncated communicative patterns, such as those encouraged by Twitter and texting, would have a potentially negative impact on the brain's language skills. He said he thought they would, but that, ironically, we as a species "were getting more intelligent" as a whole.

When it came to medicine, he said that the road to specialization had already narrowed pursuits and thought patterns, given the pressure to publish and make a name for oneself in research. This trend had more consequences in a major research center such as NIMHANS than it would in private hospitals that de-emphasized research, he thought. Within neurology itself, the divisions within imaging (MRI, fMRI, PET, SPECT, CT, EEG, etc.) and focusing upon certain types of epilepsy, and genetics, had meant that more generally trained neurologists were becoming rare. With this came the risk of "narrow thinking" and not looking systematically at the "whole of the patient," their life circumstances, general health, and sense of identity. We will recall that we heard the same concern from psychiatrists at NIMHANS. And while all seem to lament this, there does not seem to be a counter-wave being generated towards a more holistic approach within these two disciplines' training of young doctors. Where holism is invoked it seems to be in the increasing recognition of alternative AYUSH work, primarily as preventative and adjunct therapies. NIMHANS had a growing AYUSH department that received federal funding. But there was little overlap between AYUSH clinicians and therapists and biomedical specialists at NIMHANS. Nationally, the

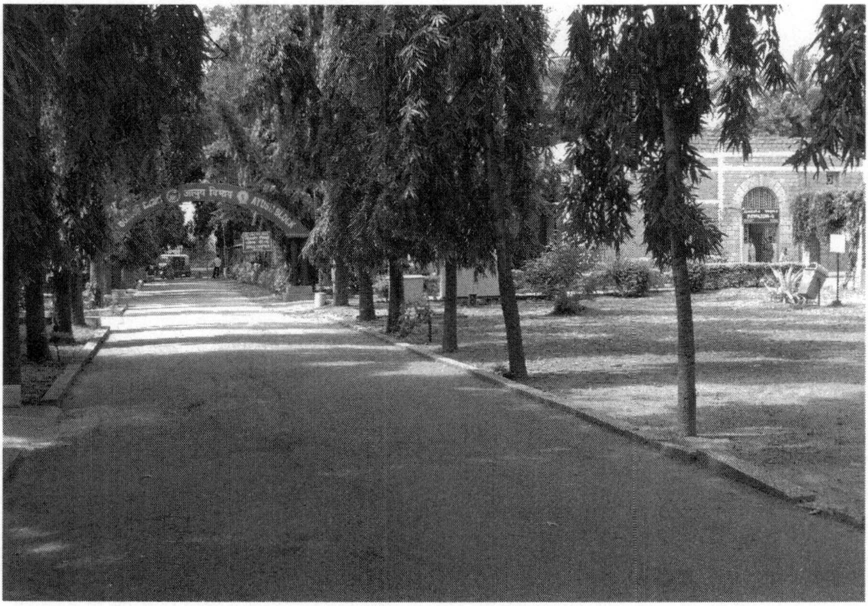

AYUSH block at NIMHANS. (Photograph by author.)

budgetary support for AYUSH treatments had increased over time and had political relevance, as support for "indigenous" non-Western medicine had a long history within anti-colonial nationalism (see Langford 2002).[10]

Another psychological clinician and professor of social work at NIMHANS had mentioned to me, on a somewhat related point, that at a time when many of the doctors were turning to the very hard sciences and searching for genetic biomarkers in psychiatry, and away from taking the beliefs of their patients into account, they, themselves, were blind to the range of traditional beliefs that they, the physicians, still harbored. These spiritual beliefs were totally compartmentalized from their hard science views of psychiatry. We might recall that some of the founding fathers of the institution were deeply immersed in Hindu philosophy (Murthy and Jain 2009; Kapur 2004; 2012), finding no apparent contradictions in scientific, philosophical, and spiritual pursuits. This was probably true in other sciences, such as in physics and engineering. Secularism and science were not prerequisites for one another in India, as had been once presumed in the rise of sciences in the West. In the context of taking culture, beliefs, and social life as important in clinical practice, this professor saw this situational amnesia among physicians as incongruous with a more holistic approach to psychiatry.

That is not to say that the doctors or psychiatrists were blind to the social. We have seen otherwise. The neurologist, the subject of this chapter, mentioned to me that NIMHANS had played a key role in the outlawing of divorce on account of epilepsy. Until recently, he explained, people could divorce their spouses if it was discovered that they had epilepsy. While it still occurred, informally, it was now illegal. As in the case just mentioned of a woman who had been divorced on account of her epilepsy, there were other instances of such abandonment that occurred and could be challenged in the courts. The law notwithstanding, the doctor did add, however, that returning a person to their parental home was seen as socially distasteful, particularly for women, who bore the brunt of social attitudes about failed marriages. Therefore, few patients would wish for this outcome. Moreover, returning a partner to a marriage that was abusive was fraught with risk, of course. Therefore, the law, while on the side of the abandoned, did not necessarily result in just resolutions for the aggrieved. At the same time, institutionalizing the patient was also less common in India, as the patient was still cared for by family members more than might be the case in North America, the doctor suggested, noting that abandonment and institutionalization by families of their ill members was still frowned upon in India, given the emotive importance of family ties in the traditional joint family. On the other hand, the quality of care received by the disabled member from the family was still an area where more education and advocacy were required, he suggested (Pinto 2014). I asked if he meant that social isolation within the family is a problem, such as when a mentally impaired or disabled person is kept out of the public eye. He said in response that this, precisely, was a big problem in India, given the fears that the ill family member would impact the marital options of other family members. In this sense, the sociocentric ideology of the "good family" (Cohen 1998; Kakar 1982; Roland 1988; Fabrega 2009) was still resonant, but countered by the potential shame brought upon the "bad" or flawed family within the wider social context. The violence of the social was palpable, and insurmountable by means of legislation alone.

The doctors at NIMHANS, in both psychiatry and neurology, were caught between idealism and pragmatism, alternatively harmonizing to the best of their abilities the competing demands of the social context in which their patients were entangled and their reformist, scientific, and rights-based aspirations for educating the public about the plight of the mentally and neurologically impaired. They were simultaneously conservative in their interventions while radical in their hopes. Caught between the rails of intransigent realities of social conservatism and the momentous changes they sought and witnessed in their own lives, they struggled with the human drama that played out every day within the sea of patients that walked through the doors of the hospital.

Conclusion

Social Dimensions of Mental Illness and Care

A common thread running throughout this study has been that of an affect *and* ascription of malevolence, oftentimes diffuse, haunting, and hard to discern. In that sense, a fractured identity, and the attempt to stabilize it—in the midst of accelerating social changes and upheaval—has had a frantic, indeed, feverish quality, desperately seeking its source of wounding, be it through tales of betrayal, haunting, or loss. But going beyond a symbolic strain model (e.g., Geertz), or an anomie model of social fracture (e.g., Durkheim), the source of malevolence has been seen, at least in part, to be a hypostatization of identity through its serialization, whether this be in the form of religions, ethnicity, gender, language, or occupational and/or bureaucratic measurements of efficiency in the changing workplace. Here identity becomes problematic through what it suppresses, be it a troublesome history or internal differences that are silenced in the name of singularity. The aporia produced by an overzealous policing of the social boundaries exacerbates already underlying psychiatric vulnerabilities, we have seen. "Hysteria," I have suggested, is one such marking of the Other's impossible demand for singular identities.

Moreover, especially critical in this study have been the traumas and subsequent wounds of history, which continue to bear traces and are "folded" into the subjectivity of the person (Pandian 2010). Given sociocentric ideologies continuing to hold sway within much of Indian society, these "folded" wounds give expression to an inner landscape that cannot express itself without symbolic work, condensation, and metaphor (Trawick 2017). This, like the hysteric's gesture, attempts a refusal of the Other's desire, but in a manner that can be immobilizing, and potentially lethal. All of this points to a rather pragmatic shift, despite the psychodynamic and deconstructive philosophical language I have deployed to move beyond cultural and social strain theories towards the subject, to the violence that inheres in the social (Siegel 2006; Thiranagama 2022; Hansen 2001), and the forces of modernity and identity politics that exacerbate it. While Anderson is rightly recognized for his understanding of nationalism as imagined, it is his attention to serialization as a form of alienating hypostatization that must be brought into dialogue with theories of mental distress. Though the theoretical language may differ at times, the psychiatrists I observed at NIMHANS were sensitive to the wounds and inequities of history, as well as the harm that monolithic and ossified demands on identity were having on already vulnerable patients.

This said, turning briefly away from philosophy and critique to more pragmatic health care concerns allows me to bring into view implications that might seem less esoteric. As a recent series in the *New England Journal of Medicine* has argued, a return to the social within medicine is both timely and necessary if we are to avoid the symptom-oriented reductionism of today's emphasis on "evidence-based medicine." Stonington, Holmes, Hansen, et al. launched the aforementioned series with a clarion call: "Much of what they [clinicians] read in clinical journals appears to corroborate the assumption that in clinical medicine, the biologic and behavioral world of the patient's body is more important than that of the social world outside it. This erasure flies in the face of increasing evidence documenting the role of social forces in determining health, disease, treatment, and recovery" (2018, 1958). While this is true for all clinical practice, it is nowhere more important than in psychiatry, clinical psychology, and the treatment of mental illness. We are at an opportune moment for a necessary rethinking of the "evidence-based psychiatry" that dominates nosology within the DSM-5 and ICD-10. Utilizing a mixed-methods approach to measuring clinical efficacy, and the incorporation of qualitative and ethnographic methods in assessing what is meaningful and experience-near to clients, is producing new insights on the social and structural determinants surrounding wellbeing, distress, and rehabilitation. This, in turn, leads to better clinical and social outcomes, providing care that is meaningful in social and cultural terms and that allows persons with mental illness to lead more productive and inclusive lives (Narasimhan et al. 2019; Luhrmann and Marrow 2016; Patel et al. 2018).

From Social Medicine and Global Mental Health to Political Psychology

A rights-based approach to care that is psychosocial in orientation, and integrates social analysis of the structural determinants of health outcomes, such as inequality, poverty, housing, comorbid health conditions, and stigma, increases empathy between clinician, social worker, and patient/client. Moreover, as research has shown (e.g., Luhrmann and Marrow 2016; Patel et al. 2018; Nakamura 2013), an emphasis on patient agency through facilitating employment, housing, and semi-independent living leads to a much better long-term prognosis. Too often, psychiatric practice focuses upon short-term measurables, such as symptom reduction and whether hospitalization was reduced through drug therapy, without capturing "culturally relevant social outcomes of recovery" (Kirmayer and Gomez-Carrillo 2018, 16) that are meaningful within the lifeworlds of the afflicted. As Kirmayer and Gomez-Carrillo suggest, "psychiatric research has tended to reduce illness experience to symptom reports, ignoring the bodily, narrative, and social embedding of illness" (2018, 16). Such symptom-oriented nosologies miss complex etiologies and the social, political, and economic forces that determine differentiated health outcomes and predict the incidence and severity of mental illness. A turn to case study methodologies that investigate the social and cultural terrain in which an individual experiences forms of structural violence, be it abuse, discrimination, stigma, or poverty, is essential for us to better understand how extreme vulnerability is contributing to degrees of mental illness. The pernicious cycle of vulnerability and illness cannot be captured through a catalogue of symptoms, but requires a more holistic intervention. Such holism within medical and social work practice contributes to the "structural humility" of the health care provider, enhances empathy, and utilizes the afflicted's, and perhaps also their community's, "own expertise and resourcefulness in resisting the structural violence that affects them" (Stonington et al. 2018, 1960). Understanding sources of resilience within individuals and communities is therefore as important as the diagnosing of symptoms, as it is through the former that medicine is made meaningful and congruent within beliefs and values that define wellbeing and allow for a capacity to aspire (Appadurai 2013).

This focus upon experience-near understandings through ethnographic work does not mean a focus upon culture above all else. Structural issues surrounding power, conflict, displacement, marginalization, inequality, and biological determinants are critical, so that comparisons across cultures and societies can be obtained, allowing for scalable models of intervention to be conceived. But attention to experience-near understandings is also critical, and they require an ethnographic approach in order to see how norms and beliefs shape illness presentations, experiences, and outcomes. As Kirmayer and Gomez-Carrillo explain, "Symptoms arise from the interaction of psychophysiological, cognitive-affective, and social processes that include culture-specific explanations of distress, and thus, are more than just indices of disorder. Symptoms are shaped and amplified by bodily, psychological, and social processes. Sensations, experiences, and events are perceived and interpreted in terms of available cultural models, as well as through ongoing interactions with others. To make sense of symptoms, clinicians therefore need to consider the specific contexts, including the clinical setting itself, in which illness experience emerges and its meanings are negotiated" (2018, 5).

Quantitative and symptom-based evidence is undoubtedly valuable, particularly as it allows for large aggregates of evidence to indicate correlations and trends. But the "seductions of quantification," to borrow a phrase from Merry (2016), can obscure what gets counted as "evidence" versus what is resonant and valid to those research participants being studied. Ethnographic accounts are critical, even when they are harder to model and quantify. They add necessary depth to the breadth addressed in survey-based aggregate data. When the patterns in qualitative and ethnographic assessments underscore key findings in large data sets, the validity of the latter is stronger. When a puzzling disjuncture emerges, however, it forces us to question whether the instruments deployed in survey-based research need recalibration or even redesign. The "evidence-based" movement in mental health research has, arguably, yet to fully grapple with the need for multidimensional analysis, inclusive of an analysis of the complex etiologies that are experiential and influenced by social and cultural dimensions of human life (Patel and Kleinman 2003; Patel et al. 2018).

Perhaps less obvious or easy to measure, the work of many anthropologists and clinicians (e.g., Obeyesekere 1985; Luhrmann and Marrow 2016; Corin 2007; Gopikumar et al. 2016) has shown the critical role that faith and traditional healing practices continue to play in establishing a sense of well-being and fortitude in the wake of the structural violence that impacted material conditions within communities and individuals. Community resilience and aspirations towards a better future are not only dependent upon assistance from outside sources, but are integrally linked to cultural and spiritual resources already established within the community. Therefore, any outside interventions and mobilization of community empowerment is more effective when conjoined to meaningful models for living that exist within communities, as aspiration and culture go hand in hand (Appadurai 2013).

Mental Health and Poverty

A World Health Organization (WHO) bulletin written by leading global mental health specialists and psychiatrists at Harvard University, Vikram Patel and Arthur Kleinman (2003), presented findings and analysis from three large global mental health reports and eleven community studies since 1990. This survey confirmed that there is a strong correlation between poverty and common mental disorders, particularly depressive- and anxiety-related disorders. The authors defined poverty as "low socioeconomic status (measured by social or income class), unemployment and low levels of education" (Patel and Kleinman 2003, 609). Patel and Kleinman indicated that income alone is not a determinative factor, whereas when it was associated with poor education and struggles for housing, the relationship with mental illness became stronger. In particular, insecurity over income, such as when a person suffers "an acute income drop in the previous six months" (Patel and Kleinman 2003, 611), raised the risk of mental disorders, noting, for example, farmer suicides in India as falling into this pattern (Vasavi 2011). Not surprisingly, they found a strong correlation, therefore, between hopelessness as a "core experience" and depression and suicide. Within this core experience of hopelessness, shame, stigma, homelessness, and humiliations associated with poverty were seen as more important than poverty itself. In urban contexts where social change associated with migration led to isolation, loneliness was another key factor leading to common mental disorders, as Émile Durkheim had long ago theorized. Trauma caused by violence, actual physical or structural, coupled with a lack of social support, played an "important role in the etiology of common mental disorders" (Patel and Kleinman 2003, 611). Gender, the authors also found, was another factor to consider, as women "bear the brunt of the adversities associated with poverty: less access to school, physical abuse from husbands, forced marriages . . . fewer job opportunities" (2003, 612). Malnutrition, lack of access to clean water and living in toxic environments, inadequate housing, and other factors associated with poor health were comorbid with mental health disorders. Moreover, the comorbid health and mental health problems presented increased costs and worsened poverty, contributing to a vicious cycle of psychosocial stress and poverty. The authors conclude, "Rather than actual income, factors such as insecurity, hopelessness, poor physical health, rapid social change and limited opportunities as a result of less education may mediate the risk of suffering from mental disorders. The most important implication of these findings is to place common mental disorders alongside other diseases associated with poverty which, on account of this association, attract attention from health policymakers and donors" (2003, 612).

A more recent survey of the epidemiological literature and ethnographic study by Luhrmann and Marrow (2016) found that the trajectory of schizophrenia, that most refractory of mental illnesses, was also influenced by experiences of "social defeat," or the repeated humiliations associated with the social violence of stigma, racism, poverty, homelessness, and interactions with a health care industry and legal bureaucracy that was oftentimes dehumanizing for the afflicted. Better prognoses were seen where housing and work was available, and "diagnostic neutrality" meant that when the emotional emphasis was lesser surrounding this medical diagnosis within the household and wider community, hope was better maintained. This study supported many earlier global studies (e.g., Hopper et al. 2007; Morgan et al. 2008) that suggested that outcomes for schizophrenia were better in many parts of the developing world as compared to the developed world due to greater diagnostic neutrality and lesser emotional investment placed in the diagnosis itself.

Kleinman has gone further in suggesting that the focus in global mental health must shift from a diagnostic model focusing on pathology versus non-pathology, towards one that addresses "social suffering" in all its multidimensional aspects, linking poverty and health in a cluster of comorbidities, in addition to understanding the psychological experience of suffering in its local and culturally shaped dimensions (2012). As such, he has a focused attention on the sometimes dehumanizing aspects of medical care, the ways it can increase social and moral defeat, despite the best intentions. Attention must be directed towards the dehumanizing treatment of the mentally ill, rather than simply expanding access to pharmaceutical treatments. In lower-resource areas, however, Kleinman points out that basic access to mental health care and counseling is often lacking. He asks, "What happens when we see the state not primarily as the source of powerful control over the mentally ill and through them society at large, but rather as fragile, constrained, and almost powerless to provide the most basic care for its most impaired and vulnerable members?" (2012, 123). In such a context, over-medicalization is not so much the issue as is alleviating the socioeconomic disparities that contribute to comorbid health and mental health problems. Health care policy, therefore, is necessarily conjoined to poverty eradication, increasing literacy, food security, potable water, infrastructural development, etc.

But creating the capacity for "aspiration" and hope, as Appadurai (2013) notes, also requires understanding the models for living the good and worthwhile life that only culture provides. Culture, obviously enough, is not only about tradition, heritage, and the past reservoir of ideas; rather, culture is a template and matrix for understanding and inducing social actions into the future. Indeed, it is about the future, as a model "of" and "for" reality, as Geertz famously argued (1973). Much of medical anthropology, Cohen (2012) notes, has aligned itself either on the side of medicine or against it, in championing locality and culture over universal public health models of illness and disease. That is, some aspects of medical and psychological anthropology have over-emphasized that illness is a cultural construct, or is "culture-bound," as in the emphasis on "culture-bound syndromes" in the literature. But Cohen, like Kleinman, has also pointed towards another reality: that the body, while cultural and local, is also produced at a confluence of structural conditions *and* local beliefs. The local body is produced, therefore, through experiences of poverty, malnutrition, and repeated social defeat, as much as it is shaped by beliefs and models for living. Or, as Pandian (2010) suggests, subjectivity "folds" historical experience upon itself, with selfhood bearing these traces. Simply put, structural and social violence is at the core of understanding any local context, in addition to how this body is experienced in symbolic or meaningful terms (also see Sunder Rajan 2017). Therefore, ethnographic case studies are invaluable in understanding context in all its symbolic, embodied, and material forms and, as such, indispensable within public health and poverty-alleviation interventions. Understanding social suffering and social defeat cannot be measured in a one-size-fits-all instrument without accounting for the experiences and voices of individuals within particular social and cultural contexts.

A Culturally Sensitive Psychiatry

While a crisis of mental health may, indeed, exist, it is a far more complicated problem than is capable of being resolved through biomedical treatment alone. Recall Murthy's admonition and warning from her perch at NIMHANS: "The practice of psychiatry in India, in its fervour to emerge as a scientific, empirical and universal science, has, in the process, become sterile and devoid of the richness of human experience." A "pill for every ill" approach to care, she warns, "is the sequestration or partitioning of professional minds" (Murthy 2018, 233). While Murthy warns of a potentially worsening trend in biomedical psychiatry, there is a critical new direction in treatment provided through the community-based model, particularly as practiced with a more holistic approach, as well as by physicians like herself and many others placed at major tertiary centers critical of the fevered use of pharmaceuticals as the "Band-Aid" applied to gaping social wounds in society. I explore this community-based approach within the Nilgiris context in the second volume of this study.

There is, as I have described in this study, a growing chorus in India among mental health care providers with similar insights and concerns. We can also draw significantly upon anthropological work on mental health and wellbeing in India, particularly work that looks at the nexus of socioeconomic precarity, familial constraints and demands in a changing economy, identity politics, and spiritual hauntings and idioms of distress through which these tensions are expressed (e.g., Nichter 1982; Obeyesekere 1981; Kakar 1982; Ecks 2014; Halliburton 2009; Sebastia 2009a; 2009b; Fabrega 2009; Corin 2007; Corin et al. 2004), and particularly in the path-breaking work by Sarah Pinto (2014; 2020a), Lawrence Cohen (1998), Saiba Varma (2020), Jocelyn Chua (2014), Lang (2018), Addlakha (2008), Luhrmann and Marrow (2016), Marrow (2022), and Veena Das (2006), all of whom look to the fractures, wounds, and everyday violence that mark the lives of those deemed mentally ill in oftentimes brilliant and provocative analyses grounded in local culture and context, but theoretically broad enough to connect their work to other parts of the world.

And while a robust cultural psychology points to the normative features with a sociocentric ideology, taking the experience of selfhood and normalcy as wholly culturally determined would miss the existential aporias and tensions within the self-imaginings that mark individuals. And with this culturalist reading, we efface the internal divisions and alterity within the self, if not the intractable symptoms that are linked to social violence and the body's agency, through symptoms, to resist, even when such resistance takes the self-defeating form of a "resistance to resistance" (Derrida 1998). Taking a radically constructivist or culturalist position, the experience of selfhood and normalcy is culturally defined, making universal claims about disease and illness impossible. But Foucault (2006) takes a constructivist and historicist argument in another direction, claiming that madness is the micro-shaping and defining of normalcy based upon workings of power through a complex set of institutional relays between cultural discourse, social practice, and embodied subjectivity (Rose 2018). Cultural determinists, however, committed to the idea of greater plasticity as an adaptive capacity, are critical of a biomedical psychiatry that affords little attention to cultural difference, whereas, in contrast, the consensus in global biomedical psychiatry argues that while symptom expression, stigma, and access to care may vary according to cultural and social forces, the underlying biomarkers for mental illness are universal, despite some variation in expression. These debates within the academy have led to productive disagreements around the emergent global mental health movement, with advocates and detractors pointing to the risks posed, alternatively, by a perceived shortage of biomedical care in the developing world as a crisis of care (Patel et al. 2018; Patel 2014) versus the pharmaceutical interests coupled with the hegemonic research paradigms in the global north that are disseminated as the global scientific standards, that are, in turn exported to the developing world (Ecks 2021; Rose 2018).

As argued in this study, an indeterminate middle ground is important, between ideas of radical difference or relativism versus universal reductionism to biochemical processes, if we are to avoid the romanticism of extreme constructivism, on the one hand, and on the other the reductionism of biomedical etiology, which ignores the social and cultural forces that impact upon wellbeing and give conscious meaning to life (Obeyesekere 1985; Kleinman 1988; 2009; Good, Subandi, and Good 2007). The doctors at NIMHANS, however, were more biocultural in their thinking and approach to caring for their patients than I had anticipated, given the purported hegemony of genomics and psycho-pharmaceutical dominance within psychiatry.

The call for "social medicine" within the *New England Journal of Medicine* and beyond is therefore timely and consistent with the pathbreaking work in community-based care and clinical interventions that are occurring in India. Still, the risk of biomedical reductionism, and its effacement of social determinants, is persistent and real, particularly given the pharmaceutical interests that drive research and treatment within global psychiatry (Rose 2018; Sunder Rajan 2017; Kirmayer and Gomez-Carrillo 2018; Ecks 2021). The sole emphasis on short-term symptom reduction is unable to address the real challenge of understanding the social determinants and culturally embodied experience of illness. A holistic, cost-effective, and sustainable model of mental health care is one in which agency, rights, and understanding are emphasized over and above short-term outcomes oriented solely around symptom reduction. It is also important to reflect, in turn, on the cultural, social, and economic determinants of biomedical practice. "Evidence-based psychiatry," as Kirmayer and Gomez-Carrillo (2018) assert, "is also cultural," bound by conventions, values, and social forces. With this humility in mind, care providers can approach the intersectional lives of the vulnerable and marginal with respect for the medical pluralism that might more meaningfully offer hope and dignity, as well as symptomatic relief. Kirmayer and Gomez-Carrillo offer this summation of the necessary disposition of a caregiver, and suggest that to "foster pluralistic mental health services that respond effectively to cultural diversity, there is a need to adapt an open-minded but critical perspective on other knowledge traditions and approaches to healing" (2018, 16). A community-based approach is urgently needed, one that can offer both an effective and a sustainable treatment model. This approach should also include a reflexive and active learning system of care, in which case studies and qualitative research reveal scalable care and valid measurements of mental health across social categories, versus those dimensions that are unique and local and, therefore, difficult to scale up without losing validity. This approach would mitigate against criticisms of the global mental health movement that have been raised (Ecks 2021; Rose 2018), whilst also addressing acute needs within segments of society where suffering is not addressed with existing local resources.

While the discussion of strategies and efficacy are of pragmatic importance if human suffering is to be reduced and the excesses of constructivism, historicism, and universalism are to be avoided, this study has centered on the affect and ascription of malevolence as one that bears the traces of history, and is, at the same time, symptomatic of the intractable dilemmas produced by modern forms of identity, be they ethnic, linguistic, or even occupational. In the political context of contemporary India, doctors I worked with at NIMHANS, we will recall, sometimes emphasized that fascistic tendencies were on the rise, producing or exacerbating, as we have witnessed, fractured identities. In several clinical cases the traumas of life were exacerbated by a profound sense of betrayal by imagined others, and the distrust that gushed forth from that betrayal. More broadly, the doctors sometimes told me that a fear of difference, of minorities, and a generalized sense of menace from a mysterious Other was increasingly conjoined to other clinical symptoms. What was this betrayal, at its root cause? The betrayals are multiple, visible and invisible, conscious and unconscious, by others and within the self, all at the same time. One name for this aporia might be, we have suggested, "hysteria," if we grant that term renewed relevance as an opening into the iniquities of modern life, and an incapacity, following Klein, of living with the "bad object." But another name we might use, I have suggested, is "archive fever," following Derrida.

But the serious and debilitating nature of the symptoms examined cannot be reduced to psychosocial strains caused by modern life. In most cases I witnessed, significant delusions, hallucinations, and cognitive impairments were influenced by a myriad of organic and non-organic factors, be they genetic or epigenetic. While my focus has been to point to shared themes as they related to predicaments of modern life, particularly the social and cultural strains brought on by rationalization and reform, I am not arguing that mental illness is simply a sociocultural construct. To do so would romanticize as resistance the suffering that each patient seemed to be enduring, with, at times, catastrophic consequences to themselves and their families.

What I am underscoring is the continuum of effects associated with the excessive hold of identity or a singular imaginary that creates or is created by legalistic demarcations of right and wrong, self and other, inside and outside, collective and individual. The attenuation of more protean and fluid lifeworlds, conjoined to latent psychiatric vulnerabilities, proved disabling, indeed, malevolent. These rigidities, in turn, were buttressed by the dangers of "betrayal," which, arguably, form the archives and supplements of difference that are further damaging to the social fabric within the family, and perhaps to the wider community. The key link, perhaps, between the psychiatric symptoms and the excessive boundaries generated by the themes of betrayal, the Law, and ethnoreligious constructs is a social and perhaps legalistic demand towards some kind of impossible and categorical singularity. These demands, of course, are buttressed by bureaucracy and material relations of power. But, against a power-centric reading,[1] in which "illness" is the mere thinking of power, we take note that the demands for singularity betray insecure origins, and are ultimately unstable. To draw a direct analogy from Derrida to Freud, we might call these economies of words that these terms signify a form of displacement, but one where effacing their traces involves an excess that is ultimately unstable and generative of further instabilities.

The question of striking a balance between the psychosocial, cultural, and organic understandings of mental illness is obviously critical. Psychiatry, in its best sense, I have observed at NIMHANS, is a creatively disruptive force, shattering false attachments and phantasmic delusions through a combination of biomedical and social analysis. How to retain this singularly disruptive and anarchic side of psychiatry in a moment when biomedical singularity and standardized diagnostic lexicons threaten to create patient "types" out of persons, and in so doing, pathologizing and producing yet another totalizing serial imaginary—that of the mental health patient? The totalizing demarcation machine of diagnostic psychiatry as conjoined to pharmaceutical interest and neoliberal governance was, in part, cautiously negotiated by the doctors at NIMHANS, who were well aware of the dangers inherent in an emergent "mental health crisis," which, while perhaps real and of great consequence, must not become singularized, standardized, and normalized within a climate of other economic and political singularities (Rose 2018).

The paralyzing idioms of distress certainly speak to the failures embedded within the sociocentric ideologies of the person and self that mark South Asian life in profound ways. The possessive force of malevolent protest against social iniquities has long been a feature of illness narratives in South Asia. In this sense, illness presentation is certainly culturally patterned and contagious as such. But biomedical psychiatry, like demonological possession, also blurs the resistance to resistance that lies embedded within the symptom, creating diagnostic lines that are potentially depoliticizing through pharmaceutical care regimes and against the implicit politics and social "knots" communicated by the symptom.[2] As one NIMHANS psychiatrist warned me, the question of today has become: "Do you hear voices, or do you think you hear voices?" In marking a clear line between delusion and hallucination, an effacement of division and the negation of the other within the symptom is potentially lost to a clinical certitude that is impossible to sustain in biomedical psychiatry, given what we know now about plasticity in both its positive and negative aspects, as well as a diagnostic lexicon that obscures social and political forms of violence, further pathologizing the sufferer. The psychotic, as opposed to the hysteric, as a diagnostic distinction in the clinic, threatens to flatten the blurring that inevitably occurs between a social and an organic symptom, as was seen in these cases. This is why hysteria matters, even if it gets called by another name. That is not to dismiss organic causation, as it has its own political valence when mitigating stigma and the normalizing violence of the sociocentric cure, be it in exorcism or drug regimes. But simply medicating a person for hallucinations as opposed to looking at the entire social context is what the doctors themselves feared when a spouse, sibling, or parent requested a "tablet" to make the patient "normal."

Hysteria or conversion disorders point to larger political and social questions, and specifically, the tensions that have in recent times been exacerbated by a sense of malevolence rising in the country,[3] as well as the targeting of those who are purported to be its provenance. Literalism, serialized and hence increasingly communalized identities,[4] economic and environmental precarity, and psychological vulnerabilities go together and must be addressed within a larger social and political field. Though a generalized sense of malevolence is witnessed in the purported mental health crises that are emergent in India, its causes are multiple,[5] though the affect of malevolence can produce political effects independent of its provenance (Massumi 2002). The psychiatrists at NIMHANS I knew were acutely aware of this, yet, when facing an acute case, were under tremendous pressures to alleviate symptoms. But they were also able to sometimes interrupt and destabilize absolutisms and harmful compulsions that were driven by an overwhelming and uncanny sway of malevolence clinically figured by the term "hysteria."

The colloquial use of this term within the clinic, and, specifically, addressed to this anthropologist, was indeed deliberative, indexing not only patient resistance and ambivalence to varied forms of excessive or malevolent figures of attachment, but also the psychiatrists' resistance to both patient and familial desires for normalization as well as their own diagnostic certitude, the "archive fever" of biomedical psychiatry. Therefore, while this study has been primarily directed at the violence of the social, as manifested in symptoms that psychiatrists linked to changing social conditions in the country, the clinic was a site of division within itself, providing symptomatic relief on the one hand and, on the other hand, an opening up of wounds and divisions that, in turn, were generative of the term "hysteria." This term has, of course, a long and complicated, if not problematic, history. This notwithstanding, it offered a kind of translatability that resisted closure or literalism.[6] Here, the clinical antiliteralism of hysteria, I suggest, resisted the increasing symptom of literalism/absolutism perceived by some psychiatrists at NIMHANS. This ambiguity, as a kind of "resistance to resistance," as Derrida (1998) argues, created the necessary cleft that kept diagnosis and analysis open, resisting the epistemic violence of biomedical psychiatry that so concerns its critics. The ambiguity of its use in the clinic also marks an inescapable undecidability at the heart of the social *and* the clinical, potentially re-aligning or divesting the afflicted from harmful attachments. This undecidability at the heart of "hysteria" within India, and probably elsewhere, can undoubtedly suppress analysis, or foreclose an etiology of social determinants, which accounts for its complicated, gendered, and violent history within psychiatry and psychoanalysis. This, in turn, is where the clinical iconoclasm of its usage in these cases leads me to deconstructive and psychoanalytic thought, though inspired by my clinician interlocutors who may not use this language.

Literalism, serial forms of identification, and the erasure of this permeable and protean possibility of identity is, however, the symptom and etiology, at the same time. That is, monocultural fantasies and ideologies of religious or ethnic singularity emergent today represent an "archive fever," in precisely Derrida's sense, but are constitutive of fevered rationalizations. Deconstructing these absolutes, however, a feature of Indian speculative and mythical thought for millennia (e.g., Trawick 2017; Smith 2006; Fabrega 2009; Shulman 1985), is mirrored uncannily in psychiatric insights about delusions and attachments, though the risk of a biomedical archive fever also lurks in the shadows of clinical care. Derrida, more precisely, I would argue, reveals that each moment, each thought, and each utterance is divided within itself, an insight that Freud radically ushered into psychiatry, but oftentimes effaced within his own scientific work. Learning to live with the ambiguities of any filial/normative order, with its contradictions and injustices, is what hysteria or any "conversion disorder" arguably paralyzes, oftentimes with tragic results.

While reciprocity and the desire to induce it animates hysteria and its demand against the Other, even its refusal can be transformative in either positive or harmful ways. Absolutism and judgement and the violence that ensues from this against the hysteric, or through the hysteric to the social field, can be one type of refused reciprocity that is harmful and immobilizing. A more positive type of withdrawal is another possibility, which, arguably, is the razor's edge that psychiatrists grapple with at NIMHANS, as they attempt to reintroduce the grey zone or ambivalence that makes life tolerable and livable for their patients caught within the intractable violence of the social.

Trawick (2017, 188–189) suggests that in Tamil, if not wider South Asian culture, a "remainder" marking the irregular must always exist for calamity to be averted. Perfection or closure is fearful in its symmetry. Hysteria or malevolent forces signify, in that sense, a remainder that cannot be squared by human hands, the law, or a definitive and determinative archive. An ethic of openness lies at the heart of hope. This is as true for mitigating against ossified and fetishized boundaries between groups, and the internal ambivalences these generate within troubled selves, haunted by inward betrayals and thwarted aspirations and desires, as it is within the biomedical and traditional healing systems that, too, must retain the indeterminate and undecidable as an ethic of care.

Excess, on the other hand, can lead to pathological fixation, feverish negation of the other, and even paralyzing hysteria. But, at the same time, a cleft or remainder is at the heart of desire, as in the dialectics of subjectivity in Lacan.[7] Desire as movement, hope, creativity, and obviously, agency and resistance persists in that gap that is never fully sutured through ideology. Yet the physicians and healers seem to identify the risk of fixation and self-harming stasis within the self. That is, living within this gap between desire and perception is becoming increasingly difficult given the demands on identity in ossified, hypostatized, and serialized form—an enumeration of types and categories generated by modern forces, such as colonialism, statecraft, and occupational roles within capitalist modernity. This risk, we might call it a fetish, freezes dialectical movement whilst also effacing traces of memory that induce feelings of betrayal. These types and categorical distinctions are sustained through an archive of the other's wrongs, exacerbating individual symptoms through amnesiac forms of "remembering" that edit, redact, and suppress. This process only heightens anxiety and uncanniness, now refigured as malevolence. An affect of malevolence is not quantifiable, but can serve political and economic ends, leading to heightened security apparatuses, profiling, medicalizing, and scapegoating, as most recently witnessed in the COVID-19 pandemic, but in a more subtle, gradual, and insidious way, perhaps, too, in the criminalizing and pathologizing of mental illness. Psychiatry, we have seen, need not be aligned to these malevolent forces of suppression. Rather, an ethic of undecidability, sustained through the imprecision of terms like "hysteria," works to untangle at least some of the intractable knots within the social.

Notes

Introduction. Two Deaths

1. Some activists and organizations that worked for Adivasi rights (e.g., Adivasi Resurgence, https://www.newindianexpress.com/states/kerala/2023/Apr/04/tribal-man-madhu-lynching-case-kerala-court-finds-14-out-of-the-16-accused-men-guilty-2562625.html) complained that many murders of tribal members had gone uninvestigated, and that witness tampering occurred in the case of Madhu's murder, as well. These complaints echo reports of atrocities against the Kurumba tribe reported in the nineteenth century, which will be discussed in the second volume.
2. See, for example, the magazine *Frontline*, August 31, 2016, for a detailed forum among experts in the field, including those from NIMHANS.
3. Ayurveda, Yoga, Unani, Siddha, and Homeopathy.
4. Sarin and Jain 2018. Sarin and Jain go further, suggesting provocatively that nineteenth-century psychiatry became preoccupied with theories of the "native mind" that were aligned with colonialism and were premised upon racial difference, citing anthropometry as one example. The implications of their argument are bolder, suggesting that the more recent intellectual forays into the native mind—advanced by, for instance, cultural psychology, structuralism, and cultural determinism, and away from a more universal humanism—could mark a retreat from the political and social.
5. NIMHANS has a large AYUSH unit, though biomedicine is their main focus of research, training, and care.
6. Patients come from all parts of the country. I saw a number of patients from Northeast India, particularly from Bengal and Assam.
7. On some occasions, this number may be as high as forty patients in one day. Dr. Sanjeev Jain, personal communication.
8. Karnataka is also thought to have a very high suicide rate among farmers who have incurred debts they cannot pay off given neoliberal agricultural policies.

9. Sarin and Jain 2018. While the political will be invoked by clinicians, it will not be given singular causal weight in the cases that follow, as each case is irreducible to political or identity-based troubling of selfhood. Rather, I point to the political as one of the important sources of othering and malevolence, as manifested symptomatically within individual cases. Many scholars, journalists, and social analysts have pointed to the encroachment of national and state-level politics surrounding religion, language, and ethnicity upon communal sentiments, pointing to intimacies between groups being troubled by increasing forms of political othering. It is my argument, as well as that of the psychiatrists whom I followed, that these forms of othering have exacerbated psychological problems, whilst effacing historical traumas that demand more attention.
10. While the city was officially named Bengaluru in 2006, following the trend of renaming cities in local languages that had been anglicized under the British, with Bombay (Mumbai), Calcutta (Kolkata), and Madras (Chennai) being other prominent examples, the name Bangalore has stuck with the general population, especially the English-speaking middle class. In my experience, Bangalore was used colloquially across all social divides more than the new name, unlike nearby Chennai, which had completely supplanted the old name, Madras. Therefore, I continue to use the old name.
11. Marrow 2008. See Marrow for a detailed study of "teeth clenching" in India as a form of conversion disorder that is culturally shaped.
12. The postcolonial ethos of NIMHANS as a progressive, non-incarcerating institution committed to holistic care of the patient resembles what Katie Kilroy-Marac (2019) describes at Fann Psychiatric Clinic in Dakar. In both cases, the idealism and eclectic nature of care, partnering with local traditional healers, and taking culture and psychosocial causation and treatment seriously in their early years was perceived by psychiatrists to be moving towards a narrower biomedical paradigm of care, and away from these "progressive" principles in favor of pharmaceutical care regimes. In both cases the critique of contemporary biomedical psychiatry came from within its own walls, to a large extent.
13. Kapur partnered with Morris Carstairs, a psychological anthropologist, to author a major and influential ethnographic and psychiatric study of a local community in coastal Karnataka, entitled *The Great Universe of the Kota* (1979).
14. With depth interviewing, I might have been able to understand the particular distress and trauma faced by individual patients, as seen, for instance, in the work of Pinto (2014), Kakar (1982), and Obeyesekere (1981). But

with the breadth of following hundreds of cases, on the other hand, certain social and even political valences of clinical practice and illness presentation appeared to be patterned. In that sense, this work, though on a less traumatic scale, is methodologically closer to Varma's (2020) recent study of Kashmiri psychiatry.

Chapter 1. Shame, Stigma, and the Normalizing Impulse

1. Diasporic Indians also returned for care to NIMHANS. I encountered cases where patients came from North America and Singapore for care, owing to the reputation of certain doctors.
2. I was not allowed to interview or contact patients outside of the clinical context at NIMHANS.
3. As we will see in several cases throughout this study, the line between epileptic and nonepileptic "fits" or "seizures" is often unclear, not just because various "hysteria"-like "fits" are labeled the same as epileptic ones, but also because the nonepileptic seizure, or "pseudo seizure," often resembles, and perhaps models, epileptic seizures, and requires neurological evaluations for determination. A later chapter will explore this in more detail.
4. In the short story by Sartre (1948), a caregiver's partner suffers from hallucinations and delusions. Over time the caregiver begins to share these same delusions.
5. Derrida (1981) describes the "pharmakon" that is the gift and poison of writing, as that which allows for forgetting, on the one hand, but also that which supplants voice and memory, on the other. In a penetrating analysis of Plato's *Phaedrus*, Derrida suggests that writing, thus, serves as the "supplement" to voice and subjective intentionality, by displacing difference as originating with writing, whereas this division and difference within the subject already exists within the subject with language and the signifier, a Freudian premise.
6. There is a good deal of clinical evidence cited from the WHO and other studies that the prognosis for schizophrenia is better in many developing countries than it is in Europe and North America (Desjarlais, Eisenberg, Good, and Kleinman 1995, Corin 2007; Waters 2010).
7. These translations from residents and fellows were an important part of the clinical process, so that some nuance and detail would not get lost in translation. It points to the complexity of providing health care in major tertiary centers, given their large catchment zones as well as India's numerous languages and dialects. The translators also allowed me to follow cases in real time, rather than to rely on doctors' commentary between patients, which also occurred but it would be too cumbersome to include all the

details. While I could get the gist of conversations in Kannada, Telugu, or Malayalam, due to knowing Tamil, I would miss large chunks of meaning in those conversations. But if the patients and their families were Tamil-speaking (or, obviously, English-speaking), I could catch most of what was said.

Chapter 2. Rebellion and Abandonment

1. I have continued to present aspects of psychological and psychiatric anthropology at NIMHANS in the years that have followed, as well as presenting the present ethnographic work in a condensed form of lecture.
2. This case was similar to one discussed in the Robert Lemelson film *The Bad Coconut*, which dealt with competing interpretations of a young man's rebellious and self-destructive behavior and the stress it caused within his Javanese family. The film and this case of Siva both probe the porous boundaries between adolescent rebellion and psychopathology.
3. My decision not to present the doctors as unique individuals, or to ostensibly write an ethnography of their clinical idiosyncrasies or personalities, was strategic depersonalization deployed to focus the narrative on the larger social critiques and cultural patterns that I became sensitive to. That is, the doctors, though fascinating and oftentimes brilliant, were not the main focus, and as such, no interviews on their background experiences, training, or worldviews were conducted. When they did, as they invariably did, offer social commentary, I included it within my fieldnotes, and hence it has found its way into this study as an important perspective, albeit presented with impersonality. Moreover, I had gained the trust of and developed a rapport with the physicians I shadowed under the condition that I was studying mental illness, its presentations and causes, at NIMHANS, and not studying the doctors themselves.
4. A limited supply of family housing was available for short-term stays at NIMHANS.
5. The doctor mentioned that Kannada and Arabic were read in different directions (left to right as opposed to right to left), and, as such, dyslexia could impact on one language more than another.
6. In contrast to the case of Catarina, analyzed by Biehl (2005) in his influential and moving book, *Vita*, Zareen's written notes were ignored, out of concern that entertaining these thoughts would harden her delusions, giving them a materiality that reinforced them. In Catarina's case, as discussed by Biehl, the "dictionary" she compiled carried within it important social critiques, as well as personal clues as to the etiology of her abandonment by her family. But in Catarina's case, as it finally

became determined, she suffered a neurological condition prior to her misdiagnosis of mental illness, though her mental condition declined in the wake of familial abandonment and institutionalization. See Nakamura (2013) and Luhrmann and Marrow (2016) for contrasting views on the clinical efficacy of engaging with patient delusions rather than silencing them.

7. For example, in Malaysia, during a festival called Adi Puram, for the Goddess, I witnessed young women, while possessed, hurling abuses and beating their mothers-in-law or husbands, only to return to deferential behavior at the conclusion of the ritual when the priest applied *vibhuti* (sacred ash) and uttered some mantras (sacred formulas).

Chapter 3. Singularities and Their Discontents

1. Anne Harrington (2020) writes of this transition to de-institutionalization and pharmaceutical dominance in the American context.
2. Wahhabi or Wahhabist Islam refers to a strict reading of Sunni Islam that prohibits, among other things, the veneration of saints, some versions of Sufi mysticism that are deemed heretical and violate doctrinal texts, and interreligious or what we might call, for lack of a better word, syncretic practices. It is named after an influential reformer and revivalist, Muhammad ibn Abd-al-Wahhab, who lived in eighteenth-century Arabia.
3. Myoclonic seizures consist of a series of rhythmic jerks, usually of the arms and legs on one side of the body.
4. A provocative book about the impact of popular culture on psychiatry by Gold and Gold (2014) argues that the film itself, as a powerful image in popular culture, proved suggestible, leading to a temporary spike of reported cases in North America.
5. Arjuna, though forgetting Krishna's divine nature, is, interestingly enough, the son of Indra, an important Vedic deity who receded in importance. This suggests, as is often the case in Hindu myth, that the gods have their limits, and often act as humans with their flaws, ignorance, and vanities (Doniger 2009).
6. One lakh is INR 100,000.
7. This idea was expressed to me by a psychiatrist during pilot research on psychiatry in Bali, Indonesia. The doctor explained to me that the Balinese were increasingly haunted by apparitions as the abortion rate had increased with modern medical procedures being easily available.
8. Some anthropologists and psychoanalysts have made an attempt to understand the concerns of pollution in India through the "culture and personality" school of thought (Carstairs 1957; Spratt 1966; Kakar 1981).

9. A major concern had to do with the prescribing of medicines. The risks of contraindicated and over-prescribed medicines by traditional medicine practitioners posed substantial risk. While in India, it is fairly easy for anyone to obtain prescription-strength medication through local pharmacies, a partnership with traditional healers and biomedical institutions, such as NIMHANS, would create potential legal liability for the latter.
10. The popular Tamil film *Chandramukhi*, starring the Tamil-film icon Rajanikanth, had dramatized the themes of possession, exorcism, and modern psychiatry, ultimately pointing to the limits of the latter and the necessity of retaining understanding of the two former. The film was first a hit in Malayalam and Hindi, entitled *Bhool Bhulaiyaa* (see Pinto 2014).
11. In Tamil Nadu, the government does not follow the national metric for the Below Poverty Card and have their own way of measuring poverty. The poverty rate is harder to measure for Tamil Nadu, NIMHANS doctors sometimes complained, and appears to be lower because the threshold of income is much higher in Tamil Nadu than in many other states.
12. Vaishnavism runs deep in Tamil history and culture, particularly with the rise of *bhakti* poets and saints known as the Alvars between the sixth and eighth centuries CE.
13. This was in response to the Gokak movement, which pushed to make all official business in the state be conducted in Kannada (Pani 2010).
14. Here I am echoing Derrida's (1998; 2015; 2002a) concern with Foucault's reading of the history of psychiatry as the thinking of power, as well as his concern with Deleuze's obviation of contradiction, division, and duality within the unconscious, in favor of a more transcendental monism.

Chapter 4. Living with Urban Stress

1. A system of yoga that involves breath control and practicing certain postures to generate "heat" in order to reduce both stress and toxins within the body.
2. Meaning he did not lose consciousness entirely, or have a tonic-clonic or "grand mal" seizure. Sometimes these are referred to as "petit mal" seizures, and can include myoclonic jerks, twitching, or absence seizures (staring without jerks).
3. This is not to discount the kinds of madness unleashed by, in this case, the Partition of the subcontinent. Indeed, part of the overall argument of this book is that the arbitrary ordering of life into cultural and social bounded categories, or what I call serial forms of identification, following Anderson, produces a kind of feverish madness to supplement the impossible claims

of difference that mark communities as purportedly separate (Willford 2014; 2018; Hansen 2001; Anderson 1998; Sarin and Jain 2018).

4. Lévi-Strauss's formulation for the efficacy and coherence of sorcery, or its opposite, healing, is based on a triadic congruence of belief between the patient/afflicted, the healer, and the "gravitational" force of the believers surrounding the patient, indexing the social. The structural logic binding these three forces together compels healing or illness, as in the placebo and nocebo effects. In a more recent article by Stengers (2009), she revisits the uncanny parallels between the charlatan's healing authority and that utilized within biomedicine to find similar structural parallels.
5. A psychiatrist, his filmmaker spouse, and another medical anthropologist based in the US.
6. These are issued as a form of welfare by the government and provide access to free medical treatment and medications within government hospitals. NIMHANS, being a national institute, fell into that category and treated thousands of patients without charge annually.
7. We saw dozens of women with a *pottu* (Tamil) or *bindi* (Hindi) on their foreheads, the "third eye" characteristic of Hindu women. Muslim women were often partially veiled and Muslim men wore traditional head gear.
8. As Vasavi (2012) argues, the precarity of small-holder farmers in rural South India has never been greater, given structural inequities associated with the liberalization of the economy, contributing to the crisis of farmer suicides. Many of the "patients" within the *dargah* came from surrounding rural areas, and thus, the agrarian crisis in India quite possibly also made healing shrines more relevant within the local social imaginary.
9. I was accompanied by two staff-persons from The Banyan and BALM, a mental health care provider, NGO, and research institution, which has its campus and two care and rehabilitative centers for the mentally ill in Kovalam. One of the staff-persons helped in making introductions and gaining for us access to staff at the shrine, whereas the other, a PhD student, conducted the fieldwork together with me, assisting in the translations as well.
10. *Taviz* involves wearing a verse from the sacred Quran around one's neck as a talisman in amulet form. Numerology is utilized to select the most efficacious verse, given the particulars of birth date and name. *Falita* involves the drinking of the verse, after it has been burned to ash. Ingesting the sacred verse drives away malignant spirits (see Flueckiger 2006).
11. This shrine is to the god Ayyapan, a fusion of Vishnu and Shiva through their offspring, the Lord Ayyapan. Vishnu, in this myth, appeared as the

female goddess Mohini and seduced Shiva, producing a child god. For a detailed study of this shrine and the pilgrimage experience it affords, see Daniel (1984). Devotees can be seen throughout South India during the time of pilgrimage. They wear black and walk barefoot towards Sabarimala.

12. In DSM-5, the manual of diagnostics less used at NIMHANS, where the ICD-10 is more commonly invoked, the five axes are: 1. Clinical disorders, 2. Personality disorders, 3. Medical or physical conditions, 4. Contributing environmental or psychosocial disorders, and 5. Global assessment of functioning.
13. The book's full title is *The Wall: (Intimacy) and Other Stories*, a collection of Sartre's short stories (1948) dealing with various forms of madness. One essay, "The Room," specifically points to the contagion of madness as it passes from husband to wife in the closed confines of their small apartment, and the room where they spend most of their time together. The wife begins to question her sanity as she starts to feel the presence of "statues" that come to life with malicious intent. These were her husband's persistent delusion. Over time, she began, in the short story, to see and feel their presence as the delusion traveled from husband to wife. The story also demonstrates the impact of the madness of the husband upon the relationship between his wife and her family, which is increasingly strained as her parents worry that their daughter's life is being enveloped and threatened by the sickness and its worsening prognosis over time.
14. By this, I refer to his involvement with the National Socialist Party (Nazis), and his subsequent silence on this after the war. The so-called Nietzsche lectures that he delivered after leaving the Party, or as he was preparing to do so, offered indirect, philosophical critique of nativism and "falling" into "tradition." In late life, in his famous and final interview in *Der Spiegel* magazine, he referred to this period of his life as his *dummheit* (stupidity). His silence on this, and his lack of a formal philosophical renunciation, angered many of his critics, whereas others have argued that he did not want to absolve or justify his actions in a pithy apology.
15. A similar concern was voiced by some of the doctors at AIIMS, the nation's premier medical college and government hospital in New Delhi (see Ruddock 2021).

Chapter 5. Seizures, "Fits," and Neurology

1. Long-term monitoring or LTM refers to the patients who are admitted and videotaped throughout the day and night together, with constant EEG leads

attached to their heads. This allows the seizures to be viewed in functional and neurological terms, simultaneously, allowing for a positive determination of epilepsy. There is a smaller subset of epileptics, however, who have both epileptic (electrical discharge) seizures and psychogenic ones. One theory that doctors share, which I had suspected and asked the doctors in the US about, was whether, in these cases, the patient has psychogenic seizures as a way to "control" the onset, type, and duration of epileptic seizures. That is, albeit unconsciously, the patient would master the trauma of uncontrollable seizures overtaking the person by the willful enactment of seizures.

2. As cases were presented in rapid fire throughout the day, my field notes reflected simple entries, without much patient information. To give a flavor of the OPD and the rhythms of the clinic, I am displaying a brief section from my fieldnotes that highlight just the illness presentation and treatment recommendations that the doctor suggested:
—a 37 yr old male. Suffered seizures for the past 17 years. Currently he had 3 seizures per month. He reported that "hot water" brought on his seizures. He was referred to NIMHANS as his seizures still "interfere with his life," though he seemed to function fine. The doctor, as was his habit, looked at his MRI early on, after hearing the quick version of his symptom presentation and glancing at his medical chart. The MRI revealed hippocampal sclerosis, a common problem with long-term seizure activity. This affects memory. He was taking Tegretol when he came but the doctor ordered a switch of medications to valproate. A new MRI and EEG was ordered.
—a female in her 70s presented with seizures. These were under control with levitracinum. An EEG was ordered. She had breast cancer and developed seizures and neuropathy as a result of the cancer and chemotherapy. But with seizure control now through medication, it is likely this was a temporary problem. She might not need to continue with the medications. The EEG will hopefully show if there are still epileptiform spikes in her brain waves.
—A 30 year-old male presented with a seizure disorder. Six years earlier he had a head injury and complained of headaches and seizures. The seizures were partial and tonic-clonic, the resident reported. There was no MRI of the injured head at the time, and it is not known whether this was an enduring brain injury. The doctor ordered a MRI and EEG to probe deeper into the seizures and headaches. The patient also complained of blurred vision. In addition to the seizures, the man had a mild stroke six months earlier. The doctor queried whether the seizures and headaches had worsened after the stroke. The family seemed to think it had been "progressively worse" from six years earlier. The patient was on valproate.

—A man in his 50s presented with seizures. They began when he was 14. He saw lines in his visual field and suffered from psychiatric problems. The MRI suggested temporal lobe epilepsy. He was having 2–3 seizures per month. He came with his wife who was worried. The doctor said he can make him "seizure free within a year," in all likelihood. But further tests were needed to see if he was a surgery candidate. His epilepsy type seemed to suggest that he might be, as temporal lobe epilepsy is more easily operated upon than is parietal lobe epilepsy. He was on risperidone for his psychiatric problems.

—A college age male started having seizures at four years of age—this, after a febrile illness. They were now "complex partial seizures" (patient retained some consciousness) and only occurred once per month. At the onset of the seizure, the patient experienced fear and a loss of hearing as his "aura" (symptoms just prior to the seizure). Then he became "unaware and began smacking his lips" for two to three minutes. Sometimes he would just have the aura without the loss of consciousness. The EEG showed no obvious epileptiform waves. But the suspected area was the right temporal lobe, according to the doctor. This made him a reasonable candidate for surgery. The doctor ordered that the EEG be redone. The doctor explained to me later that while one per month is not too bad, they do the year-long workup towards surgery so as to line up the pieces in the event that the patient's condition progresses. It typically took a year, evidently, to complete all tests and to get onto the surgery schedule at NIMHANS. During this time, the patient will also receive some counseling. So being put on the surgery track doesn't necessarily mean a high likelihood of surgery, he explained.

3. As mentioned, I was impressed by the doctor's stamina as I watched him for about four or five hours of his OPD time without break, whereas he was actually in the OPD for more than ten hours. While I felt exhausted trying to note details of each case, he seemed attentive to the smallest of details and asked incisive but reassuringly calm questions throughout the day, without any visible fluctuation of energy.
4. I saw one or two patients in the OPD who came from North America, but had family in India. In another case, I saw a patient of Indian origin who traveled from Singapore for psychiatric care at NIMHANS. Medical tourism was more popular in private clinics where heart surgeries were a specialty in India. There was also the more dubious organ trade that drew people to India, particularly for kidney transplantation (see Cohen 2010).
5. I heard neurologists and epileptologists in the US also suggest this was the case, so my interpretation was hardly novel or insightful.

6. I have personal experience with this, as a family member with epilepsy had been evaluated for surgery four or five separate times at leading hospitals for neurosurgery in the US, in each case being told that uncertainty persisted, and therefore surgery was not advised.
7. This was different from the occasional two-week stays I saw in the US. Most epilepsy centers in the US would advise a five- to ten-day admission within the LTM so that a sufficient number of seizures and their types were captured. A patient, for instance, might have both epileptic and psychogenic seizures; therefore it was important to capture a range of seizures from the same patient.
8. MTS occurs in the hippocampus region of the brain, which is associated with long-term memory. MTS is caused by long-term seizure activity, and is one of the worst effects that epilepsy produces in patients with intractable seizures.
9. *Taviz* amulets contain Quranic verses within them to protect individuals from supernatural malignant forces, such as those caused by sorcery or *jinn* possession.
10. Some of the doctors suggested to me that the rise of Hindu nationalism in the country had also stimulated interest in "traditional" medicine and support for AYUSH research and treatments at major research institutions such as NIMHANS.

Conclusion. Social Dimensions of Mental Illness and Care

1. Here I am echoing Derrida's concern with Foucault's reading of the history of psychiatry as the thinking of power, as well as his concern with Deleuze's obviation of contradiction, division, and duality within the unconscious, in favor of a more transcendental monism (see Derrida 2015).
2. Pandolfo 2018.
3. Taneja 2018; Vasavi 2020.
4. Hansen 2001; Ghassem-Fachandi 2012; Menon 2022.
5. Thiranagama 2022; Pinto 2014.
6. See Pinto 2022.
7. In Lacan's varied and complex corpus of work (e.g., 1977; 2014), the influence of Heidegger on his clinical thinking is ubiquitous, as are the citations of the former's work on anxiety, uncanniness, and being-unto-death. While for Heidegger the sense of fundamental anxiety as to our individual mortality, as an existential condition of humanity, is the path towards authentic Being, as opposed to just being another animal among animals in this world, the overwhelming sway of the uncanny can also trigger its opposite motion, a "fall" into tradition, the values of the "they" and an ensnarement

within the technologies and apparatuses of measurement, picturing, figuring, and turning humans into the ultimate "standing reserve" (e.g., 2000; 1996; 1992; 1977). Thus, the sovereignty of man, in Heidegger's diagnosis of the modern age, is an illusory sovereignty, built upon an edifice of measurements that perpetually haunt subjectivity. The influence of Heidegger's notion of illusory sovereignty, the being who, while claiming to seize and control his objectifying and measurable world, is seized and controlled, in his fallen and ensnared state, by the technologies of control, has particular resonance in all of Derrida's work, as well. The notion of the archive that I have cited in this study as a key analytic, taken from Derrida, could be described as a technology that seizes, ensnares, and fixates the subject, when provoked by the inner betrayals induced by the very same technology. Derrida, in his last seminar (2002a), however, critiqued Heidegger's categorical distinction between the human and the animal, suggesting that for all of his critique and diagnosis of the modern age, this distinction recuperates an intractable and harmful division between humanity, animals, and nature, rearticulating a metaphysical sovereignty of authentic being despite unmasking and deconstructing the sources of ensnarement and fixation. Derrida (1998; 2002a), in turn, has made a similar critique of Lacan's complex and universalizing systems of analysis. But this critique of both acknowledges his debt to their thinking, all the same. One could say the same of Freud's relationship to Derrida. In all three cases, it might be fair to say that it was their brilliance and radicality that was being called out by Derrida, in showing that their insights, precisely, did not allow for the definitive and authoritative claims they, in turn, made in philosophy and psychoanalysis. And while critics of Derrida would accuse him of a kind of nihilist hall of mirrors approach to knowledge, his admirers pointed to the ethics of openness and hospitality to alterity and difference as life-affirming (Critchley 2014).

References

Addlakha, Renu. 2008. *Deconstructing Mental Illness: An Ethnography of Psychiatry, Women, and the Family*. New Delhi: Zubaan.

Al-Kassim, Dina. 2007. "Resistance, Terminable and Interminable." In *Derrida, Deleuze, Psychoanalysis*, edited by Gabriele Schwab. New York: Columbia University Press.

Anderson, Benedict. 1998. "Nationalism, Identity, and the Logic of Seriality." In *The Spectre of Comparisons*. London: Verso.

Appadurai, Arjun. 2000. "Dead Certainty: Ethnic Violence in the Era of Globalization." In *Globalization and Identity*, edited by Birgit Meyer and Peter Geschierre. London: Blackwell.

Appadurai, Arjun. 2013. *The Future as Cultural Fact: Essays on the Global Condition*. London: Verso.

Aretxaga, Begonia. 2008. "Madness and the Politically Real: Reflections on Violence in Postdictatorial Spain." In *Postcolonial Disorders*, edited by Mary-Jo DelVecchio Good, Sandra Hyde, Sarah Pinto, and Byron Good. Berkeley: University of California Press.

Bateson, Gregory. 1977. *Steps to an Ecology of Mind*. New York: Ballantine.

Benedict, Ruth. 1934. *Patterns of Culture*. New York: Houghton Mifflin Co.

Benjamin, Walter. 1968. "The Storyteller." In *Illuminations*, edited by Hannah Arendt. New York: Schocken.

Biehl, João. 2005.*Vita: Life in a Zone of Social Abandonment*. Berkeley: University of California Press.

Biehl, João, and Amy Moran Thomas. 2009. "Symptoms, Subjectivities, Social Ills, Technologies." *Annual Review of Anthropology* 38: 267–288.

Birbeau, Gilles, and Ellen Corin. 2009. "Afterword: Turning Many into One: Mental Health at the Junction of Classic Hindu Texts, Religious Practices, and Modern Psychiatric Knowledge." In *Restoring Mental Health in India*, edited by Brigitte Sebastia. New Delhi: Oxford University Press.

Bourdieu, Pierre. 1977. *Outline of a Theory of Practice*. Cambridge: Cambridge University Press.

Carstairs, G. Morris. 1957. *The Twice Born: A Study of a Community of High-Caste Hindus.* London: Hogarth Press.

Carstairs, G. M., and R. L. Kapur. 1979. *The Great Universe of the Kota.* Berkeley: University of California Press.

Chandrasekhar, C. R. 2008. *Gods, Ghosts, Witchcraft and the Mind.* Bangalore: Navakarnataka Publications.

Chua, Jocelyn Lim. 2014. *In Pursuit of the Good Life: Aspiration and Suicide in Globalizing South India.* Berkeley: University of California Press.

Clinton, Chelsea, and Devi Shridhar. 2017. *Governing Global Health: Who Runs the World and Why?* Oxford: Oxford University Press.

Clothey, Fred W. 1978. *The Many Faces of Murugan: The History and Meaning of a South Indian God.* The Hague: Mouton.

Cohen, Alex, Arthur Kleinman, and Benedetto Saraceno. 2002. *World Mental Health Casebook: Social and Mental Health Programs in Low-Income Countries.* New York: Kluwer Academic/Plenum.

Cohen, Lawrence. 1998. *No Aging in India: Alzheimer's, the Bad Family, and Other Modern Things.* Berkeley: University of California Press.

Cohen, Lawrence. 2010. "Ethical Publicity: On Transplant Victims, Wounded Communities, and the Moral Demands of Dreaming." In *Ethical Life in South Asia*, edited by Anand Pandian and Daud Ali. New Delhi: Oxford University Press.

Cohen, Lawrence. 2012. "Making Peasants Protestants and Other Projects: Medical Anthropology and Its Global Condition." In *Medical Anthropology at the Intersections: Histories, Activisms, and Futures*, edited by Marcia Inhorn and Emily Wentzell. Durham: Duke University Press.

Cohen, Lawrence. 2022. "The Duplicate Malady: Repositioning Hysteria in South Asia." *South Asia: The Journal of South Asian Studies* 45 (February 2022). https://doi.org/10.1080/00856401.2022.2020021.

Colebrook, Claire. 2006. *Deleuze: A Guide for the Perplexed.* London: Bloomsbury.

Comaroff, John L., and Jean Comaroff. 2006. "Law and Disorder in the Postcolony: An Introduction." In *Law and Disorder in the Postcolony*, edited by John L. Comaroff and Jean Comaroff. Chicago: University of Chicago Press.

Comaroff, John L., and Jean Comaroff. 2009. *Ethnicity, Inc.* Chicago: University of Chicago Press.

Corin, Ellen. 2007. "The 'Other' of Culture in Psychosis: The Ex-Centricity of the Subject." In *Subjectivity: Ethnographic Investigations*, edited by João Biehl, Byron Good, and Arthur Kleinman. Berkeley: University of California Press.

Corin, Ellen, Rangaswami Thara, and Ramachandran Padmavati. 2004. "Living Through a Staggering World: The Play of Signifiers in Early Psychosis in South India." In *Schizophrenia, Culture, and Subjectivity: The Edge of Experience*, edited by Janice Jenkins and Robert Barret. Cambridge: Cambridge University Press.

Critchley, Simon. 2014. *The Ethics of Deconstruction: Derrida and Levinas*. Edinburgh: University of Edinburgh Press.

Daniel, E. Valentine. 1984. *Fluid Signs: Being a Person the Tamil Way*. Berkeley: University of California Press.

Das, Veena. 2006. *Life and Words: Violence and the Descent into the Ordinary*. Berkeley: University of California Press.

Das, Veena. 2015. *Affliction: Health, Disease, Poverty*. New York: Fordham University Press.

Datta, Damayanti. 2015. "The Great Depression." *India Today*, March 2, 2015.

Davar, Bhargavi, and Madhura Lohokare. 2012. "Recovering from Psychosocial Traumas: The Place of Dargahs in Maharashra." In *Medical Pluralism in Contemporary India*, edited by V. Sujatha and Leena Abrahman. Delhi: Orient BlackSwan.

Deleuze, Gilles. 1994. *Difference and Repetition*. New York: Columbia University Press.

Deleuze, Gilles. 1998. *Essays: Critical and Clinical*. Minneapolis: University of Minnesota Press.

Deleuze, Gilles, and Felix Guattari. 1972. *Anti-Oedipus: Capitalism and Schizophrenia*. Minneapolis: University of Minnesota Press.

Deleuze, Gilles, and Felix Guattari. 1987. *A Thousand Plateaus: Capitalism and Schizophrenia*. Minneapolis: University of Minnesota Press.

Derrida, Jacques. 1976. *Of Grammatology*. Baltimore: Johns Hopkins University Press.

Derrida, Jacques. 1981. *Dissemination*. Chicago: University of Chicago Press.

Derrida, Jacques. 1995. *Archive Fever: A Freudian Impression*. Translated by Eric Prenowitz. Chicago: University of Chicago Press.

Derrida, Jacques. 1998. *Resistances of Psychoanalysis*. Stanford: Stanford University Press.

Derrida, Jacques. 2002a. "Psychoanalysis Searches the States of Its Soul: The Impossible Beyond of a Sovereign Cruelty." In *Without Alibi*, translated and edited by Peggy Kamuf. Stanford: Stanford University Press.

Derrida, Jacques. 2002b. "Force of Law." In *Acts of Religion*. London: Routledge.

Derrida, Jacques. 2007. "Geopsychoanalysis 'and the Rest of the World.'" In *Psyche: Inventions of the Other*. Vol. 1, edited by Peggy Kamuf and Elizabeth Rottenberg. Stanford: Stanford University Press.

Derrida, Jacques. 2015. "Beyond the Power Principle." Translated by Elizabeth Rottenberg. *The Undecidable Unconscious: A Journal of Deconstruction and Psychoanalysis* 2: 7–17.

Desjarlais, Robert, Leon Eisenberg, Byron Good, and Arthur Kleinman. 1995. *World Mental Health: Problems and Priorities in Low-Income Countries*. New York: Oxford University Press.

Devereux, George. 1980. *Basic Problems of Ethnopsychiatry*. Chicago: University of Chicago Press.

D'Mello, Marisa, and Sundeep Sahay. 2008. "Betwixt and Between? Exploring Mobilities in a Global Workplace in India." In *In an Outpost of the Global Economy: Work and Workers in India's Information Technology Industry*, edited by Carol Upadhya and A. S. Vasavi. New Delhi: Routledge.

Doniger, Wendy. 2010. *The Hindus: An Alternative History.* New York: Penguin.

Dumont, Louis. 1970. *Homo Hierarchicus.* Chicago: University of Chicago Press.

Ecks, Stefan. 2013. *Eating Drugs: Psychopharmaceutical Pluralism in India.* New York: New York University Press.

Ecks, Stefan. 2021. "Mental Ills for All: Genealogies for the Movement for Global Mental Health." In *The Movement for Global Mental Health: Critical Views from South and Southeast Asia*, edited by William Sax and Claudia Lang. Amsterdam: Amsterdam University Press.

Ewing, Katherine. 1997. *Arguing Sainthood: Modernity, Psychoanalysis, Islam.* Durham: Duke University Press.

Fabrega, Horatio. 2009. *History of Mental Illness in India: A Cultural Psychiatry Retrospective.* New Delhi: Motilal Banarsidas.

Fassin, Didier, and Richard Rechtman. 2009. *The Empire of Trauma: An Inquiry into the Condition of Victimhood.* Princeton: Princeton University Press.

Favret-Saada, Jeanne. 2015. *The Anti-Witch.* Chicago: HAU Books.

Fink, Bruce. 1995. *The Lacanian Subject: Between Language and Jouissance.* Princeton: Princeton University Press.

Flaxman, Gregory. 2011. *Gilles Deleuze and the Fabulation of Philosophy.* Minneapolis: University of Minnesota Press.

Flueckiger, Joyce. 2006. *In Amma's Healing Room: Gender and Vernacular Islam in South India.* Bloomington: Indiana University Press.

Foucault, Michel. 1994. "Psychiatric Power." In *Ethics: Subjectivity, and Truth*, edited by Paul Rabinow. New York: The New Press.

Foucault, Michel. 2003. "The Subject and Power," "About the Concept of the 'Dangerous Individual' in Nineteenth-Century Legal Psychiatry," and "Madness and Society." In *The Essential Foucault*, edited by Paul Rabinow. New York: The New Press.

Foucault, Michel. 2006. *History of Madness.* Translated by Jean Khalfa. Oxford: Routledge.

Freud, Sigmund. 1961. *Beyond the Pleasure Principle.* New York: Norton.

Freud, Sigmund. 1997. "The Uncanny." In *Writings on Art and Literature*. Stanford: Stanford University Press.

Funahashi, Daena. 2023. *Untimely Sacrifices: Work and Death in Finland.* Ithaca: Cornell University Press.

Ganesalingam, Shaalini, and Abhinaya Devi. 2018. "Loss of Land and Identity: An Indigenous Health Story." *Current Conservation*, October 30, 2018. https://

www.currentconservation.org/loss-of-land-and-identity-an-indigenous-health-story/.

Geertz, Clifford. 1973. *The Interpretation of Cultures.* New York: Basic Books.

Ghassem-Fachandi, Parvis. 2012. *Pogrom in Gujarat: Hindu Nationalism and Anti-Muslim Violence in India.* Princeton: Princeton University Press.

Goel, D. S., S. P. Agarwal, R. L. Ichhpujani, and S. Shrivastava. 2004. "Mental Health 2003: The Indian Scene." In *Mental Health: An Indian Perspective*, edited by S. P. Agarwal. New Delhi: Directorate General of Health Services, Ministry of Health and Family Welfare.

Gold, Ann Grodzins. 2014. "Sweetness and Light: The Bright Side of Pluralism in a Rajasthan Town." In *Religious Pluralism, State and Society in Asia*, edited by Chiara Formichi. London: Routledge.

Gold, Joel, and Ian Gold. 2014. *Suspicious Minds: How Culture Shapes Madness.* New York: Free Press.

Gomez-Carrillo, Ana, Laurence J. Kirmayer, et al. 2023. "Integrating Neuroscience in Psychiatry: A Cultural–Ecosocial Systemic Approach." *Lancet* 10 (2023): 296–304.

Good, Byron, Subandi, and Mary-Jo DelVecchio Good. 2007. "The Subject of Mental Illness: Psychosis, Mad Violence, and Subjectivity in Indonesia." In *Subjectivity: Ethnographic Investigations*, edited by João Biehl, Byron Good, and Arthur Kleinman. Berkeley: University of California Press.

Gopikumar, V., K. V. Kishore Kumar, Alok Sarin, and Sanjeev Jain. 2016. "How Centers of Faith Can Help Provide Better Mental Healthcare in India." *Scroll.in*, September 23, 2016. https://scroll.in/article/815852.

Gopikumar, V., D. Padgett, A. Sarin, R. Mezzina, A. Willford, and S. Jain. 2020. "Mental Health and the Coronavirus: A Global Perspective." *World Social Psychiatry* 2: 88–93.

Gottschalk, Peter. 2000. *Beyond Hindu and Muslim: Multiple Identity in Narratives from Village India.* New York: Oxford University Press.

Grosz, Elizabeth. 2005. *Time Travels: Feminism, Nature, Power.* Durham: Duke University Press.

Gupta, Akhil. 1998. *Postcolonial Developments: Agriculture in the Making of Modern India.* Durham: Duke University Press.

Gupta, Akhil. 2012. *Red Tape, Bureaucracy, Structural Violence, and Poverty in India.* Durham: Duke University Press.

Guyer, Sara. 2007. "Buccality." In *Derrida, Deleuze, Psychoanalysis*, edited by Gabriele Schwab. New York: Columbia University Press.

Halliburton, Murphy. 2009. *Mudpacks and Prozac: Experiencing Ayurvedic, Biomedical and Religious Healing.* Walnut Creek: Left Coast Press.

Halliburton, Murphy. 2017. *India and the Patent Wars: Pharmaceuticals in the New Intellectual Property Regime.* Ithaca: ILR Cornell University Press.

Hallowell, A. Irving. 1955. *Culture and Experience.* Philadelphia: University of Pennsylvania.

Hansen, Thomas. 1999. *The Saffron Wave: Democracy and Hindu Nationalism in Modern India.* Princeton: Princeton University Press.

Hansen, Thomas. 2001. *The Wages of Violence.* Princeton: Princeton University Press.

Harrington, Anne. 2020. *Mind Fixers: Psychiatry's Troubled Search for the Biology of Mental Illness.* New York: Norton.

Hart, George L. 1975. *The Poems of Ancient Tamil: Their Milieu and Their Sanskrit Counterparts.* Berkeley: University of California Press.

Hart, George L. 1979. *Poets of the Tamil Anthologies: Ancient Poems of Love and War.* Princeton: Princeton University Press.

Hegel, G. W. F. 1977. *Hegel's Phenomenology of Spirit.* Oxford: Oxford University Press.

Heidegger, Martin. 1977. "The Age of the World Picture." In *The Question Concerning Technology and Other Essays*, translated by William Lovitt. New York: Harper Torchbook.

Heidegger, Martin. 1992. *History of the Concept of Time.* Translated by Theodore Kisiel. Bloomington: Indiana University Press.

Heidegger, Martin. 1996. *Being and Time.* Translated by Joan Stambaugh. Albany: State University of New York Press.

Heidegger, Martin. 2000. *Introduction to Metaphysics.* Translated by Gregory Fried and Richard Polt. New Haven: Yale University Press.

Hiltebeitel, Alf, and Kathleen Erndl, eds. 2000. *Is the Goddess a Feminist? The Politics of South Asian Goddesses.* New York: New York University Press.

Hopper, Kim, Glynn Harrison, Aleksandar Janca, and Norman Sartorius, eds. 2007. *Recovery from Schizophrenia: A Report from the WHO Collaborative Project, The International Study of Schizophrenia.* Oxford: Oxford University Press.

Horwitz, Allan. 2002. *Creating Mental Illness.* Chicago: University of Chicago Press.

Irschick, Eugene F. 1994. *Dialogue and History: Constructing South India, 1795–1895.* Berkeley: University of California Press.

Iype, George. 2004. "South India: World's Suicide Capital." Rediff.com, April 15, 2004. https://www.rediff.com/news/2004/apr/15spec.htm.

Jaffrelot, Christophe. 2021. *Modi's India: Hindu Nationalism and the Rise of Ethnic Democracy.* Princeton: Princeton University Press.

Kakar, Sudhir. 1981. *The Inner World.* Delhi: Oxford University Press.

Kakar, Sudhir. 1982. *Shamans, Mystics, and Doctors.* Delhi: Oxford University Press.

Kakar, Sudhir. 1996. *The Colors of Violence.* Chicago: Oxford University Press.

Kapur, R. L. 2004. "The Story of Community Mental Health in India." In *Mental Health: An Indian Perspective*, edited by S. P. Agarwal. New Delhi: Directorate General of Health Services, Ministry of Health and Family Welfare.

Kapur, R. L. 2012. *Another Way to Live: A Psychiatrist Among Indian Ascetics.* New Delhi: Viking.

Kardiner, Abram. 1939. *The Individual and Society.* New York: Columbia University Press.

Kaviraj, Sudipta. 1991. "The Imaginary Institution of India." In *Subaltern Studies 7*, edited by Partha Chatterjee and Gyanendra Pandey. Delhi: Oxford University Press.

Keane, Webb. 1997. *Signs of Recognition: Powers and Hazards of Representation in an Indonesian Society.* Berkeley: University of California Press.

Kilroy-Marac, Katie. 2019. *An Impossible Inheritance: Postcolonial Psychiatry and the Work of Memory in a West African Clinic.* Berkeley: University of California Press.

Kinsley, David. 1986. *Hindu Goddesses.* Berkeley: University of California Press.

Kirmayer, Laurence, and Ana Gomez-Carrillo. 2018. "Culturally Responsive Clinical Psychology and Psychiatry." In *Cultural Clinical Psychology and PTSD*, edited by Andreas Maercker, Eva Heim, and Laurence Kirmayer. Gottingen: Hogrefe.

Kirmayer, Laurence, Robert Lemelson, and Constance Cummings, eds. 2015. *Re-Visioning Psychiatry: Cultural Phenomenology, Critical Neuroscience, and Global Mental Health.* Cambridge: Cambridge University Press.

Klein, Melanie. 1986. *The Selected Melanie Klein.* New York: Free Press.

Kleinman, Arthur. 1988. *Rethinking Psychiatry.* New York: Free Press.

Kleinman, Arthur. 2012. "Medical Anthropology and Mental Health: Five Questions for the Next Fifty Years." In *Medical Anthropology at the Intersections: Histories, Activisms, and Futures*, edited by Marcia Inhorn and Emily Wentzell. Durham: Duke University Press.

Kohrt, Brandon A., and Emily Mendenhall. 2015. "Introduction" and "Conclusion." In *Global Mental Health: Anthropological Perspectives*, edited by Brandon A. Kohrt and Emily Mendenhall. New York: Routledge.

Koschorke, Mirja, R. Padmavati, S. Kumar, et al. 2014. "Experiences of Stigma and Discrimination of People with Schizophrenia in India." *Social Science and Medicine* 123 (2014): 149–159.

Kurtz, Stanley. 1992. *All the Mothers Are One: Hindu India and the Cultural Reshaping of Psychoanalysis.* New York: Columbia University Press.

Lacan, Jacques. 1977. *Ecrits: A Selection.* Translated by Alan Sheridan. New York: Norton.

Lacan, Jacques. 1981. *The Four Fundamental Concepts of Psychoanalysis: The Seminar of Jacques Lacan, Book XI.* Translated by Alan Sheridan, edited by Jacques Alain-Miller. New York: Norton.

Lacan, Jacques. 1992. *The Ethics of Psychoanalysis: The Seminar of Jacques Lacan, Book VII.* Translated by Dennis Porter, edited by Jacques Alain-Miller. New York: Norton.

Lacan, Jacques. 1993. *The Psychoses: The Seminar of Jacques Lacan, Book III.* Translated by Russell Brigg, edited by Jacques Alain-Miller. New York: Norton.

Lacan, Jacques. 2014. *Anxiety: The Seminar of Jacques Lacan, Book X.* Translated by A. R. Price, edited by Jacques Alain-Miller. Cambridge: Polity.

Lang, Claudia. 2018. *Depression in Kerala: Ayurveda and Mental Health Care in 21st Century India.* London: Routledge.

Langford, Jean. 2002. *Fluent Bodies: Ayurvedic Remedies for Postcolonial Imbalance.* Durham: Duke University Press.

Lévi-Strauss, Claude. 1973. "The Sorcerer and His Magic." In *Structural Anthropology.* New York: Basic Books.

Lewis, I. M. 1989. *Ecstatic Religion: An Anthropological Study of Spirit Possession and Shamanism.* New Orleans: Pelican Press.

Luhrmann, Tanya Marie. 2000. *Of Two Minds: An Anthropologist Looks at American Psychiatry.* New York: Alfred Knopf.

Luhrmann, Tanya Marie. 2016. "Introduction." In *Our Most Troubling Madness: Case Studies in Schizophrenia Across Cultures*, edited by Tanya Luhrmann and Jocelyn Marrow. Berkeley: University of California Press.

Luhrmann, Tanya, and Jocelyn Marrow, eds. 2016. *Our Most Troubling Madness: Case Studies in Schizophrenia Across Cultures.* Berkeley: University of California Press.

Luhrmann, T. M., and R. Padmavati. "Voices that Are More Benign: The Experience of Auditory Hallucinations in Chennai." In *Our Most Troubling Madness: Case Studies in Schizophrenia Across Cultures*, edited by Tanya Luhrmann and Jocelyn Marrow. Berkeley: University of California Press.

Malabou, Catherine. 2012. *Ontology of the Accident: An Essay on Destructive Plasticity.* Cambridge: Polity.

Mankekar, Purnima, and Akhil Gupta. 2017. "Future Tense: Capital, Labor, and Technology in a Service Industry." *HAU: Journal of Ethnographic Theory* 7 (3). https://doi.org/10.14318/hau7.3.004.

Marcuse, Herbert. 1964. *One-Dimensional Man: Studies in the Ideology of Advanced Industrial Society.* Boston: Beacon Press.

Marriott, McKim. 1976. "Hindu Transactions: Diversity without Dualism." In *Transaction and Meaning: Directions in the Anthropology of Exchange and Symbolic Behavior*, edited by Bruce Kapferer. Philadelphia: Institute for the Study of Human Issues.

Marrow, Jocelyn. 2008. *Psychiatry, Modernity, and Family Values: Clenched Teeth Illness in North India.* PhD diss., Departments of Psychology and Human Development. University of Chicago.

Marrow, Jocelyn. 2016. "Vulnerable Transitions in a World of Kin: In the Shadow of Good Wifeliness in North India." In *Our Most Troubling Madness: Case Studies in Schizophrenia Across Cultures*, edited by Tanya Luhrmann and Jocelyn Marrow. Berkeley: University of California Press.

Marrow, Jocelyn. 2022. "Hysteria Narratives and Love-in-Separation (*Viraha*) in North India." *South Asia: The Journal of South Asian Studies* 45 (January 2022). https://doi.org/10.1080/00856401.2022.2014123.

Marrow, Jocelyn, and Tanya Marie Luhrmann. 2016. "Conclusion." In *Our Most Troubling Madness: Case Studies in Schizophrenia Across Cultures*, edited by Tanya Luhrmann and Jocelyn Marrow. Berkeley: University of California Press.

Martin, Emily. 2007. *Bipolar Expeditions: Mania and Depression in American Culture.* Princeton: Princeton University Press.

Massumi, Brian. 2002. *Parables for the Virtual.* Durham: Duke University Press.

Mauss, Marcel. 1902. Reprint, Routledge, 2002. *A General Theory of Magic.* London: Routledge.

Mazza, Giulia. 2016. "Work and Respect in Chennai." In *Our Most Troubling Madness: Case Studies in Schizophrenia Across Cultures*, edited by Tanya Luhrmann and Jocelyn Marrow. Berkeley: University of California Press.

Menon, Kalyani. 2010. *Everyday Nationalism: Women of the Hindu Right in India.* Philadelphia: University of Pennsylvania Press.

Menon, Kalyani. 2022. *Making Place for Muslims in Contemporary India.* Ithaca: Cornell University Press.

Merry, Sally. 2016. *The Seductions of Quantification: Measuring Human Rights, Gender Violence and Sex Trafficking.* Chicago: University of Chicago Press.

Mitchell, Juliet. 1986. "Introduction." In *The Selected Melanie Klein*, edited by Juliet Mitchell. New York: Free Press.

Mitchell, Juliet. 2000. *Madmen and Medusas: Reclaiming Hysteria.* New York: Basic Books.

Mohammad, Abdul Hafeez. 2017. "The Biography of Hazrat Tamim Ansari, Chennai." https://www.calameo.com/read/00030938201a47690a443.

Morgan, Craig, Kwame McKenzie, and Paul Fearon, eds. 2008. *Society and Psychosis.* Cambridge: Cambridge University Press.

Morris, Rosalind. 2000. *In the Place of Origins.* Durham: Duke University Press.

Morris, Rosalind. 2017. "After de Brosses: Fetishism, Translation, Comparativism, Critique." In *The Returns of Fetishism: Charles de Brosses and the Afterlives of an Idea*, edited by Rosalind Morris and Daniel Leonard. Chicago: University of Chicago Press.

Mukherjee, Sanjukta. 2008. "Producing the Knowledge Professional: Gendered Geographies of Alienation in India's New High-Tech Workplace." In *In an Outpost of the Global Economy: Work and Workers in India's Information Technology Industry*, edited by Carol Upadhya and A. S. Vasavi. New Delhi: Routledge.

Murthy, Pratima. 2018. "Looking Within, Looking Without." In *The Psychological Impact of the Partition of India*, edited by Sanjeev Jain and Alok Sarin. New Delhi: Sage.

Murthy, Pratima, and Sanjeev Jain. 2009. "Diagnosis and Treatment Approaches at the Asylum in Bangalore." In *Restoring Mental Health in India*, edited by Brigitte Sebastia. New Delhi: Oxford University Press.

Nabokov, Isabelle. 2000. *Religion Against the Self: An Ethnography of Tamil Rituals.* Oxford: Oxford University Press.

Nagaraja, D., and Pratima Murthy. 2008. "Future Directions for Mental Health Care in India." In *Mental Health Care and Human Rights*, edited by D. Nagaraja and Pratima Murthy. New Delhi: National Human Rights Commission.

Nair, Janaki. 2005. *The Promise of the Metropolis: Bangalore's Twentieth Century.* Delhi: Oxford University Press.

Nakamura, Karen. 2013. *A Disability of the Soul: An Ethnography of Schizophrenia and Mental Illness in Contemporary Japan.* Ithaca: Cornell University Press.

Nandy, Ashis. 1983. *The Intimate Enemy: Loss and Recovery of Self Under Colonialism.* Delhi: Oxford University Press.

Narasimhan, Lakshmi, Vandana Gopikumar, Vaishnavi Jayakumar, Joske Bunders, and Barbara Regeer. 2019. "Responsive Mental Health Systems to Address the Poverty, Homelessness, and Mental Illness Nexus: The Banyan Experience from India." *International Journal of Mental Health Systems* 13 (54). https://doi.org/10.1186/s13033-019-0313-8.

Nichter, Mark. 1982. "Idioms of Distress: Alternatives in the Expression of Psychosocial Distress: A Case Study from South India." *Medicine, Culture, and Psychiatry* 5 (4): 379–408.

NIMHANS. 2009. District Mental Health Programme. Originally published 1996.

Obeyesekere, Gananath. 1981. *Medusa's Hair: An Essay on Personal Symbols and Religious Experience.* Chicago: University of Chicago Press.

Obeyesekere, Gananath. 1985. *The Work of Culture: Symbolic Transformation in Psychoanalysis and Anthropology.* Chicago: University of Chicago Press.

Ortner, Sherry. 1979. "On Key Symbols." In *Reader in Comparative Religion: An Anthropological Approach*, edited by William Lessa and Evan Vogt. New York: Harper & Row.

Pandian, Anand. 2010. "Interior Horizons: An Ethical Space of Selfhood in South India." *Journal of the Royal Anthropological Institute* 16: 64–83.

Pandolfo, Stefania. 2018. *Knot of the Soul: Madness, Psychoanalysis, Islam.* Chicago: University of Chicago Press.

Pani, Narendar. 2010. "Imaginations of Bengaluru." In *Bengaluru, Bangalore, Bengaluru: Imaginations and Their Times*, edited by Narendar Pani, Sindhu Radhakrishna, and Kishor G. Bhat. New Delhi: Sage.

Patel, Vikram, and Arthur Kleinman. 2003. "Poverty and Common Mental Disorders in Developing Countries." *Bulletin of the World Health Organization* 81 (8): 609–615.

Patel, Vikram, Shekhar Saxena, C. Lund, et al. 2018. "The *Lancet* Commission on Global Mental Health and Sustainable Development," and "Supplementary Index." *The Lancet*, October 9, 2018. https://doi.org/10.1016/S0140-6736(18)31612-X.

Pinto, Sarah. 2014. *Daughters of Parvati: Women and Madness in Contemporary India*. Philadelphia: University of Pennsylvania Press.

Pinto, Sarah. 2020a. *The Doctor and Mrs. A: Ethics and Counter-Ethics in an Indian Dream Analysis*. New York: Fordham University Press.

Pinto, Sarah. 2020b. "Madness: Recursive Ethnography and the Critical Uses of Psychopathology." *Annual Reviews of Anthropology* 49: 299–316.

Pinto, Sarah. 2022. "Hysteria: A South Asian History of Global Medicine." *South Asia: The Journal of South Asian Studies* 45.

Povinelli, Elizabeth. 2016. *Geontologies: A Requiem to Late Liberalism*. Durham: Duke University Press.

Powis, Laura, Samsuda Khem-Nguad, and Halammal Rangasamy. 2015. "Exploring Kurumba Health Perspectives." Kotagiri: unpublished research paper.

Radhika, P., Pratima Murthy, and Sanjeev Jain. 2015. *Mindscape and Landscape: An Illustrated History of NIMHANS 1850–2014*. Bangalore: National Institute of Mental Health and Neuro Sciences.

Raguram, R., Mitchell G. Weiss, S. M. Channabasavanna, and Gerald Devins. 1996. "Stigma, Depression, and Somatization in South India." *American Journal of Psychiatry* 153 (8): 1043–1049.

Raguram, R., A. Vekateswaran, Jayashree Ramakrishna, and Mitchell G. Weiss. 2002. "Traditional Community Resources for Mental Health: A Report of Temple Healing from India." *BMJ* 325 (July 6, 2002): 38–40.

Ram, Kalpana. 2013. *Fertile Disorder: Spirit Possession and Its Provocation of the Modern*. Honolulu: University of Hawaii Press.

Ramanujam, A. K. 1973. *Speaking of Siva*. Baltimore: Penguin Books.

Ramanujam, A. K. 1997. *A Flowering Tree, and Other Folk Tales from India*. Gurgaon: Penguin Books.

Ramberg, Lucinda. 2014. *Given to the Goddess: South Indian Devadasis and the Sexuality of Religion*. Durham: Duke University Press.

Reyes-Foster, Beatriz. 2018. *Psychiatric Encounters: Madness and Modernity in Yucatan, Mexico*. New Brunswick: Rutgers University Press.

Robbins, Joel. 2004. *Becoming Sinners: Christianity and Moral Torment in a Papua New Guinea Society*. Berkeley: University of California Press.

Roland, Alan. 1988. *In Search of Self in India and Japan: Towards a Cross-Cultural Psychology*. Princeton: Princeton University Press.

Rosaldo, Michelle. 1984. "Toward an Anthropology of Self and Feeling." In *Culture Theory: Essays on Mind, Self, and Emotion*, edited by Richard Shweder and Robert LeVine. Cambridge: Cambridge University Press.

Rose, Nikolas. 2018. *Our Psychiatric Future.* London: Polity.

Ruddock, Anna. 2021. *Special Treatment: Student Doctors at the All Indian Institute of Medical Sciences.* Stanford: Stanford University Press.

Sapir, Edward. 2010. "The Psychology of Culture." In *Psychological Anthropology: A Reader in Self and Culture*, edited by Robert LeVine. Oxford: Wiley-Blackwell.

Sarin, Alok, and Sanjeev Jain. 2018. "Setting the Stage: The Partition of India and the Silences of Psychiatry." In *The Psychological Impact of the Partition of India*, edited by Sanjeev Jain and Alok Sarin. New Delhi: Sage.

Sartre, Jean-Paul. 1948. *The Wall: (Intimacy) and Other Stories.* New York: New Directions.

Sastri, Nilakanta. 1975. *A History of South India.* Madras: Oxford University Press.

Schechter, Kate. 2014. *Illusions of the Future: Psychoanalysis and the Biopolitics of Desire.* Durham: Duke University Press.

Seale-Feldman, Aidan. 2022. "The Possibility of Translation: Turning Ghosts into Psychosomatic Disorders in Nepal." *South Asia: The Journal of South Asian Studies* 45.

Sebastia, Brigitte. 2009a. "Restoring Mental Health." In *Restoring Mental Health in India: Pluralistic Therapies and Concepts*, edited by Brigitte Sebastia. New Delhi: Oxford University Press.

Sebastia, Brigitte. 2009b. "The Last Resort: Why Patients with Severe Mental Disorders Go to Therapeutic Shrines in India." In *Restoring Mental Health in India: Pluralistic Therapies and Concepts*, edited by Brigitte Sebastia. New Delhi: Oxford University Press.

Sen, Priyardarshini. 2015. "The Grey Side of the Moon: Why Is the 'Mentally Ill' Label So Safe for Abuse." *Outlook*, July 20, 2015.

Shrubsall, Marius, Nisha Vinayak, Andrew Willford, et al. 2021. *Impact of COVID-19 on Ultra-Vulnerable Groups: The Banyan Experience.* A Report for the World Health Organization. Chennai: BALM.

Shulman, David Dean. 1980. *Tamil Temple Myths: Sacrifice and Divine Marriage in South Indian Saiva Tradition.* Princeton: Princeton University Press.

Shulman, David Dean. 1985. *The King and the Clown in South Indian Myth and Poetry.* Princeton: Princeton University Press.

Shulman, David Dean. 2016. *Tamil: A Biography.* Cambridge: Belknap Press of Harvard University Press.

Shweder, Richard. 1984. "Anthropology's Romantic Rebellion Against the Enlightenment, or There Is More to Thinking than Reason and Evidence." In *Culture Theory: Essays on Mind, Self, and Emotion*, edited by Richard Shweder and Robert LeVine. Cambridge: Cambridge University Press.

Siegel, James T. 2006. *Naming the Witch.* Stanford: Stanford University Press.

Simmel, Georg. 1971. "The Metropolis and Mental Life." In *On Individuality and Social Forms*, edited by Donald Levin. Chicago: University of Chicago Press.

Singh, Bhrigupati. 2015. *Poverty and the Quest for Life: Spiritual and Material Striving in Rural India.* Chicago: University of Chicago Press.

Smith, Frederick. 2006. *The Self Possessed: Deity and Spirit Possession in South Asian Literature and Civilization.* New York: Columbia University Press.

Sood, Anubha. 2016. "Madness Experienced as Faith: Temple Healing in North India." In *Our Most Troubling Madness: Case Studies in Schizophrenia Across Cultures*, edited by Tanya Luhrmann and Jocelyn Marrow. Berkeley: University of California Press.

Spiro, Melford. 1984. "Some Reflections on Cultural Determinism and Relativism with Special Reference to Emotion and Reason." In *Culture Theory: Essays on Mind, Self, and Emotion*, edited by Richard Shweder and Robert LeVine. Cambridge: Cambridge University Press.

Spratt, Philip. 1966. *Hindu Culture and Personality: A Psycho-Analytic Study.* Bombay: Manaktalas.

Srinivas, Smriti. 2001. *Landscapes of Urban Memory: The Sacred and the Civic in India's High-Tech City.* Minneapolis: University of Minnesota Press.

Srinivas, Tulsi. 2018. *The Cow in the Elevator: An Anthropology of Wonder.* Durham: Duke University Press.

Stengers, Isabelle. 2003. "The Doctor and the Charlatan." *Cultural Studies Review* 9 (2): 11–36.

Stonington, Scott, Seth Holmes, Helena Hansen, et al. 2018. "Case Studies in Social Medicine: Attending to Structural Forces in Clinical Practice." *The New England Journal of Medicine* 379, no. 20 (Nov. 15, 2018): 1958–1961.

Subramanian, Ajantha. 2019. *Caste of Merit: Engineering Education in India.* Cambridge: Harvard University Press.

Sujatha, V., and Leena Abraham. 2012. "Introduction." In *Medical Pluralism in Contemporary India*, edited by V. Sujatha and Leena Abraham. Delhi: Orient BlackSwan.

Sunder Rajan, Kaushik. 2017. *Pharmocracy: Value, Politics, and Knowledge in Global Biomedicine.* Durham: Duke University Press.

Taneja, Anand. 2018. *Jinnealogy: Time, Islam, and Ecological Thought in the Medieval Ruins of Delhi.* Stanford: Stanford University Press.

Thippaiah, S. M., M. S. Najappa, and S. Bada Nath. 2019. "Suicide in India: A Preventable Epidemic." *Indian Journal of Medical Research* 150 (October 2019): 324–327.

Thiranagama, Sharika. 2022. "Figures of Menace: Militarisation in Post-War Sri Lanka." *South Asia: The Journal of South Asian Studies* 45. https://doi.org/10.1080/00856401.2022.2017231.

Trawick, Margaret. 1992. "Death and Nurturance in Indian Systems of Healing." In *Paths to Asian Medical Knowledge*, edited by Charles Leslie and Allan Young. Berkeley: University of California Press.

Trawick, Margaret. 2017. *Death, Beauty, Struggle: Untouchable Women Create the World*. Philadelphia: University of Pennsylvania Press.

Turner, Victor. 1974. *Dramas, Fields, and Metaphors: Symbolic Action in Human Society*. Ithaca: Cornell University Press.

Upadhya, Carol, and A. R. Vasavi. 2008. "Outposts of the Global Information Economy: Work and Workers in India's Outsourcing Industry." In *In an Outpost of the Global Economy: Work and Workers in India's Information Technology Industry*, edited by Carol Upadhya and A. R. Vasavi. New Delhi: Routledge.

Varma, Saiba. 2020. *The Occupied Clinic: Militarism and Care in Kashmir*. Durham: Duke University Press.

Vasavi, A. R. 2012. *Shadow Spaces: Suicides and the Predicament of Rural India*. Gurgaon: Three Essays Collective.

Vasavi, A. R. 2020. "The Tiger and the Tube Well: Malevolence in Rural India." *Critical Asian Studies* 52 (3). https://doi.org/10.1080/14672715.2020.1764855.

Waters, Ethan. 2010. *Crazy Like Us: The Globalization of the American Psyche*. New York: Free Press.

Weiss, Mitchel G., R. Raguram, and S. M. Channabasavanna. 1995. "Cultural Dimensions of Psychiatric Diagnosis: A Comparison of DSM-III-R and Illness Explanatory Models in South India." *British Journal of Psychiatry* 166: 353–359.

Willford, Andrew. 2006. *Cage of Freedom: Tamil Identity and the Ethnic Fetish in Malaysia*. Ann Arbor: University of Michigan Press.

Willford, Andrew. 2014. *Tamils and the Haunting of Justice: History and Recognition in Malaysia's Plantations*. Honolulu: University of Hawaii Press.

Willford, Andrew. 2018. *The Future of Bangalore's Cosmopolitan Pasts: Civility and Difference in a Global City*. Honolulu: University of Hawaii Press.

Willford, Andrew. 2022. "'Do You Hear Voices, or Do You Think You Hear Voices?': Malevolence and Modernity in the Psychiatric Clinic." *South Asia: Journal of South Asian Studies* 45: 164–182. https://doi.org/10.1080/00856401.2022.2018639.

Young, Allan. 1995. *The Harmony of Illusions: Inventing Post-Traumatic Stress Disorder*. Princeton: Princeton University Press.

Young, Allan. 2007. "America's Transient Mental Illness." In *Subjectivity*, edited by João Biehl, Byron Good, and Arthur Kleinman. Berkeley: University of California Press.

Zimmerman, Francis. 1987. *The Jungle and the Aroma of Meats: An Ecological Theme in Hindu Medicine*. Berkeley: University of California Press.

Zizek, Slavoj. 1993. *Tarrying with the Negative*. Durham: Duke University Press.

Zizek, Slavoj. 2004. *Organs without Bodies: On Deleuze and Consequences*. London: Routledge.

Index

Page numbers in boldface type refer to figures and maps.

About the Author

Andrew C. Willford's work characteristically explores aspects of selfhood, identity, and subjectivity within a field of power and statecraft. He was recently awarded the Fulbright-Nehru Distinguished Chair Fellowship for teaching and research in India (2022). He has previously held Fulbright Senior Fellowships in India (2014–2015) and Malaysia (2003–2004), as well as the American Institute of Indian Studies Senior Fellowship for India (2015). He is the author of *The Future of Bangalore's Cosmopolitan Pasts: Civility and Difference in a Global City* (University of Hawaii Press, 2018), *Tamils and the Haunting of Justice: History and Recognition in Malaysia's Plantations* (University of Hawaii Press, 2014), and *Cage of Freedom: Tamil Identity and the Ethnic Fetish in Malaysia* (University of Michigan Press, 2006), and coeditor of *Spirited Politics: Religion and Public Life in Contemporary Southeast Asia*, Andrew Willford and Kenneth George, eds. (Southeast Asia Program Publications, Cornell University, 2005), and *Clio/Anthropos: Exploring the Boundaries Between History and Anthropology*, Andrew Willford and Eric Tagliacozzo, eds. (Stanford University Press, 2009).